Diabetes Education Curriculum

A Guide to Successful Self-Management

Second Edition

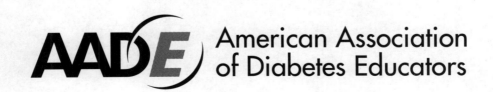

©2015, American Association of Diabetes Educators, Chicago, Illinois.

First Edition: 2009, American Association of Diabetes Educators, Chicago, Illinois.

All rights reserved. No part of this publication may be reproduced electronically or mechanically, stored in a retrieval system, or transmitted in any form or by any means. The information contained in these files may not be copied to a diskette, mounted to a server, or otherwise distributed in any form without the express written permission of the American Association of Diabetes Educators. Printed and bound in the United States of America.

The views expressed in this publication are those of the authors and do not necessarily reflect the policies and/or official positions of the American Association of Diabetes Educators. Mention of product names in this publication does not constitute endorsement by the authors or by the American Association of Diabetes Educators. The American Association of Diabetes Educators and its officers, directors, employees, agents, and members assume no liability whatsoever for any personal or other injury, loss, or damage that may result from the application of the information contained herein.

10 9 8 7 6 5 4 3 2 1   15 16 17 18 19 20 21 22 23 24

Table of Contents

Acknowledgments v

Implementation Guide 1

Module 1   Introduction to Diabetes and Prediabetes 17

Module 2   Healthy Eating 23

Module 3   Being Active 73

Module 4   Taking Medication 101

Module 5   Monitoring 171

Module 6   Problem Solving 211

Module 7   Healthy Coping 249

Module 8   Reducing Risks 289

Supplement   Sexual Dysfunction 371

Appendix   Diabetes Resources 393

Index 397

Acknowledgments

The American Association of Diabetes Educators (AADE) thanks the following individuals for their extensive contributions to the development of the *Diabetes Education Curriculum: A Guide to Successful Self-Management*, Second Edition:

David K. Miller, BSN, MSEd, RN, CDE, FAADE, Editor-in-Chief
Mary M. Austin, MA, RD, CDE, FAADE, Module 5: Monitoring
Sheri R. Colberg, PhD, FACSM, Module 3: Being Active
Ann Constance, MA, RD, CDE, FAADE, Module 8: Reducing Risks
Dave L. Dixon, PharmD, BCPS, CDE, Module 4: Taking Medication
Janice MacLeod, MA, RD, LD, CDE, Module 5: Monitoring
Shelley Mesznik, MA, RD, CDE, CDN, Module 6: Problem Solving and Module 7: Healthy Coping
Lois Moss-Barnwell, MS, RD, LDN, CDE, Module 2: Healthy Eating
Alyce Thomas, RD, All modules: Gestational Diabetes and Pregnancy and Preexisting Diabetes

Implementation Guide

Table of Contents

AIM 2

RATIONALE 2

INTENDED AUDIENCE 2

CURRICULUM FOUNDATION 3

    AADE Standards for Outcomes Measurement of Diabetes Self-Management Education 3

    Curriculum's Relationship to Other Standards 5

METHODOLOGY 7

    Principles of Adult Learning. 7

    Theory of Multiple Intelligences 7

    Behavior Change Theories 9

READABILITY. 10

MODULE ORGANIZATION 10

    An Educator's Overview 10

        AADE Systematic Review of the Literature 10

        Background Information and Instructions for the Educator 11

    Learning Objectives 11

    Behavioral Objectives 11

    Instructional Plan 11

        Questions to Ask Participants. 11

        Questions to Anticipate From Participants. 12

        Notes to Educator 12

        Teaching and Learning. 12

        Survival Skills. 12

        Advanced Detail. 12

    Identifying Barriers/Reality Scenarios 12

    Identifying Facilitators 13

2   Diabetes Education Curriculum

Setting a SMART Goal. 13

Follow-up/Outcomes Measurement. 13

References. 14

Module Resources. 14

Diabetes Resources Appendix. 14

DESCRIPTION OF MODULES. 14

Module 1: Introduction to Diabetes and Prediabetes 14

Module 2: Healthy Eating 14

Module 3: Being Active 15

Module 4: Taking Medication 15

Module 5: Monitoring. 15

Module 6: Problem Solving 15

Module 7: Healthy Coping 15

Module 8: Reducing Risks 15

REFERENCES 16

AIM

The purpose of this curriculum is to support diabetes educators in the teaching of self-management concepts, with the ultimate goal of helping patients achieve the behavioral changes necessary to manage their health condition(s).

RATIONALE

This aim is worth achieving because people with diabetes and related conditions make myriad daily decisions about their self-care that ultimately impact their clinical outcomes and overall health status. Self-management education is key to their success in making the decisions that will best serve them. Effective self-management includes not only the acquisition of knowledge, attitude, and skills but also the adoption of behavior change strategies. In fact, acquisition of knowledge without behavior change is futile; behavior change without knowledge acquisition is unlikely. Thus, this curriculum places equal emphasis on the content to be taught and the facilitation of behavior change.

INTENDED AUDIENCE

The intended audience for this curriculum is people with prediabetes or diabetes and related conditions, and their significant others. Patients present for self-management education with varying levels of prior knowledge and skill. Additionally, patients' health beliefs, attitudes, and levels of readiness to learn and change may vary widely. Educators are challenged to structure their services to maximize the educational opportunity for participants: whether to offer individual consultation or groups, whether to group the newly diagnosed together with those with long-standing diabetes, and whether to separate type 1 diabetes from type 2 diabetes.

American Association of Diabetes Educators©

CURRICULUM FOUNDATION

The AADE Standards for Outcomes Measurement of Diabetes Self-Management Education (DSME)[1]

The AADE Standards for Outcomes Measurement of Diabetes Self-Management Education (2003) provide the foundation for this curriculum (see Figure I.1). The following overview of outcomes is important in order to clarify the influence of the AADE Standards for Outcomes Measurement of DSME on the practice of diabetes education in general, and on this curriculum in particular.

More than 30 years ago, physician Avedis Donebedian proposed a model for assessing healthcare quality based on structures, processes and outcomes.[2] Many of the continuous quality improvement (CQI) efforts that have been adopted in US health care have been drawn from this model, including the National Standards for DSME Programs.[3] According to Donebedian, **a health outcome is defined as "a measurable product . . . the changed state or condition of an individual as a consequence of healthcare over time."**[2]

Over the years, diabetes education programs have used a variety of measures, including A1C, in an attempt to show whether their interventions changed health outcomes. Metabolic outcomes like A1C, however, are impacted by a variety of interventions by other members of the healthcare team. For example, a change in a patient's diabetes medication, which is prescriber-driven, can improve the A1C. So, it was not always clear whether the educational intervention made a *unique contribution* to such an improved health outcome.

The development of the AADE Standards for Outcomes Measurement of DSME in 2003 provided a framework for educators to answer the question, "Does the educational intervention make a difference?" A more detailed discussion of the outcomes standards answers that question.

Standard: **Behavior change is the unique outcome measurement for DSME.**

Behavior change is directly affected by the diabetes education experience, which involves self-care training and ongoing support. To continue the example cited above—the patient whose A1C improved after a change in diabetes medication—the *behavior of taking the medication* had to be sufficiently mastered in order for the medication to have its desired effect. Behavior change is just one outcome on a continuum of outcomes categories (see Figure I.2).

Standard: **The continuum of outcomes, including learning, behavioral, clinical, and health status, should be assessed to demonstrate the interrelationship between DSME and behavior change in the care of individuals with diabetes.**

Learning is an immediate outcome, which can be measured at the time of the educational intervention. Questions that probe for patient understanding of a concept just taught can reveal whether learning has occurred, as can

---

1. Behavior change is the unique outcome measurement for DSME.

2. Seven diabetes self-care behavior measures determine the effectiveness of DSME at individual participant and population levels.

3. Diabetes self-care behaviors should be evaluated at baseline and then at regular intervals after the education program.

4. The continuum of outcomes, including learning, behavioral, clinical, and health status, should be assessed to demonstrate the interrelationship between DSME and behavior change in the care of individuals with diabetes.

5. Individual patient outcomes are used to guide the intervention and improve care for that patient. Aggregate population outcomes are used to guide programmatic services and for continuous quality improvement activities for the DSME and the population it serves.

FIGURE I.1 AADE Standards for Outcomes Measurement of Diabetes Self-Management Education (DSME)

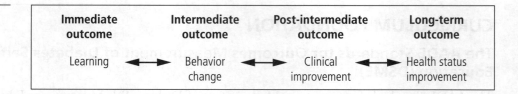

FIGURE I.2 Continuum of Outcomes Categories

knowledge tests and return demonstration of a self-care skill. Identification of facilitators and barriers, as well as strategies to overcome barriers, is also an immediate outcome of learning. Questions are embedded throughout this curriculum that will help the educator determine patient understanding, as well as assist patients in identifying barriers to appropriate self-care.

Behavior change is an intermediate outcome. It requires more than a single measurement and must be measured over time. Intermediate outcomes are measured after the educational encounter and once the patient has had adequate time to implement newly learned behaviors in a real-life setting. Behavior change can be subjectively measured through patient self-report of behaviors at follow-up (eg, "I have been monitoring my blood sugar twice a day"), and it can be objectively measured through review of documented records (eg, glucose logbook results, meter data). *Clinical improvement is a post-intermediate outcome*, which results from the interaction of diabetes education, the patient's self-management efforts, and the provider's clinical management. A1C reduction, improved blood pressure, and weight loss are all examples of post-intermediate outcomes. *Improved health status is a long-term outcome* and can be measured by changes in quality of life, reductions in healthcare costs, and increased productivity (such as fewer missed days of work). Ideally, education programs should measure all outcomes categories, but the diabetes educator's skills and influence most directly impact the first two—learning and behavior change.

Standard: Seven diabetes self-care behavior measures determine the effectiveness of DSME at individual participant and population levels.

The curriculum's instructional content is centered around the AADE7 Self-Care Behaviors™ (see Figure I.3).

Standard: Diabetes self-care behaviors should be evaluated at baseline and then at regular intervals after the education program.

Each module in the curriculum includes sections entitled "Setting a SMART Goal" and "Follow-up/Outcomes Measurement." In "Setting a SMART Goal," the educator is prompted to help the patient develop an individual goal for behavior change. In keeping with principles of adult learning, the patient should be involved in selection of goals, but only once he or she is at a point of readiness to attempt the change in behavior. The acronym SMART helps ensure the goal is **S**pecific, **M**easurable, **A**ttainable, **R**ealistic, and has a **T**imeline. In "Follow-up/Outcomes Measurement," the educator is guided in the measurement of immediate and intermediate outcomes at baseline and follow-up intervals. The method of goal setting and outcomes measurement is compatible with use of the AADE7™ Goal Sheets and the AADE7™ System, which can help educators efficiently and accurately track and measure behavior change.

Healthy eating
Being active
Taking medication
Monitoring
Problem solving
Healthy coping
Reducing risks

FIGURE I.3 AADE7 Self-Care Behaviors™

Standard: Individual patient outcomes are used to guide the intervention and improve care for that patient. Aggregate population outcomes are used to guide programmatic services and for continuous quality improvement activities for the DSME and the population it serves.

At follow-up, the educator assesses the patient's progress with behavior change. Barriers faced and attempts at problem solving should be discussed. The patient and the educator should collaborate to develop a plan for future behavior change. In the "Follow-up/Outcomes Measurement" section of each module, the steps discussed above are outlined, specific to each behavior. At the population level, aggregate outcomes data should be used by the program to determine effectiveness and identify areas needing improvement. The CQI process is then followed.

Curriculum's Relationship to Other Standards

In addition to meeting the AADE Standards for Outcomes Measurement of DSME, this curriculum meets many of the guiding principles published in other practice documents important to the specialty of diabetes education:

- ◆ **The AADE Standards for Outcomes Measurement of Diabetes Self-Management Education (DSME):** In 2015, a joint position statement, Diabetes Self-Management Education and Support in Type 2 Diabetes, was issued by the American Diabetes Association, the American Association of Diabetes Educators, and the Academy of Nutrition and Dietetics. The joint position statement noted that diabetes self-management education and support (DSME/S) provides the foundation to help people with diabetes navigate daily self-management decisions and activities and has been shown to improve health outcomes.[4]

  Diabetes self-management support (DSMS) refers to the support that is required for implementing and sustaining coping skills and behaviors needed to self-manage on an ongoing basis.[4]

  A patient-centered approach to DSME/S at diagnosis provides the foundation for current and future needs. Ongoing DSME/S can help the person with diabetes overcome barriers and cope with the ongoing challenges in order to facilitate changes during the course of treatment and life transitions[4] (see Figure I.4).

  The diabetes education algorithm provides an evidence-based visual depiction of when to identify and refer individuals with type 2 diabetes to DSME/S.[4] The algorithm defines 4 critical points for the delivery and key information on the self-management skills that are necessary. The algorithm relies on 5 guiding principles and represents how DSME/S should be provided through[4]:

  —Patient engagement

  —Information sharing

  —Psychosocial and behavioral support

  —Integration with other therapies

  —Coordinated care across specialty care, facility-based care, and community organizations

- ◆ **National Standards for DSME/S (NSDSME/S)** define quality diabetes education programs. These standards focus on the *structure* of the program, the *process* of providing DSME, and *outcomes* of the educational process.[3] This curriculum specifically addresses standards 6, 7, 8, 9, and 10.

  —**Standard 6/Curriculum:** A written curriculum reflecting current evidence and practice guidelines, with criteria for evaluating outcomes, will serve as the framework for the provision of DSME. The needs of the individual participant will determine which parts of the curriculum will be provided to that individual.

  —**Standard 7/Individualization:** The diabetes self-management, education, and support needs of each participant will be assessed by one or more instructors. The participant and instructor(s) will then together develop an individualized education and support plan focused on behavior change.

  —**Standard 8/Ongoing Support:** The participant and instructor(s) will together develop a personalized follow-up plan for ongoing self-management support. The participant's outcomes and goals and the plan for ongoing self-management support will be communicated to other members of the healthcare team.

  —**Standard 9/Patient Progress:** The provider(s) of DSME and DSMS will monitor whether participants are achieving their personal diabetes self-management goals and other outcome(s) as a way to evaluate the effectiveness of the educational intervention(s), using appropriate measurement techniques.

  —**Standard 10/Quality Improvement:** The provider(s) of DSME will measure the effectiveness of the education and support and look for ways to improve any identified gaps in services or service quality, using a systematic review of process and outcome data.

American Association of Diabetes Educators©

6 Diabetes Education Curriculum

ADA *Standards of Medical Care in Diabetes* recommends all patients be assessed and referred for:		
Nutrition Registered dietitian for medical nutrition therapy ⟷	**Education** Diabetes self-management education and support ⟷	**Emotional health** Mental health professional, if needed

Four critical times to assess, provide, and adjust diabetes self-management education and support:			
1 **At diagnosis**	**2** **Annual** assessment of education, nutrition, and emotional needs	**3** When new **complicating factors** influence self-management	**4** When **transitions** in care occur

When primary care provider or specialist should consider referral:			
☐ Newly diagnosed. All newly diagnosed individuals with type 2 diabetes should receive DSME/S. ☐ Ensure that both nutrition and emotional health are appropriately addressed in education or make separate referrals.	☐ Needs review of knowledge, skills, and behaviors ☐ Long-standing diabetes with limited prior education ☐ Change in medication, activity, or nutritional intake ☐ HbA1C out of target ☐ Maintain positive health outcomes ☐ Unexplained hypoglycemia or hyperglycemia ☐ Planning pregnancy or pregnant ☐ For support to attain and sustain behavior change(s) ☐ Weight or other nutrition concerns ☐ New life situations and competing demands	Change in: ☐ Health conditions such as renal disease and stroke, need for steroid or complicated medication regimen ☐ Physical limitations such as visual impairment, dexterity issues, movement restrictions ☐ Emotional factors such as anxiety and clinical depression ☐ Basic living needs such as access to food, financial limitations	Change in: ☐ Living situation such as inpatient or outpatient rehabilitation or now living alone ☐ Medical care team ☐ Insurance coverage that results in treatment change ☐ Age-related changes affecting cognition, self-care, etc.

FIGURE I.4 Algorithm of Care

⬥ **AADE Standards of Practice for Diabetes Educators** define nationally accepted standards of practice for diabetes educators and ensure quality and accountability in the practice of diabetes education.[5] This curriculum specifically addresses standards 2, 3, 4, 5, and 6 (and selected measurement criteria).

—**Standard 2/Goal Setting:** The diabetes educator works with the person with or at risk for diabetes to identify mutually acceptable goals. The goals reflect information obtained through the assessment process. Goals should be specific, measurable, attainable, realistic, and timely.

—**Standard 3/Planning:** The diabetes educator develops the DSME/T plan to attain the mutually defined goals to achieve desired outcomes. The plan integrates current diabetes care practices and established principles of teaching and learning. The plan is coordinated among the diabetes healthcare team

American Association of Diabetes Educators©

members, the person with or at risk for diabetes, his or her family, significant others, other relevant support systems, and the referring provider.

— **Standard 4/Implementation:** The diabetes educator provides DSME/T according to the defined plan and desired goals and outcomes. Implementation may involve collaboration with other professional and community resources and services.

— **Standard 5/Evaluation:** The diabetes educator evaluates individual outcome measures for each person with diabetes, aggregate outcome measures for the program, and the quality and outcomes of DSME/T according to the 5 Standards for Outcomes Measurement defined by AADE.

— **Standard 6/Documentation:** The diabetes educator establishes a complete and accurate record of the client's DSME/T experience and follow-up DSMS.

METHODOLOGY

This curriculum is not based on one single methodology. Instead, its theoretical base and underlying principles are derived from a variety of sources: Knowles's principles of adult learning,[6-8] Gardner's theory of multiple intelligences,[9] and behavior change models and theories, including the patient empowerment model, the health belief model, and social cognitive theory.

Principles of Adult Learning

Established principles of teaching and learning theory are reflected in the curriculum's design. According to Malcolm Knowles, the "father of adult education," learning should be an active process which draws on the learners' experiences, and the information should fill an immediate need and be presented in a problem-oriented format. Table I.1 shows how these principles are applied within the curriculum.

Knowles urges educators to view adult learners as mutual partners in the learning endeavor. He proposes that addressing the needs and interests of learners is the most efficient way to teach.[6,7] Lessons should be developed from the responses of students, and not from a previously determined logical structure. If the educator's priority is to deal with the participants' responses to problems—the kinds of questions they will ask, the obstacles they will face, their attitudes, and the possible solutions they will offer—there is no compelling need to "cover ground," eg, check off all the required topic areas.[8]

Theory of Multiple Intelligences

This curriculum has been developed in accordance with Knowles's philosophy for adult education. Callout boxes that highlight teaching and learning principles are sprinkled throughout the instructional plan to remind the educator to use educational approaches that enhance adult learning. These "teaching and learning" boxes also incorporate Howard Gardner's theory of multiple intelligences.[9] This theory argues that the traditional definition of intelligence does not adequately encompass the full spectrum of human abilities. It suggests that every person possesses each of 7 core intelligences in varying degrees, as outlined in Table I.2. The different categories of intelligence give educators a variety of platforms from which to present content, thus allowing learners to grasp new concepts in ways that resonate with their abilities.

However, as Gardner himself has noted in the preface of the third edition of his book *Frames of Mind: The Theory of Multiple Intelligences*:

Multiple intelligences should not—in and of itself—be an educational goal. To the extent possible, an educator should teach and assess in ways that bring out that [person's] capacities. . . . The educator should decide on which topics, concepts, or ideas are of the greatest importance, and should then present them in

American Association of Diabetes Educators©

8 Diabetes Education Curriculum

TABLE I.1 Application of the Principles of Adult Learning

Principles of Adult Learning*	Application Within Curriculum
The learning experience should be active and not passive.	Questions to ask participants are included throughout the curriculum to assess their assumptions, attitudes, beliefs, and knowledge level concerning the various aspects of self-management. Learners are actively engaged in the learning experience.
The information should fill an immediate need. It should be meaningful to learners and support their "need to know."	Learners are involved in deciding on the content that will be covered. Questions at the beginning of every module serve to identify what they want to learn. Educators are directed to base teaching on participants' identified concerns.
	The educator will note that the instructional plan in this curriculum is laid out in a logical progression of information. This arrangement of content, however, is not meant to provide a static basis for lecture from start to finish within each topic area. In order for the information to be meaningful to participants, their queries should guide what content is delivered by the educator. So, even though the educator may believe that the learner "needs to know" everything in the instructional plan, participants ultimately decide what they "need to know" at that particular encounter.
	In certain cases, participants will need some direction. They may not know what to ask because the experience of living with diabetes is so new. When participants lack the required skills and knowledge to be self-directed, the educator should provide appropriate information, then allow subsequent participant questions to drive the experience further.[†]
Adults are problem-oriented learners; therefore, information should be presented in a problem-oriented format.	While educators are typically fascinated by diabetes as an academic subject, participants want to learn about how it will affect their lives from day to day. A certain amount of time, naturally, should be spent teaching the basic pathophysiology of diabetes, so that learners can grasp the rationale for self-care. The majority of time with learners, though, should be spent attending to the real-life issues—emotional, relational, and physical—involved in living with diabetes.
	Reality scenarios and problem-solving exercises are included in which participants are encouraged to brainstorm, to determine multiple possible solutions to self-care barriers. The emphasis in the curriculum is applying the content to everyday life with diabetes, translating knowledge of the topic into a behavioral action.
The educational process should incorporate learners' personal experiences. Adults have a rich reservoir of experiences that can serve as a resource for learning. Learners feel valued and respected for the experiences and perspectives they bring to the learning situation. New material should be related to what learners already know.	Probing questions are included in each module, intended to draw on participants' experience. Participants who have successfully overcome difficulties are invited to share with other learners in the group. It encourages the development of improved problem-solving skills because they can draw on situations they have encountered or are likely to encounter.

*M Knowles, "Introduction: The Art and Science of Helping Adults Learn," in MS Knowles, ed, *Androgagy in Action: Applying Modern Principles of Adult Learning* (San Francisco: Jossey-Bass, 1984); M Knowles, *The Modern Practice of Adult Education*, rev. ed. (Chicago: Association Press/Follett, 1980); DS Greene, BP Beardin, JM Bryan, "Addressing attitudes during diabetes education: suggestions from adult education," *Diabetes Educ* 17, no. 6 (1991): 470-3; EA Walker, "Characteristics of the adult learner," *Diabetes Educ* 25 (1999): 16-24.
[†] DD Pratt, "Andragogy as a relational construct," *Adult Education Quarterly* 38, no. 3 (1988): 160-72.

a variety of ways. . . . When a topic is taught in multiple ways, one reaches more students. Additionally, the multiple modes of delivery convey what it *means* to understand something well. When one has a thorough understanding of a topic, one can typically think of it in several ways, thereby making use of one's multiple intelligences. Conversely, if one is restricted to a single mode of conceptualization and presentation, one's own understanding (whether teacher or student) is likely to be tenuous.[9(pxvii)]

American Association of Diabetes Educators©

TABLE I.2	Multiple Intelligences
Category of Intelligence	Learning Is Enhanced By:
Verbal-linguistic	Well-developed verbal skills and sensitivity to the sounds, meanings, and rhythms of words
Mathematical-logical	Ability to think conceptually and abstractly, and capacity to discern logical and numerical patterns
Musical	Ability to produce and appreciate rhythm, pitch, and timber
Visual-spatial	Capacity to think in images and pictures, to visualize accurately and abstractly
Bodily-kinesthetic	Ability to control one's body movements and to handle objects skillfully
Interpersonal	Capacity to detect and respond appropriately to the moods, motivations, and desires of others
Naturalist	Ability to recognize and categorize plants, animals, and other objects in nature
Existential	Sensitivity and capacity to tackle deep questions about human existence, such as What is the meaning of life? Why do we die? How did we get here?

Behavior Change Theories

Useful precepts from a variety of behavior change theories and models are embedded in this curriculum, including the following:

◈ **Patient Empowerment Model.**[10,11] People with diabetes are in control of their own self-management. They make the choices that have the most impact on their outcomes. Because they live with the consequences of their decisions, they have the right and the responsibility to be the primary decision-maker in their diabetes management. The empowerment approach requires willing participation. It is best implemented after basic survival skills have been acquired.

In this curriculum, the empowerment model is evident by the inclusion of questions that help patients more clearly define their self-management problems as well as identify their feelings surrounding the problem. Anticipating barriers, formulating strategies, and setting goals for behavior change are a consistent approach within the curriculum. Having patients evaluate their experience after putting the plan into action, and revising for future goal-setting, is encouraged. Educators can use the "Problem-Solving Activity Script" in Module 7: Healthy Coping to help participants begin to address self-care problems in an incremental manner.

◈ **Health Belief Model.**[12] A person's health-related behavior depends on his or her perception of 4 areas: the seriousness (severity) of his or her condition, how vulnerable (susceptible) one believes he or she is to developing problems, the benefits of taking action, and the barriers (costs or hassles) related to taking action. One's confidence in his or her ability to take action (self-efficacy), the degree to which he or she is convinced that taking action is necessary, and cues to action are all influential on behavior.

This curriculum incorporates the health belief model by its suggested use of reminders to provide cues to action, as well as probing questions that the educator can ask to uncover participants' beliefs about severity susceptibility, benefits, and barriers. The "Goal-Setting Activity" in Module 6: Problem Solving can be used to help participants learn how to set appropriate behavior change goals based on their health beliefs. In the same module, "Tips for the Educator: Using Motivational Interviewing Techniques to Enhance Confidence and Conviction" provides educators a guide to using confidence and conviction scales with patients. In Module 7: Healthy Coping, the "Costs Versus Benefits Learning Activity" helps learners become more aware of their values and motivators for behavior.

◈ **Social Cognitive Theory.**[12] Behavior is affected by environmental influences such as family, friends, the workplace, and the community. One's level of self-efficacy and expectation about performing a behavior (*what's in it for me?*) are important determinants for making a change. People draw on the experiences of others as a way to shape their own behavior. Future performance of a specific behavior is based in part on one's experience with the behavior, whether it is positive or negative.

American Association of Diabetes Educators©

10   Diabetes Education Curriculum

In this curriculum, credible participants in group settings are invited to share their experiences with classmates in an effort to model targeted behaviors. Self-efficacy is enhanced by providing clear instruction and approaching behavior change in small incremental steps. Patients are encouraged to use self-initiated rewards and incentives to reinforce new behaviors.

READABILITY[13]

It is understood that participants will not be *reading* the curriculum content. When providing DSME/T, however, the educator must *translate the written content into the spoken word*. One known barrier to health literacy is when healthcare professionals speak at a level of language that is comfortable to them but not clear to patients. In an effort to promote participant understanding, the curriculum's instructional plan content has been written at a seventh-grade level. Educators should assess their clients' literacy levels and adjust their communication accordingly.

Flesch-Kincaid readability statistics were calculated for each module's instructional plan content to determine the level of understandability and grade level. The Flesch Reading Ease score bases its rating on the *average number of syllables per word* and the *average number of words per sentence*. According to Flesch, a reading ease score of 60 to 70 is recommended for most documents. The average reading ease score for the instructional plan of this curriculum is 62. Although a person's years of education do not necessarily predict literacy, the content was also evaluated for grade level. The Flesch-Kincaid Grade Level test recommends aiming for a score of 7.0 to 8.0 for most documents. The average grade level score for the curriculum's instructional plan content is 7.6.

It is hoped that this approach will remind educators to speak to participants on a layman's level that will be understood by most. For some curriculum content, the use of multisyllabic words (eg, carbohydrate, hypoglycemia, retinopathy, pioglitazone) was unavoidable and may have inflated the scores. In such cases, the word is defined with its first use, as should educators when instructing patients.

The narrative voice of the curriculum instructional content is mostly written in the *second person*. **A second-person narrative voice is intended to make the information more personal to the intended audience, as compared with third-person narrative voice.** An illustration of the difference is: "You should have a blood test to check your kidneys before starting metformin therapy" (second person) versus "People with diabetes should have a blood test to check their kidneys before starting metformin therapy" (third person).

MODULE ORGANIZATION

The curriculum begins with Introduction to Diabetes. This introductory module focuses on the risk factors and pathophysiology of type 1 diabetes, type 2 diabetes, and prediabetes. Its purpose is to give participants a basic foundation upon which to begin learning about the self-care behaviors involved in the management or prevention of diabetes. Following this introduction is a module for each of the AADE7 Self-Care Behaviors™ (refer to Figure I.3). With few exceptions, the modules are structured as follows.

An Educator's Overview

AADE Systematic Review of the Literature

For each of the AADE7 Self-Care Behaviors™, the growing body of evidence has been systematically reviewed by a team of researchers engaged by the American Association of Diabetes Educators (AADE).[14-20] Key points and

American Association of Diabetes Educators©

conclusions of these reviews are outlined in this section, providing support for DSME interventions that have been integrated into the curriculum's instructional plan.

Background Information and Instructions for the Educator

Salient background information and relevant instructions prepare the educator to instruct and counsel participants about each self-care behavior. Educators are encouraged to read this section prior to using the instructional plan with participants.

Learning Objectives

Prior to instruction, an assessment should be performed. An educator's review of the assessment will reveal which areas of self-care the participant needs to learn about. When using the empowerment approach, however, the participant's interests determine which topics areas are covered and when. Since there is usually a great deal that needs to be learned, it is not realistic to assume each participant will successfully meet every listed objective in a session. The educator and the participant will need to prioritize which learning objectives can be met in each encounter. At the beginning of each module, a range of potential learning objectives are listed. These objectives are measurable statements that indicate what the participant could potentially learn if the entire instructional plan were covered.

Behavioral Objectives

Behavioral objectives are developed collaboratively between the educator and the participant *after* the instructional encounter(s). Because they are personalized, every participant's behavioral objectives will be unique, different from those of other participants. At the beginning of each module is a statement that the participant will set a behavioral goal for the specific self-care behavior. See "Setting a SMART Goal" for details on how behavioral goals are developed.

Instructional Plan

One traditional educational approach is to deliver instructional content in a lecture format, in a set order of topics, and from basic to advanced level, followed by a question-and-answer period. Experience with the patient empowerment approach, however, has shown that this is not necessarily the most effective method for educating adults. **Addressing psychosocial concerns first stimulates participant interaction.** It shows them that the educator respects their experiences and perspectives. By focusing on the day-to-day problems of living with diabetes, the educator can then center the instruction around the participants' interests. While this approach may require educators to stretch their comfort zone and change their program structure, this practical approach enhances learning and promotes behavior change.

Questions to Ask Participants

Each module in this curriculum begins with a list of questions the educator may ask participants. These queries are intended to encourage active discussion, keep learners engaged, probe for understanding, and assess reasoning and critical thinking skills. Additional questions appear throughout the module.

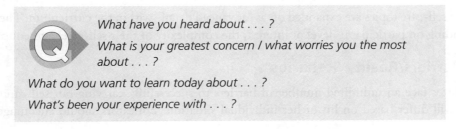

Questions to Anticipate From Participants

Throughout most modules there are common questions the educator may anticipate from participants, followed by the answers. If they are not asked by participants, the educator may choose to pose these questions to the participants to enhance the learning experience.

Is it safe for a person with diabetes to have a pedicure?

Notes to Educator

These notes are tips for the educator for how to best use particular material in the curriculum.

Be sure to make the point that *blood glucose is the same as blood sugar.* Don't assume that participants know these terms are synonymous. Whichever term you choose to use, though, it helps to be consistent so as to avoid confusion.

Teaching and Learning

A variety of principles of adult learning are highlighted in teaching and learning boxes, and distributed throughout the modules as reminders to the educator.

Adults learn best when the learning experience is active and not passive. **Keep participants engaged with questions like "Can you list . . . ?"**

Survival Skills Survival Skill

When faced with the prospect of teaching "survival skills," many educators wonder where to draw the line. Opinions may vary on what topics to include in survival skills, as well as the depth of instruction. Most educators agree that, at the very least, survival skills should include prevention, recognition, and treatment of hypoglycemia for at-risk persons (eg, those taking insulin or oral insulin secretagogues); recognition and treatment of hyperglycemia; how to safely take prescribed diabetes medication, and recognition of side effects that should be reported; healthy food choices and basic meal planning; glucose monitoring and proper care of testing supplies; target blood glucose levels; and when to call the healthcare team for help. Red survival skills tags appear throughout the curriculum to identify potential survival skills topics.

Advanced Detail

Various aspects of self-care topics are expanded on as "advanced detail" within the curriculum. These are to be used as needed, depending on participants' level of interest, the complexity of their self-care, and educator preference.

Identifying Barriers/Reality Scenarios

People with diabetes face an unlimited number of barriers to successfully carrying out self-care behaviors. Each person's barriers will differ based on his or her individual situation. Educators should encourage participants to identify barriers that will likely disrupt their self-care. To help activate this process, common barriers to self-care are listed in most modules, along with possible solutions. This section provides a springboard for discussion about barriers, used at the discretion of the educator. Rather than passively offering solutions to participants, however, the educator is challenged to actively engage them in the problem-solving process. The sample solutions included for each Reality Scenario may not apply or be useful for each participant. In group education sessions, invite the participants to brainstorm together and learn from each other's experiences.

Identifying Facilitators

As important as it is to identify barriers, educators often forget about the facilitators to self-care, the potential positives in the situation. This module section calls attention to the facilitators—the people, resources, and activities that can help participants adhere to their self-care plan. The educator can help them identify the people in their lives who may be supportive of their efforts, and help them maximize that support. A list of resources appears at the end of the module and can be copied and given to participants as a handout. This list includes many useful national resources. Depending on the self-care behavior, available local community resources should be explored with participants. Activating reminder systems and cues to behavior may be helpful for those starting new behaviors. Instituting a reward system can help reinforce behaviors.

Setting a SMART Goal

Collaborative setting of behavior change goals (behavioral objectives) should take place after instruction. Educators are prompted to use the SMART acronym as a guide to help participants set goals. Goals should be:

S—Specific, not vague
M—Measurable (eg, how much, for how long, how often)
A—Attainable; challenging but not out of reach
R—Realistic; given the person's situation, can it be done?
T—Timeline; short-term, over the next week or two

There is a newer version of the acronym SMART, used in both health care and corporate management. In this alternative version, *Realistic* is replaced by *Relevant*. *Realistic* is seen as too similar to *Attainable*, while *Relevant* is seen as more patient-focused (ie, is the goal relevant to the patient?).

Educators may find it tempting, in the interest of time, to set goals for the participant. This approach will likely backfire, however, since it is not patient-driven. Goals should be selected based on what the participant feels is important and needed. He or she must understand what is needed to make the change in behavior, have the confidence to do it, and believe that it will lead to an improvement in health or quality of life. A date should be set for follow-up, in order to evaluate progress with the selected behavior change.

Documentation of behavior change goals represents standard practice and is a requirement for program accreditation. Educators can develop their own tools for documenting the setting of goals or use a tool such as the AADE7™ Goal Sheets or the AADE7 System™. Visit the AADE Web site to order goal sheets in English or Spanish: http://www.diabeteseducator.org/product/K712. For more on the electronic AADE7 System™, see the AADE Web site: https://www.diabeteseducator.org/practice/aade7-system.

Follow-up/Outcomes Measurement

The process for measuring outcomes is delineated at the end of each module. Learning—acquiring knowledge and skills—is an immediate outcomes measure, meaning that it can be measured immediately after the education session. Additionally, learning outcomes should be measured at follow-up encounters. This provides the educator an opportunity to assess for gaps in knowledge and skills and educate accordingly.

American Association of Diabetes Educators©

14   Diabetes Education Curriculum

As an intermediate outcome, behavior change requires measurement over at least 2 points in time. The status of the behavior is measured at baseline (after the education session) and again after the patient has had time to implement the new behavior.

According to the AADE Standards for Outcomes Measurement of Diabetes Self-Management Education, the first follow-up should ideally be conducted within 2 to 4 weeks after the teaching session. Subsequent follow-up is recommended at 3- to 6-month intervals thereafter.[1] Measurement of outcomes may be objective or subjective. Subjective measurement includes patient report. If it can be directly observed by the educator, measurement is objective.

References

Throughout the curriculum, self-care recommendations are supported by available evidence, and statements of fact are referenced.

Module Resources

Resources relevant to each self-care behavior are included in each of the 7 behavior modules. Any of these resources may be copied and shared with class participants. If you wish to use these resources in any other manner aside from providing them to class participants free of charge, you will need to contact AADE, Copyrights & Permissions.

Diabetes Resources Appendix

The appendix at the end of the book provides additional resources to enhance the educator's effectiveness and/or serve as a resource for the participant. The information may be copied and used as participant handouts as needed, following the same rules of use as described for module resources.

DESCRIPTION OF MODULES

This edition has a greater emphasis on pregnancy. You will notice that each module addresses issues related to pregnancy and provides recommendations for that population.

Module 1: Introduction to Diabetes and Prediabetes

Module 1 addresses concerns common among those newly diagnosed with diabetes or prediabetes. Risk factors are discussed to help answer the "why me, why now?" questions. Information is included about how the diagnosis is made and classified (type 1 diabetes, type 2 diabetes, prediabetes). Basic pathophysiology is described. The natural progression of the condition, and resulting need for therapy change, is emphasized in the section on type 2 diabetes. The pathophysiology content is intended to give participants a foundation upon which to begin learning about the self-care behaviors involved in the management or prevention of diabetes.

Module 2: Healthy Eating

Module 2 provides information about goals for healthy eating, basic nutrition concepts and terms, and food and nutrient groups. Other practical activities include learning how to read food labels, how to measure food, and strategies for eating out. Participants benefit by having an individualized meal plan developed collaboratively with the registered dietitian.

American Association of Diabetes Educators©

Module 3: Being Active

Module 3 focuses on increasing physical activity, from a lifestyle approach to a structured approach, according to participant ability. Recommended types of physical activity for people with diabetes, safety issues, and special considerations are discussed.

Module 4: Taking Medication

In Module 4, content centers around safe medication-taking behavior. Medications available for the management of diabetes are described, with a focus on how they work, how to take them, precautions, and important side effects. For injectable medications, information on storage guidelines, injection technique, and disposal of needles is included. Participants starting injectable medications should be given hands-on practice time with appropriate privacy. This module also contains an "Advanced Detail" section about vitamins and minerals, as well as complementary and alternative medicine.

Module 5: Monitoring

The benefits of monitoring glucose and other health parameters are introduced in Module 5, along with target glucose levels. Selecting a glucose meter and guidelines for monitoring are included. The educator should provide an opportunity for hands-on practice of the monitoring technique. Emphasis is placed on timing and frequency of monitoring, and how to interpret and respond to the results in the self-management of diabetes.

Module 6: Problem Solving

Module 6 is divided into 2 sections:

- The first section centers on the development of problem-solving skills, which can be applied to any self-care behavior. Problem-solving and goal-setting activities are included to help strengthen these important skills.
- The intent of the second section is to help participants develop problem-solving skills pertaining to hypoglycemia, hyperglycemia, and sick-day management. Strategies for recognizing these conditions, understanding their causes, and treating and preventing them are included.

Module 7: Healthy Coping

Coping with the demands of diabetes transcends any one self-care behavior. Thus, the information in this module can be integrated into all the others. Topics discussed in this module include responding to the diagnosis of diabetes, recognizing and dealing with depression and anxiety, exploring feelings related to diabetes, problem solving, motivation for self-care, relapse prevention, stress management, and strategies for getting support from family, friends, healthcare providers, and the community. Several participant activities are included: "Exploring Feelings and Attitudes About Diabetes," "Costs Versus Benefits Learning Activity," "Problem-Solving Role-Playing Activity," and "Getting Support Participant Activity."

Module 8: Reducing Risks

The American Diabetes Association's Standards of Medical Care for People With Diabetes is used as a template to organize this module's information on risk reduction strategies for cardiovascular, kidney, eye, and nerve health; foot, skin, and dental care; and preventive immunizations. Additionally, awareness of sleep apnea is included, as this is a growing comorbidity of diabetes. Other areas of risk reduction are also covered, including before and during pregnancy, while traveling, and during disaster conditions. The module includes a supplement focusing on sexual dysfunction.

American Association of Diabetes Educators©

16   Diabetes Education Curriculum

REFERENCES

1. Mulcahy K, Maryniuk M, Peeples M, et al. Standards for outcomes measurement of diabetes self-management education (position statement). Diabetes Educ. 2003;29(5):804-16.

2. Donebedian A. The Definition of Quality: A Conceptual Exploration. Ann Arbor, Mich: Health Administration Press; 1980.

3. Hass L, Maryniuk M, Beck J, et al. National standards for diabetes self-management education and support. Diabetes Educ. 2012;38:619-29.

4. Powers MA, Bardsley J, Cypress M, et al. Diabetes self-management education and support in type 2 diabetes: a joint position statement of the American Diabetes Association, the American Association of Diabetes Educators, and the Academy of Nutrition and Dietetics. J Acad Nutr Diet. 2015 Jun 2;pii: S2212-2672(15)00549-3 (cited 2015 July 19). On the Internet at: https://www.diabeteseducator.org/practice/practice-documents/practice-statements.

5. Kocurek B, Hammons T, Lierman P, et al. The scope of practice, standards of practice, and standards of professional performance for diabetes educators. 2011 update (cited 2015 July 19). On the Internet at: https://www.diabetes educator.org/practice/practice-documents/scope-standards.

6. Knowles M. Introduction: the art and science of helping adults learn. In: Androgagy in Action: Applying Modern Principles of Adult Learning. San Francisco: Jossey-Bass; 1984:1-21.

7. Knowles M. The Modern Practice of Adult Education. Rev ed. Chicago: Association Press/Follett; 1980.

8. Knowles M, Holton EF, Swanson RA, eds. The Adult Learner: The Definitive Classic in Adult Education and Human Resource Development. 6th ed. Burlington, Mass: Elsevier; 2005.

9. Gardner H. Frames of Mind: The Theory of Multiple Intelligences. 3rd ed. New York: Basic Books; 2011.

10. Anderson RM, Funnell MM. The Art of Empowerment: Stories and Strategies for Diabetes Educators. 2nd ed. Alexandria, Va: American Diabetes Association; 2005.

11. Funnell MM, Anderson RM, Arnold MS, et al. Empowerment: an idea whose time has come in diabetes education. Diabetes Educ. 1991;17:37-41.

12. US Department of Health and Human Services, National Institutes of Health. Theory at a glance: a guide for health promotion practice. 2nd ed. Publication no. 05-3896. Washington, D.C.; 2005.

13. DuBay WH. The Principles of Readability. Costa Mesa, Calif: Impact Information; 2004.

14. Povey RC, Clark-Carter D. Diabetes and healthy eating: a systematic review of the literature. Diabetes Educ. 2007;33(6):931-59.

15. Kavookjian J, Elswick BM, Whetsel T. Interventions for being active among individuals with diabetes: a systematic review of the literature. Diabetes Educ. 2007;33(6):962-88.

16. McAndrew L, Schneider SH, Burns E, et al. Does patient blood glucose monitoring improve diabetes control? A systematic review of the literature. Diabetes Educ. 2007;33(6):991-1011.

17. Odegard PS, Capoccia K. Medication taking and diabetes: a systematic review of the literature. Diabetes Educ. 2007;33(6):1014-29.

18. Hill-Briggs F, Gemmell L. Problem solving in diabetes self-management and control: a systematic review of the literature. Diabetes Educ. 2007;33(6):1032-50.

19. Boren SA, Gunlock TL, Schaefer J, et al. Reducing risks in diabetes self-management: a systematic review of the literature. Diabetes Educ. 2007;33(6):1053-77.

20. Fisher EB, Thorpe CT, McEvoy B, et al. Healthy coping, negative emotions, and diabetes management: a systematic review and appraisal. Diabetes Educ. 2007;33(6):1080-103.

American Association of Diabetes Educators©

MODULE 1

Introduction to Diabetes and Prediabetes

Table of Contents

LEARNING OBJECTIVES 17

INTRODUCTION TO DIABETES AND PREDIABETES: INSTRUCTIONAL PLAN. 18

    Identifying Participant Thoughts and Feelings About Diabetes. 18

    Why Now? Why Me? What's Happening in My Body? 18

        Fuel Metabolism Before the Diagnosis of Diabetes. 18

        Diabetes. 19

    How Is the Diagnosis Made? 21

        Ways to Diagnose Prediabetes 21

        Ways to Diagnose Type 1 or Type 2 Diabetes. 21

        Ways to Diagnose Gestational Diabetes 22

    I Have Diabetes: Now What? 22

REFERENCES 22

LEARNING OBJECTIVES

- ◆ The participant will define diabetes in basic terms.
- ◆ The participant will state what type of diabetes he or she has.
- ◆ The participant will list the main self-care behaviors involved in diabetes self-management.

INTRODUCTION TO DIABETES AND PREDIABETES: INSTRUCTIONAL PLAN

Identifying Participant Thoughts and Feelings About Diabetes

What have you heard about diabetes?
How did you feel when you were first diagnosed with diabetes?
Were you surprised to learn you had diabetes? Why or why not?
What types of diabetes have you heard about?

Adults learn best when they feel valued and respected for the experiences and perspectives they bring. **Use probing questions to elicit learners' experiences and perspectives.**

Why Now? Why Me? What's Happening in My Body?

For some people, the diagnosis of diabetes comes as a complete surprise. For others, it's an expected event that was "just a matter of time." There are factors that cause you to be at higher risk for getting certain types of diabetes. As the module takes a closer look at what's happening in the body with diabetes, these risk factors will be pointed out. Diabetes is a problem with how your body uses food for energy. To better understand diabetes, it helps to know what happens in the body normally.

Be sure to make the point that *blood glucose is the same as blood sugar*. Don't assume that participants know these terms are synonymous. Whichever term you choose to use, though, it helps to be consistent so as to avoid confusion.

Fuel Metabolism Before the Diagnosis of Diabetes

Most of the food you eat breaks down into glucose, which is the same thing as sugar. As you digest the food, glucose passes from your intestines into your bloodstream. You need glucose. It's your body's main source of energy. But to use glucose for energy, it must first get into your body cells. Glucose can't move into the cells by itself. It needs insulin to help. Insulin is a hormone made by the pancreas, which is the organ behind your stomach.

Most of the time, the pancreas releases just a small steady stream of insulin. But after a meal, your pancreas releases a *burst* of insulin. If you eat a big meal, the pancreas releases a big burst of insulin; if you eat a smaller amount, the pancreas releases a smaller burst of insulin. Insulin allows the glucose to move from your bloodstream into your body cells.

When you are fasting (meaning you haven't eaten in the past 8 hours), the normal blood glucose range is below 100 mg/dL (5.6 mmol/L). After you eat a meal, food causes the blood glucose to rise, but it will stay under 140 mg/dL (7.8 mmol/L) within the 2 hours after a meal. As insulin moves the glucose into the cells, your blood glucose level begins to go down again.

If your blood glucose level ever drops too low (<70 mg/dL or <3.9 mmol/L), your body automatically takes steps to correct the problem. Your liver holds an extra store of glucose just in case you ever need it. For example, if you go too long without eating, your liver will release some of this stored glucose back into the bloodstream. This glucose is the fuel that gives you energy until you can eat a meal.

American Association of Diabetes Educators©

Adults learn best when they can relate new information to what they already know. Consider using an analogy such as the following to explain how insulin works to transport glucose:

Are you familiar with those parking lots that require a card key to enter? To enter the lot, you drive up to the gate, insert a card key into a slot, and wait for the gate to open. After it opens you can drive into the lot. If you don't have a card, or if the slot won't accept your card, you can't drive into the lot. Cars will begin to stack up behind you.

Think of the card key as insulin. Insulin must be present to open the cell door (the gate) so that glucose (your car) can move into your body cell (the lot). If you have little or no insulin, or if your body cells won't properly accept insulin, glucose can't move into your body cells. That's diabetes.

Be creative and come up with one of your own that will work with your patient population.

So, to summarize the normal process: The right amount of insulin from the pancreas keeps your blood glucose level from going too high. Glucose stored in the liver keeps your blood glucose level from dropping too low. The blood glucose level normally stays between 70 and 99 mg/dL (3.9 to 5.5 mmol/L) before eating, and is less than 140 mg/dL (7.8 mmol/L) within the 2 hours after a meal.

Diabetes

When diabetes occurs, your pancreas makes little or no insulin, or your body cells don't respond to the insulin that is produced. In either case, glucose cannot properly move into the body cells. Glucose builds to high levels in the bloodstream. Even though glucose is available in your blood, your body cells can't use it. Your cells now lack the energy they need to keep your body working properly.

There are 3 main types of diabetes:

- type 1 diabetes
- type 2 diabetes
- gestational diabetes

Focus discussion time on the type(s) of diabetes relevant to the participant(s).

Type 1 Diabetes

In type 1 diabetes, little or no insulin is released by the pancreas. The body's immune system turns against itself, destroying the pancreas cells that produce insulin. Normally, the immune system only attacks and destroys invaders like infection. Scientists don't know exactly why the immune system attacks the pancreas, but it's believed that it may be triggered by a virus. Genetic tendencies and the environment may also play a role in why a person gets type 1 diabetes. People with type 1 diabetes usually present with elevated blood glucose. If undiagnosed or untreated, the person will experience weight loss, polyuria, and polydipsia. This will progress with marked elevated blood glucose and development of ketoacidosis. Coma and death can result from delayed diagnosis or treatment. Without insulin, glucose continues to build up in the bloodstream. Some of the excess glucose leaves the body through the urine, taking lots of water along with it. This causes the person to be very thirsty. Since the cells are not getting energy from glucose, body fat is used for energy. This accounts for the sudden weight loss, even though the person is constantly hungry and eating. Burning a lot of fat very quickly causes a buildup of acids called *ketones*. If ketones become excessive, it can lead to a life-threatening condition called *diabetic ketoacidosis* or *DKA*.

20   Diabetes Education Curriculum

Only about 10% of all people with diabetes have type 1. A person with type 1 diabetes must take insulin every day to stay alive. Type 1 diabetes can develop at any age but is usually diagnosed before the age of 30. About 75% of type 1 diabetes cases are diagnosed by the age of 18.

Type 2 Diabetes

The most common form of diabetes is type 2, accounting for about 90% of all diabetes cases.[1] It tends to occur later in life, but can occur earlier if certain risk factors are present. Onset of type 2 diabetes in adolescence is becoming more common as obesity rates rise among youth. There are usually not symptoms at the time of diagnosis. This can be due to absence of symptoms or attributing symptoms to other causes. A person is more likely to develop type 2 diabetes if he or she has the following risk factors:

- Family history of diabetes
- Overweight or obese
- History of gestational diabetes or having had a baby weighing more than 9 lb
- Inactive lifestyle
- Race/ethnicity background:
  - African American
  - Asian American
  - Hispanic/Latino
  - American Indian
  - Native Hawaiian or other Pacific Islander

As type 2 diabetes develops, the pancreas is still producing some insulin. But the body cells don't respond as they should. This is called *insulin resistance*. When the body cells are resistant, it takes more and more insulin to move glucose into the cells. So the pancreas begins to release a higher than normal amount of insulin. This extra insulin production may keep the blood glucose normal, or close to normal, for many years.

Type 2 diabetes is a progressive condition. Eventually, the pancreas cannot keep up with the demand. Insulin production starts to decline. When there is no longer enough insulin released from the pancreas, the blood glucose level rises too high. Over the years, the pancreas may eventually stop making insulin altogether. Also, in type 2 diabetes, the liver releases extra glucose into the bloodstream, raising the glucose level even higher.

As mentioned earlier, some people have no symptoms when their blood glucose level is high. Others may have symptoms such as:

- tiredness
- increased thirst
- increased hunger
- blurred vision
- weight loss
- slow healing
- sexual problems
- numbness or tingling in the feet or hands

Prediabetes

During prediabetes, the blood glucose level is above normal, but not high enough for the person to be diagnosed with diabetes. The pancreas is still producing insulin, but the body cells don't respond as they should. This is called *insulin resistance*. When the body cells are resistant, it takes more and more insulin to move glucose into the cells. So the pancreas begins to release a higher than normal amount of insulin. This extra insulin production keeps the blood glucose normal, or just above normal. This can go on for many years, without causing symptoms.

American Association of Diabetes Educators©

Module 1   *Introduction to Diabetes and Prediabetes*   21

Fortunately, people with prediabetes can do something to prevent or delay the onset of type 2 diabetes. Studies show that a person can lower the risk by losing about 5% to 7% of his or her body weight. For a person who weighs 200 lb, that amounts to about a 10- to 14-lb weight loss. In one study, people who lost this amount of weight lowered their risk of type 2 diabetes by 60%. They lost the weight by eating less fat and fewer calories and by walking at least 30 minutes five days a week.[2] Identifying people at risk for diabetes is the first step in preventing the disease.

Gestational Diabetes

Some women develop gestational diabetes in the last 3 months of pregnancy. In this form of diabetes, the hormones of pregnancy cause insulin resistance. If the woman's pancreas cannot supply enough insulin to overcome this resistance, the blood glucose levels rise too high. High blood glucose levels during pregnancy can result in a very large baby and other birth complications.

After the baby is born, gestational diabetes usually goes away. Women with gestational diabetes are at high risk for developing type 2 diabetes. Up to half of all women with gestational diabetes will develop type 2 diabetes over the next 5 to 10 years. They may be able to lower this risk by maintaining a reasonable body weight and staying physically active.

How Is the Diagnosis Made?[3]

Ways to Diagnose Prediabetes

Unless a person has unmistakable symptoms of high blood glucose, positive test results must be followed by a **repeat test** on another day to confirm the diagnosis. Diagnostic tests for prediabetes include the following:

- **Fasting Plasma Glucose Test** (preferred method). For this test, a person fasts overnight. Blood is drawn from the vein and tested. If the glucose level is between 100 and 125 mg/dL (5.6 to 6.9 mmol/L), this is positive for prediabetes. It is also called impaired fasting glucose (IFG).

- **Oral Glucose Tolerance Test** (OGTT). For this test, a person fasts overnight. After the person drinks a solution of 75 g of glucose dissolved in water, blood is drawn from the vein and tested. If the glucose level is between 140 and 199 mg/dL (7.8 to 11.1 mmol/L), this is positive for prediabetes. It is also called impaired glucose tolerance (IGT).

- **A1C.** For this test, there is no fasting. Blood is drawn from the vein and tested. If the A1C results are 5.7% to 6.4% this is positive for prediabetes. It is important to understand that A1C tests may not be reliable in a variety of circumstances.

Ways to Diagnose Type 1 or Type 2 Diabetes

Unless a person has unmistakable symptoms of high blood glucose, positive test results must be followed by a **repeat test** on another day to confirm the diagnosis. Diagnostic tests for type 1 or type 2 diabetes include the following:

- **Fasting Plasma Glucose Test** (preferred method). For this test, a person fasts overnight. Blood is drawn from the vein and tested. If the glucose level is 126 mg/dL (7.0 mmol/L) or higher, this is considered positive for diabetes.

- **Oral Glucose Tolerance Test** (OGTT). For this test, a person fasts overnight. After the person drinks a solution of 75 g of glucose dissolved in water, blood is drawn from the vein and tested. If the glucose level is 200 mg/dL (11.1 mmol/L) or higher, this is positive for diabetes.

- **Random Blood Glucose Test.** For this test, it does not matter if the person has eaten recently or not. It can be done anytime. Blood is drawn from the vein and tested. If the glucose level is 200 mg/dL (11.1 mmol/L) or higher *and* the person has the classic symptoms of diabetes (excessive thirst, urination, and weight loss), this is positive for diabetes.

- **A1C.** For this test, there is no fasting. Blood is drawn from the vein and tested. If the A1C result is >6.5% this is positive for diabetes. It is important to understand that A1C tests may not be reliable in a variety of circumstances.

American Association of Diabetes Educators©

22   Diabetes Education Curriculum

Ways to Diagnose Gestational Diabetes

- **Oral Glucose Tolerance Test** (OGTT). For this test, a woman fasts overnight. After she drinks a solution of 100 g of glucose dissolved in water, blood is drawn from the vein and tested. The woman must remain seated and should not smoke during this test. If 2 or more of the following glucose levels are met or exceeded, this is positive for gestational diabetes:

    —Fasting: 95 mg/dL (5.3 mmol/L)

    —1-hour: 180 mg/dL (10.0 mmol/L)

    —2-hour: 155 mg/dL (8.6 mmol/L)

    —3-hour: 140 mg/dL (7.8 mmol/L)

I Have Diabetes: Now What?[4]

Living with diabetes is not easy. The choices you make will have an impact on your blood glucose level each day. And what happens each day will affect your future health. But diabetes can be managed if you *partner together* with your diabetes educator.

Diabetes educators are here to offer you the information you need to make the best choices about your self-care. While diabetes educators know a lot about diabetes and its treatment, *you* are the expert about your own life. *You* know better than anyone else what you are able to do to manage your diabetes. Work with your diabetes educator to combine what educators know about diabetes and what you know about yourself to develop a workable plan. Sometimes the plan may not work out like you want it to. That just means you and your diabetes educator need to keep trying until a workable plan is developed.

Diabetes is a self-managed disease. Taking care of your diabetes means making healthy food choices, being physically active, monitoring your glucose, and taking your medication, if needed. Your provider will prescribe medication according to your individual needs. All people with type 1 diabetes will need insulin. Most people with type 2 diabetes will need some form of diabetes medication to help keep glucose levels in the target range. *Remember the progressive nature of type 2 diabetes*—as time goes on and your pancreas changes, your treatment will need to change too. This may include taking several types of oral medications or even injections. Fortunately, today there are more options than ever before to manage diabetes.

The goal of taking care of your diabetes is to feel well today and to avoid complications in the future. By doing what you can to get your glucose close to normal, these goals are attainable. Your provider may suggest a blood glucose target range for you. Goals should be individualized, and lower goals may be reasonable based on benefit-risk assessment. The American Diabetes Association recommends these general targets for people with diabetes[3]:

- Fasting: 70 to 130 mg/dL (3.9 to 7.2 mmol/L)

- 1 to 2 hours after eating: below 180 mg/dL (10.0 mmol/L)

- A1C <7%

REFERENCES

1. Centers for Disease Control and Prevention. Diabetes (cited 2015 Sept 22). On the Internet at: http://www.cdc.gov/media/presskits/aahd/diabetes.pdf.

2. Diabetes Prevention Program Research Group. Reduction in the incidence of type 2 diabetes with lifestyle intervention or metformin. N Engl J Med. 2002;346(6):393-403.

3. American Diabetes Association. Standards of medical care in diabetes—2009. Diabetes Care. 2009;32 Suppl 1:S13-61.

4. Funnell MM, Anderson RM. Empowerment and self-management of diabetes. Clin Diabetes. 2004;22(3):123-7.

American Association of Diabetes Educators©

MODULE 2

Healthy Eating

Table of Contents

HEALTHY EATING: AN EDUCATOR'S OVERVIEW 25

    AADE Systematic Review of the Literature 25

    Background Information and Instructions for the Educator 25

    Learning Objectives 26

        Knowledge 26

        Skills 26

        Barriers and Facilitators 26

    Behavioral Objective 27

HEALTHY EATING: INSTRUCTIONAL PLAN 27

    Identifying Participant Thoughts and Feelings About Eating 27

    Healthy Eating: Facts Versus Fiction 27

    Goals for Healthy Eating and Meal Planning 27

        Healthy Eating and Metabolism 28

        Healthy Eating and Blood Glucose Control 28

        Healthy Eating and Blood Pressure Control 28

        Healthy Eating and Lipids 28

        Healthy Eating and Weight 28

    What's a Healthy Weight? 29

        Measuring Waist Circumference 31

        Risk Factors for Conditions Linked to Obesity 31

        Weighing In 31

        Daily Calorie Needs 31

    Common Nutrition Terms 32

        Meal Plan 32

        Portion 33

        Portion Control 33

24 Diabetes Education Curriculum

Serving 33

Serving Size 33

Food and Nutrient Groups 34

Carbohydrates 35

Starch 36

Fruits 36

Milk 38

Sweets 38

Mix and Match 39

Nonstarchy Vegetables 40

Protein 42

Fats 42

Sweeteners 46

Free Foods 48

Snacks 49

Fiber and Whole Grains 50

Water 51

Sodium 52

Alcohol 53

Reading Food Labels 54

Serving Size 55

Number of Servings in the Container 55

Calories per Serving 55

Fat per Serving 55

Cholesterol per Serving 55

Sodium per Serving 55

Potassium 56

Total Carbohydrate Content 56

Protein 57

Vitamins A and C, Calcium, and Iron 57

Percent Daily Value 57

List of Ingredients 57

Eating Out and Reading Restaurant Menus 58

Identifying Barriers to Healthy Eating 59

Identifying Facilitators for Healthy Eating 60

Common Facilitators 60

Setting a SMART Goal for Healthy Eating 61

Follow-up/Outcomes Measurement 61

REFERENCES 62

HEALTHY EATING: RESOURCES 65

American Association of Diabetes Educators©

Module 2 *Healthy Eating* 25

HEALTHY EATING: AN EDUCATOR'S OVERVIEW

AADE Systematic Review of the Literature

A systematic review of the literature was conducted by the American Association of Diabetes Educators (AADE) to "examine interventions that have been designed to promote healthy eating in people with diabetes."[1] Noted in the review was a tendency for successful interventions to include the dimension of physical activity as well as group work among participants. Therefore, diabetes educators may wish to consider the inclusion of physical exercise and group work in interventions designed to help patients lower their calorie and fat intake and lose weight.

Background Information and Instructions for the Educator

Healthy eating is one of the 7 self-care behaviors to which people with diabetes (or prediabetes) can aspire. The educator's goal when providing nutrition intervention should not merely be to transfer information to the patient. Rather, the highest priority should be to help the patient make, and sustain, behavior changes that will positively impact diabetes and its comorbidities. Behavior changes in the realm of eating are intended to improve the patient's clinical status and, ultimately, lead to an improvement in overall health status.[2]

Every person with diabetes should have a meal plan that is designed with his or her unique needs in mind. After conducting a thorough nutrition assessment, the educator should develop a nutrition plan, collaboratively negotiating short-term goals with the patient. The focus of goal-setting may be on any number of eating behaviors: moderating the intake of carbohydrates, reducing fat or calories, increasing fiber, adjusting the timing and distribution of meals and snacks, controlling portion size, or coordinating meals with activity and medications. The meal planning approaches used by the educator may vary widely between patients (from very simple to extremely sophisticated), as the approach should be based on patients' individual capabilities, lifestyle, and resources, as well as their level of motivation and willingness to make changes. Barriers or road blocks to behavior change must be considered when developing the meal plan. Such barriers may include emotions, financial concerns, environmental triggers for eating, the patient's role within the family, and cultural expectations related to eating and food preparation.

At the beginning of nutrition education sessions, educators should encourage patients to take the lead by asking open-ended questions such as "What would you like to work on today?" Starting with the patient's agenda fosters empowerment and focuses the session time on what is valuable to the patient. Educators should avoid referring to the meal plan as a *diet*, as this term is fraught with negativity. Use terms such as *healthy eating program* or *meal plan*.

Eating habits are steeped in family tradition and cultural identity. Therefore, educators should make every effort to include the patient's significant others (eg, family, cohabitants, caretakers) when providing nutrition education. Prior to educating patients of diverse cultural backgrounds, particularly those new to the United States, the educator should first ascertain the patient's cultural background and level of acculturation. Educators should research commonly eaten foods relevant to the culture and ethnicity of the patient. Inclusion of familiar and preferred foods in the meal plan demonstrates respect and acceptance of cultural differences.[3-5] It should also be noted that certain foods, such as raw eggs, unpasteurized milk, certain fish, and deli meats (unless heated until steaming hot), should not be consumed during pregnancy. Consuming these foods may increase the risk of food-borne illnesses, such as listeriosis or salmonella.

Evidence-based nutrition practice guidelines (NPGs) developed by the Academy of Nutrition and Dietetics provide diabetes educators a framework (nutrition care process) for delivering medical nutrition therapy (MNT).[6] The AADE supports the provision of MNT following evidence-based guidelines.[2] These NPGs give detailed guidance as to the following elements:

◆ Nutrition assessment—medical history, laboratory data, food and nutrition history, level of physical activity, and anthropometric measures, including height, weight, waist-to-hip ratio, body mass index (BMI), and body composition. In pregnancy, this would also include weight gain and nutrient supplementation

American Association of Diabetes Educators©

26   Diabetes Education Curriculum

(prenatal vitamins, iron). Assessment should also include the patient's level of knowledge and skills, motivation and attitudes, and readiness to learn. The presence of barriers related to cultural identity, lifestyle, health, and beliefs should be assessed, as well as facilitators, such as the patient's support system.

- Nutrition diagnosis, nutrition intervention (education and counseling), and nutrition monitoring and evaluation. Ongoing follow-up to support long-term lifestyle changes, evaluate outcomes, and modify interventions as needed.[7]
- Length of visits—45 to 90 minutes.
- Frequency of sessions—an initial series of 3 or 4 encounters; more if needed.
- Time between encounters—initial series of encounters completed within 3 to 6 months of diagnosis or time of first referral; at least 1 follow-up encounter annually to reinforce lifestyle changes and monitor need for MNT or medication changes.[7]
- Clinical and behavioral outcomes to measure.

The consistent measurement of outcomes is essential to show the effectiveness of the nutrition education intervention, not only for the individual patient but for the population of patients frequenting the diabetes education program.[2]

Although the entire healthcare team has a role in diabetes care, the registered dietitian (RD)/registered dietitian nutritionist (RDN) is the clinician with the greatest expertise in providing MNT. Studies demonstrate that when NPGs were implemented by RDs/RDNs, A1C was reduced by an average of 1% to 2%.[8-10] All members of the healthcare team should reinforce the principles taught by the RD/RDN.

Learning Objectives

Knowledge

The participant will:

- state the effect of different foods and beverages on blood glucose levels
- describe the meal plan (the type of food choices, the amount of food/beverage, the timing of meals and snacks, responses to special situations, etc) that is appropriate for his or her nutritional goals
- state the recommended weight gain guideline for her prepregnancy BMI (if applicable)

Skills

The participant will:

- correctly demonstrate how to measure/weigh food portions
- accurately demonstrate how to count carbohydrates
- accurately interpret relevant information on food labels
- correctly identify menu items that are appropriate for his or her meal plan/nutritional goals
- collaboratively develop a meal plan with the educator and make adjustments as needed

Barriers and Facilitators

The participant will:

- identify potential barriers and facilitators that may affect his or her ability to implement a meal plan for healthy eating
- develop strategies for reducing barriers and increasing facilitators in order to successfully implement a meal plan for healthy eating

American Association of Diabetes Educators©

Module 2 *Healthy Eating* 27

Behavioral Objective

- The participant will set realistic, measurable, and sustainable individual goals for healthy eating.

HEALTHY EATING: INSTRUCTIONAL PLAN

Identifying Participant Thoughts and Feelings About Eating

What does the word "diet" mean to you?
How do you feel about making changes in your eating habits?
What do you want to learn today about healthy eating?
What is your greatest concern about healthy eating?
What is the hardest part about healthy eating for you?
What is the best part about healthy eating for you?
What have you heard about the benefits of healthy eating?
How do you think your eating habits will affect your pregnancy?

Adults learn best when they feel valued and respected for the experiences and perspectives they bring. Use probing questions to elicit learners' experiences and perspectives.

Healthy Eating: Facts Versus Fiction

The word *diet* refers to all the food a person eats plus the beverages he or she drinks. However, when most people hear the word *diet*, they think of restrictions to what they can eat. You may think that a diet is a list of good foods versus bad foods—some foods are OK to choose, and others are forbidden. If the word *diet* has come to have a negative tone in your mind, it may help to think of dietary changes as *healthy eating*.

Healthy eating is a good plan for a lifetime. Eating healthfully gives you balanced nutrition throughout the phases of your life. It changes as your needs change. It's about variety, flexibility, and choice, so that you can maintain healthy eating over the course of your life.

A plan for healthy eating needs to be individualized to match your needs. One plan does not fit all people. An RD/RDN can help you customize a meal plan to fit your lifestyle. Your likes and dislikes, your cultural identity, and your schedule are all considered in an individualized meal plan. A plan for healthy eating may require you to rethink a lifetime of eating habits or to learn new ways. Like any new habit, it will take a while to get used to as you incorporate small changes into your life. But the payoff will be better nutrition for you and even for your family.

You probably don't want to prepare 2 meals: one for yourself and another for your family. That would be too hard, and it's unrealistic. The main ideas behind healthy eating for diabetes are also good for the entire family. And since type 2 diabetes runs in families, healthy eating is one tool in the prevention of diabetes.

Goals for Healthy Eating and Meal Planning

One goal for healthy eating is to prevent the long-term complications of diabetes. If a person has already developed a diabetes complication, healthy eating can aid in its treatment. Healthy eating, along with physical

American Association of Diabetes Educators©

28   Diabetes Education Curriculum

activity, lowers the risk for getting type 2 diabetes in some people.[7] Successful approaches should also include behavioral intervention to help sustain a healthier lifestyle. A plan for healthy eating should help control blood glucose, blood pressure, body weight, and lipids (blood fats) to prevent or delay secondary complications.[11] Healthy eating also helps support your metabolism. Let's look briefly at how eating habits affect each of these areas.

In pregnancy, healthy eating has 4 important goals: assist in gaining appropriate weight, help to avoid developing maternal ketosis, provide for adequate nutrition for maternal and fetal health, and minimize blood glucose elevations.

Healthy Eating and Metabolism `Survival Skill`

It is important to space your meals throughout the day. Going too long without eating may result in excessive hunger, which can lead to overeating later on. Eating every 4 to 5 hours or so during the waking hours keeps your body cells energized and helps prevent hypoglycemia (low blood glucose). If you go too many hours without eating, your metabolism starts to slow down in order to save energy. A slower metabolism promotes storage of fat. *Skipping breakfast is a good way to gain weight.* On the other hand, eating breakfast every day jump-starts your metabolism and begins the calorie-burning process. Including small snacks between meals as part of your daily intake helps keep your metabolism going. If you are pregnant with diabetes, whether gestational or preexisting, you may benefit by eating snacks to avoid between-meal hunger and overeating at meals.

Healthy Eating and Blood Glucose Control `Survival Skill`

Certain foods raise the blood glucose level more than others. Foods/choices from the carbohydrate group have the greatest effect on blood glucose after eating. So, choosing the right type and amount of carbohydrates at each meal and snack can help you control your blood glucose level. Also, these carbohydrates should be spaced throughout the day to help keep your glucose level steady. If you are pregnant, you may need to restrict or reduce certain high-carbohydrate foods to control your blood glucose level.

Healthy Eating and Blood Pressure Control `Survival Skill`

Gradually decreasing the amount of sodium (salt) in your diet can help control blood pressure. Regular table salt is about 40% sodium and contains 2400 mg sodium per teaspoon. There are many ways to reduce the amount of dietary sodium in cooking, at the table, in prepared grocery products, and while dining out. (More details on sodium intake are provided later in this module.)

Healthy Eating and Lipids

Lipid refers to the cholesterol and triglycerides in the blood. Abnormal lipid levels increase the risk for heart disease. Losing weight, reducing carbohydrate intake, and choosing healthy fats while avoiding unhealthy fats have a positive effect on lipid levels.[7]

Healthy Eating and Weight

For people with prediabetes and those in the early stages of type 2 diabetes, moderate weight loss can help the body use insulin better. A moderate weight loss means losing 5% to 10% of body weight. Weight loss also helps control blood pressure and blood fats (lipids) and lowers the risk of getting breast, colon, or kidney cancer. Keep in mind, weight loss is not recommended during pregnancy.

Physical activity should always be part of any weight loss effort, along with a healthful eating plan and behavior change goals. Studies show that slow weight loss of one half to 2 pounds per week is kept off more easily than rapid weight loss. Quick weight loss is usually regained—plus losing more than 3 pounds per week for more than a few weeks increases the risk of developing gallstones.[12]

American Association of Diabetes Educators©

What's a Healthy Weight?[13]

To assess your weight and whether it is healthy, you must look at 3 measures:

1. BMI
2. Waist circumference
3. Risk factors for conditions linked to obesity

Body mass index is a measure of body fat based on your weight relative to your height and differs between men and women. The amount of total body fat is related to the risk for diseases and death. Body mass index is not a perfect measure, but it is a good screening tool. In muscular people or athletes, the BMI may overestimate body fat. In elderly people or those who have lost muscle mass, the BMI may underestimate body fat. Look at the BMI scale to learn your measurement. An online government resource for BMI calculation is found at the Web site of the National Heart, Lung, and Blood Institute US Department of Health & Human Services: http://www.nhlbi.nih.gov/health/educational/lose_wt/BMI/bmicalc.htm. (A BMI chart is included in the "Resources" section of this module and may be used as a patient handout.) The following scores assign the weight category for BMI for adults only, 20 years and older:

BMI (kg/m^2)	Weight Category
Below 18.5	Underweight
18.5–24.9	Normal* (Asian American adults 18.5–22.9)
25–29.9	Overweight* (Asian American adults 23–29.9)
30–39.9	Obese
40 and higher	Extreme obesity

*The 2015 ADA Standards of Medical Care in Diabetes revised the BMI cut point for screening overweight or obese Asian Americans for prediabetes and type 2 diabetes to 23 kg/m^2. BMI cut point for screening remains at 25 kg/m^2 for all other adults. Asian Americans develop diabetes at a lower BMI than the general population's guideline of 25. This doesn't define overweight, just the BMI cut point for screening diabetes.

The above BMI chart **does not apply** to infants, children, or teens through 19 years of age. For information about BMI for children see the Centers for Disease Control and Prevention (CDC) Healthy Weight link: http://www.cdc.gov/healthyweight/assessing/bmi/childrens_bmi/about_childrens_bmi.html.

Of course, when you are pregnant, your waist circumference can't be measured! Instead, the Institute of Medicine (IOM) has established guidelines to help determine the appropriate amount of weight to be gained during your pregnancy. This is based on your BMI before pregnancy. The recommended ranges are listed in Table 2.1. You

TABLE 2.1 Recommended Ranges of Weight Gain for Pregnant Women by Prepregnancy BMI		
BMI Category	Recommended Total Weight Gain (Single Gestation)	Recommended Total Weight Gain (Twin Gestation)
Underweight (<18.6)	28–40 lb (12.7–18.2 kg)	
Normal weight (18.6–24.9)	25–35 lb (11.3–16 kg)	37–54 lb (16.8–24.5 kg)
Overweight (25–29.9)	15–25 lb (6.8–11.3 kg)	31–50 lb (14.1–22.7 kg)
Obese (≥30)	11–20 lb (4.5–9 kg)	25–42 lb (11.3–19.1 kg)

Source: Institute of Medicine, *Weight Gain During Pregnancy: Reexamining the Guidelines* (Washington, DC: Institute of Medicine, 2009), 2.

American Association of Diabetes Educators©

should try to stay within the amount of weight for your BMI. If you gain more weight than what is recommended, your baby may be too large and you may have a more difficult time losing the extra weight after the pregnancy.

 Adults learn best when the content is meaningful to their experience and fills a perceived need. Distributing the BMI chart to participants can help them quantify their need for weight management.

Waist circumference is the distance around your waist. This measurement is an indicator of abdominal or belly fat. Studies in recent years have shown that belly fat is a reliable predictor of the risk for developing certain conditions, including diabetes, high blood pressure, elevated blood fats, and heart disease.[14] If the waist circumference is more than 40 inches in men and over 35 inches in women, the risk increases. If the BMI is above normal *and* the waist circumference is above 40 inches for men/above 35 inches for women, the risk for developing other diseases goes up even more.

Updated research shows the measurement of waist-to-hip ratio provides no advantage over waist circumference alone.[14] Using BMI and waist circumference together is adequate to assess body fat. (See Figure 2.1.) The waist/hip ratio (WHR) can still be used as an indicator of risk for developing heart disease as an added measure. To check WHR, measure your waist, then your hips (at the widest part). Divide the waist measurement by the hip measurement. If the WHR is >0.9 for men or >0.85 in women, the risk for heart disease is increased.

The good news is that research also shows that losing a few inches off your waist can have great benefits.

 Have tape measures on hand for those who wish to assess their waist circumference and/or WHR (see next section). Note: Disposable paper tape measures may be purchased in bulk from a number of resources. Do an Internet search on "disposable tape measures."

FIGURE 2.1 Measuring Waist Circumference

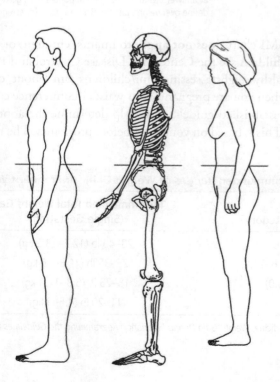

Measuring Waist Circumference

To measure waist circumference, locate the upper hip bone and the top of the right iliac crest. Place a measuring tape in a horizontal plane around the abdomen at the level of the iliac crest. Before reading the tape measure, ensure that the tape is snug, does not compress the skin, and is parallel to the floor. The measurement is made at the end of a normal expiration.[13]

Risk Factors for Conditions Linked to Obesity

If you are overweight or obese *and* you have 2 or more of the following risk factors, you should lose weight:

- High blood pressure
- High LDL ("bad") cholesterol
- Low HDL ("good") cholesterol
- High triglycerides (blood fats)
- High blood glucose
- Family history of early heart disease
- Sedentary lifestyle
- Smoker

Even losing just 5% to 10% of your current weight will lower your risk. If you are overweight but have fewer than 2 risk factors, you should at least prevent further weight gain.

 Have charts available for participants who want to plot their weight by date. See the "Resources" section of this module for a handout for your class participants.

Weighing In

If you are trying to lose weight, regular monitoring of your weight is important. It's not necessary to weigh yourself every day. Today's weight is not a true measure of yesterday's eating. Tomorrow's weight won't accurately reflect your eating today. This is because water weight in your body changes from day to day. Some people tend to retain more water weight than other people. This is especially related to how your body handles sodium. Weight loss is geared toward losing fat, not water. Fat weight does not change measurably in the space of 1 day.

When you do weigh in, keep in mind that scales can differ in their measurement. Try to use the same scale each time to get more accurate weight trends. You may find it useful to track your weight each week on a graph. A graph will work better than a list to show you the change in weight.

In pregnancy, a prenatal weight gain grid will show if you are gaining too much, too little, or the recommended amount of weight.

Daily Calorie Needs

Adult calorie needs can vary and are based on current body weight, body composition, sex, age, activity level, health status, desired weight change, etc. To lose 1 lb of body fat per week, total calorie deficit needs to be 500 calories daily through reduced calorie intake and/or increased calories used through physical activity. See Table 2.2 for estimated calorie requirements for male and female adults.

Calories for children and teens should be adequate to provide for normal growth and development in addition to daily metabolic needs. To determine normal growth and weight profiles, growth of children and adolescents should be monitored on a CDC or similar height-weight growth chart (http://www.cdc.gov/growthcharts/clinical_charts.htm) at regular intervals. Children's calorie needs should be based not only on the CDC chart but

32   Diabetes Education Curriculum

TABLE 2.2   Estimated Calorie Requirements (in Kilocalories) for Each Gender and Age Group at 3 Levels of Physical Activity*

Gender	Age (Years)	Activity Level		
		Sedentary	Moderately Active	Active
Child	2–3	1000	1000–1400	1000–1400
Female	4–8	1200	1400–1600	1400–1800
Female	9–13	1600	1600–2000	1800–2000
Female	14–18	1800	2000	2400
Female	19–30	2000	2000–2200	2400
Female	31–50	1800	2000	2200
Female	51+	1600	1800	2000–2200
Male	4–8	1400	1400–1600	1600–2000
Male	9–13	1800	1800–2200	2000–2600
Male	14–18	2200	2400–2800	2800–3200
Male	19–30	2400	2600–2800	3000
Male	31–50	2200	2400–2600	2800–3000
Male	51+	2000	2200–2400	2400–2800

Notes:

a. These levels are based on estimated energy requirements from the IOM Dietary Reference Intakes macronutrients report (2002), calculated by gender, age, and activity level for reference-sized individuals. "Reference size," as determined by IOM, is based on median height and weight for ages up to 18 and median height and weight for that height to give a BMI of 21.5 for adult females and 22.5 for adult males.

b. Sedentary means a lifestyle that includes only the light physical activity associated with typical day-to-day life.

c. Moderately active means a lifestyle that includes physical activity equivalent to walking about 1.5 to 3 miles per day at 3 to 4 miles per hour, in addition to the light physical activity associated with typical day-to-day life.

d. Active means a lifestyle that includes physical activity equivalent to walking more than 3 miles per day at 3 to 4 miles per hour, in addition to the light physical activity associated with typical day-to-day life.

e. The calorie ranges shown are to accommodate needs of different ages within the group. For children and adolescents, more calories are needed at older ages. For adults, fewer calories are needed at older ages.

*This calorie requirement chart presents estimated amounts of calories needed to maintain energy balance (and a healthy body weight) for various gender and age groups at 3 levels of physical activity. The estimates are rounded to the nearest 200 calories and were determined using an equation from the Institute of Medicine.

Source: US Department of Health and Human Services and US Department of Agriculture, *Dietary Guidelines for Americans, 2005*, 6th ed (Washington, DC: US Government Printing Office, 2005).

also on the results of a diet history. The meal plan should not restrict calories but should ensure a consistent, nutritionally balanced diet. Parents of young children and adolescents need to adjust insulin rather than restricting food and beverages to allow for enjoyment and healthy growth patterns. See Table 2.2 for estimated calorie requirements for children and teens.

Common Nutrition Terms

Words like *meal plan, calories, portion, serving, choice,* and *serving size* are often used in discussions of nutrition. This section defines each of these terms.

Meal Plan

Survival Skill A *meal plan* is a guide for healthy eating. It should be balanced nutritionally throughout the day. A balanced meal plan includes the right amount of the 3 main nutrients found in food: carbohydrate, protein, and fat. They each supply energy for your body but are used in different ways. Getting enough vitamins, minerals, and water from all foods and beverages consumed is also an important part of your overall meal plan.

American Association of Diabetes Educators©

The energy from the 3 major nutrients or macronutrients—carbohydrate, protein, and fat—in foods and beverages is measured in *calories or kilocalories (kcals)*. Some nutrients provide more energy than others. Carbohydrate is the primary immediate source of fuel for the body, providing 4 calories per gram. Protein, a slower fuel source, builds and repairs tissue and also provides 4 calories per gram. Fat is a concentrated energy source serving as a storage depot for future energy needs. Fat provides 9 calories per gram, about twice as many calories per gram as carbohydrate or protein. Alcohol, though not a nutrient, provides 7 calories per gram.[15]

A meal plan should include enough calories for your energy needs. If you take in fewer calories than you need, you will lose weight. If you take in more calories than you need, you will gain weight. Each person's calorie needs vary. Children require more calories because they are still growing and are more active. Men usually need more calories than women as they are generally larger and have more muscle mass to support. Pregnant women will need more calories than nonpregnant women.

A meal plan should be developed with your individual needs in mind. Several things may be considered: your age, sex, activity level, height and weight, whether you are pregnant, and any other health conditions. A meal plan can be very detailed, or it can be very simple, based on your preference. There is no one meal plan for every person with diabetes. Your meal plan should be one that works for *you*. There are different approaches to meal planning you may want to consider.

Recent evidence suggests there is no "ideal" eating pattern or distribution of carbohydrate, protein, and fat that is expected to benefit all individuals with diabetes. A variety of combinations of different foods and food groups are acceptable for diabetes management. Total energy intake (total calories) and portion size are important to consider with all eating patterns. A variety of eating patterns, in addition to the traditional, have been shown to be modestly effective in managing diabetes, including Mediterranean style, Dietary Approaches to Stop Hypertension (DASH), plant based (vegan or vegetarian), lower fat, and lower carbohydrate patterns. Collaborative goals, including behavior and other lifestyle changes, should also be developed with the individual with diabetes.[7,11,16]

Portion `Survival Skill`

The amount of a food you eat is called a *portion*. The portion you eat may actually be several servings, based on the serving size on the Nutrition Facts[17] panel of the label.

Portion Control `Survival Skill`

Part of managing diabetes is to practice *portion control*. There is more than one way you can approach portion control. Your meal plan may list how many *servings* of a food equals 1 portion. Or, your meal plan may tell you how much of your plate should be filled with foods from different groups.

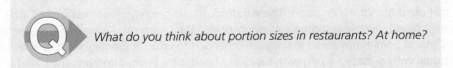

What do you think about portion sizes in restaurants? At home?

Serving `Survival Skill`

A *serving* is a specific amount of food. Your meal plan may include 1, 2, or 3 servings of a certain food within a meal or snack. Because food comes in a variety of shapes and consistencies, *serving sizes* are measured in different ways. Servings are referred to as *choices*.

Serving Size

Liquids and soft foods can be measured using a measuring cup or spoon. Fruit or vegetables can be measured in a variety of ways, based on how you prepare them. If you eat a food whole, it's measured by the size of the piece. If you chop up a food, it's measured in a cup. Meat can be measured by the ounce with a food scale or portion of the package weight. Protein choices are based on cooked or ready-to-eat portions, so allow for shrinkage from raw.

Another way to measure food is to compare average serving sizes to everyday items. For example, 3 ounces of meat is the size of a deck of cards. See "Measuring Food With Everyday Items as a Guide" in the "Resources" section for other comparisons.

Your meal plan may call for more than 1 serving (choice) of a specific food at a meal. For example, breakfast may include 2 servings (choices) of starch. If 1 slice of toast is a single serving, this means you could have 2 slices of toast, or you could have 1 slice of toast plus a half cup of oatmeal. Dinner on your meal plan may include 3 servings (choices) of meat. If you know that a serving is 1 ounce, this means you could eat 3 ounces of meat.

Your individualized meal plan will tell you how many daily servings (choices) you should eat from the different food groups. Everyone's needs are different, so the meal plan will vary from person to person. Ask for a referral to an RD/RDN, who can help you determine what approach is right for you, provide guidance and support, and help you set goals.

Let's look at food's main nutrients—carbohydrate, protein, and fat—in more detail.

Show everyday items that compare in size to average serving sizes. This technique is particularly helpful for those with visual/spatial intelligence. You can also use food models or real food as appropriate, such as dry cereal in a bowl.

Advanced Detail

Carb Counting—Getting Started and Match Your Insulin

For all individuals with diabetes, the right type of food in the right amount and at the right time helps match their available insulin, whether internal or external, to their needs. Carb counting, a method of keeping track of the grams of carbohydrate consumed at meals and in snacks, is one form of meal planning. Individuals using MNT alone or along with glucose-lowering medications or fixed insulin doses at meals and snacks should be consistently consuming evenly distributed carbohydrates throughout the day.

Though there is no ideal carbohydrate intake for people with diabetes, general suggestions for meals are as follows: breakfast, 2 or 3 carb choices (30 to 45 g carbohydrate); lunch and dinner, 3 or 4 carb choices (45 to 60 g carbohydrate) each; plus snacks, 1 or 2 carb choices (15 to 30 g carbohydrate) each. Men may need an additional carb choice at breakfast as well as at lunch and dinner. This method can be referred to as basic carb counting.[15]

Those individuals with type 1 or type 2 diabetes who adjust their mealtime insulin doses or are on an insulin pump therapy generally use an advanced carbohydrate counting method. This method adjusts their insulin dose to match their carbohydrate intake in grams. These individuals are given an individualized I:Carb (insulin to carb) ratio based on their blood glucose response to carbohydrate. The I:Carb ratio covers carbohydrate consumed at a meal or in a snack. Sometimes additional insulin is needed to lower a premeal glucose level back to a goal range. The individual with diabetes, along with his or her healthcare team, interprets the blood glucose pattern and responses to determine the specific I:Carb ratio, such as 1:15, 1:10, etc. Protein and fat content plus total energy intake are also important considerations.[15,16]

Food and Nutrient Groups

Adults learn best when the learning experience is active and not passive. Keep participants engaged with questions like *Can anyone list some grains? Who can name some starchy vegetables?*

Carbohydrates `Survival Skill`

When carbohydrate foods are eaten, they break down into glucose. *Glucose* is the medical word for *sugar*. During digestion, this sugar passes through the walls of the intestine and enters the bloodstream, causing the blood glucose level to go up after eating. Carbohydrate-rich foods have the greatest immediate effect on the blood glucose level. For this reason, they should be spread out throughout the day, depending on your individualized meal plan. Remember, there is no ideal amount of carbohydrate for all people with diabetes, so monitoring carbohydrate intake along with blood sugar levels is key to achieving blood glucose control.[11]

Carbohydrate choices include starch, fruit, milk, and sweets. The amount of carbohydrate in food is measured in *grams*. For good health, carbohydrates from vegetables, fruits, whole grains, legumes, and dairy products are your best choices.[11] See Table 2.3 for examples of carbohydrates and their single serving sizes.

Spreading out carbohydrate-rich foods throughout the day is especially important in pregnancy. In women who had diabetes before pregnancy, the amount and distribution of calories and carbohydrates are individualized and based on the woman's food preferences, blood glucose log, and physical activity level. The mealtime insulin must match the amount of carbohydrates at mealtime to keep her blood glucose levels in the target range before and after eating.

The Academy of Nutrition and Dietetics' Evidence-Based Nutrition Practice Guidelines suggest that women with gestational diabetes divide their carbohydrate into 3 small-to-moderate meals with 2 to 4 snacks. The initial meal plan *may* look like this:

- Breakfast: 15 to 45 g
- Lunch and dinner: 45 to 75 g
- Snacks: 15 to 45 g

The breakfast carbohydrate amount is usually lower than the lunch and dinner amount because of higher hormonal levels in the morning, which may cause more insulin resistance than at other times during the day. The types of carbohydrates may also be restricted or reduced. Breakfast cereals may be discouraged as well as highly processed foods and sweetened beverages. However, the total amount of carbohydrates is more significant than the type. Certain foods, such as milk or fruit, may need to be eaten at snack time so that a more normal amount of carbohydrates can be consumed at meals.

Keep in mind that all women need some extra carbohydrates in pregnancy in order to provide additional glucose for the baby's growth. The *minimum* amount of carbohydrate needed in pregnancy is 175 g each day. The RD will help in your meal planning to ensure you get the necessary amount of carbohydrates.

TABLE 2.3 Carbohydrate Choices (Whole Grain Preferred) and Their Serving Sizes

Bagel, ¼ regular or ½ Bagel Thin/Skinny Bagel/Biali	Pasta, ⅓ cup
Bread or roll, 1 slice or 1 small roll	Pita bread, ½ of 6-inch piece
Cooked dry beans or peas, ½ cup	Polenta, ⅓ cup
Corn, ½ cup	Popcorn, 3 cups (popped)
Crackers, 6 Saltines; 3 graham-type 2½-inch squares	Potatoes, ½ cup or 1 small
Dry cereal (varies), ½ to 1½ cup	Rice, ⅓ cup
English muffin, ½ muffin	Rice cakes, 2
Grits or Cream of Wheat, ½ cup (cooked)	Tortilla (corn or flour), 1 (6 inches across)
Hamburger bun, ½ bun	Yams, ½ cup
Hot dog bun, ½ bun	Waffle, 1 (4 inches across)
Oatmeal, ½ cup (cooked)	

Sources: Academy of Nutrition and Dietetics and American Diabetes Association, *Choose Your Foods: Food Lists for Diabetes* (Chicago and Alexandria, Va: Academy of Nutrition and Dietetics and American Diabetes Association, 2014); US Department of Agriculture, "What's in the foods you eat search tool, 2011-2012" (cited 2015 July 15), on the Internet at: http://www.ars.usda.gov/News/docs.htm?docid=17032.

American Association of Diabetes Educators©

Starch `Survival Skill`

Starches include grain foods, starchy vegetables, lentils, and dried beans.

Grains include wheat, oats, rice, barley, and rye. These grains are usually used in making breads, cereals, crackers, and pasta. Starchy vegetables include corn, potatoes, lima beans, and peas. Most starches also contain varying amounts of fiber. Each serving (choice) of food from this group contains **about 15 g** of carbohydrate. Your individualized meal plan will tell you how many starch servings (choices) are recommended for you.

What other starches are commonly eaten in your culture/family?

Cultural competency enhances the educator-patient relationship.
- Become familiar with the foods commonly eaten by patients of cultural/ethnic groups other than your own. See Table 2.4 for examples of starches commonly used in international cuisine.
- Update the list of starches as needed to reflect your patients' food choices.
- Be aware of which foods are not recommended during pregnancy.

Fruits `Survival Skill`

Fruits are packed with vitamins and minerals. They are a good source of fiber, especially if you eat the whole fruit. Each serving of food from this group contains about 15 g of carbohydrate. The carbohydrate from a serving of fruit juice is absorbed more quickly than the carbohydrate from a serving of whole fruit. A serving (choice) of fruit juice is sometimes used for treatment of low blood sugar (hypoglycemia). A balanced meal plan includes at least 2 servings of fruit per day. Your individualized meal plan will tell you how many fruit servings (choices) are recommended for you. See Table 2.5 for examples of fruits and their single serving sizes.

TABLE 2.4 Starches Commonly Used in International Cuisine

Food Item	Region
Bulgur wheat, ½ cup (cooked)	ME, MED
Cassava (yucca), ⅓ cup (cooked)	A, AF, CA, CAR, SA
Chapatti, 1 small (6 inches across)	AF, IN
Couscous (kuskus, maftoul), ⅓ cup (cooked)	AF, ME, MED
Kasha (buckwheat groats), ½ cup (cooked)	EE
Quinoa, ⅓ cup (cooked)	ME, SA
Naan bread (nan, non, nan bya), ¼ of large (8 × 2-inch) piece	IN
Plantain, ⅓ cup (cooked)	A, AF, CA, CAR, SA
Tabbouleh (tabouleh, tabouli, tipili), ½ cup (prepared)	ME, MED

Region Legend

A = Asia, AF = Africa, CA = Central America, CAR = Caribbean, EE = Eastern Europe, IN = India, ME = Middle East, MED = Mediterranean, SA = South America

TABLE 2.5 Fruit Choices and Their Serving Sizes

Apples, 1 small (4 ounces)	Honeydew, 1 cup cubes	Tangerine, 2 small
Apricots, 4 whole or 8 dried halves	Kiwi, 1 large piece	Watermelon, 1¼ cup cubes
Bananas, extra small or a 6-inch piece	Oranges, 1	
Blackberries, ¾ cup	Peaches, 1 medium	*Fruit juices:*
Blueberries, ¾ cup	Pears, 1 medium	Apple, ½ cup
Cantaloupe, 1 cup cubes	Pineapple, ¾ cup	Grape, ⅓ cup
Cherries, 12	Plums, 2 (2⅛ inches across)	Grapefruit, ½ cup
Cranberries, raisins, 2 tablespoons (dried)	Pomegranate, ½ (3⅜ inches across)	Orange, ½ cup
Figs, 2 medium (2¼ inches across)	Prunes, 3 (dried)	Pineapple, ½ cup
Grapefruit, ½	Raspberries, 1 cup	Pomegranate, ½ cup
Grapes, 17	Strawberries, 1¼ cup whole	Prune, ⅓ cup

Note: Fruits are in raw, fresh form unless otherwise specified.

Sources: Academy of Nutrition and Dietetics and American Diabetes Association, *Choose Your Foods: Food Lists for Diabetes* (Chicago and Alexandria, Va: Academy of Nutrition and Dietetics and American Diabetes Association, 2014); US Department of Agriculture, "What's in the foods you eat search tool, 2011-2012" (cited 2015 July 15), on the Internet at: http://www.ars.usda.gov/News/docs.htm?docid=17032.

Are there other fruits that are commonly eaten in your culture/family?

Cultural competency enhances the educator-patient relationship.

- Show and tell: Ask patients to bring in an example of fruit commonly eaten in their culture/ethnic group but with which you are unfamiliar.
- See Table 2.6 for fruits commonly used in international cuisine.

TABLE 2.6 Fruit Choices Commonly Used in International Cuisine

Food Item	Region	Food Item	Region
Akee	CAR	Mango, ½ cup	A, CA, CAR, IN, SA
Breadfruit (pana), ¼ cup	A, CAR, PI	Papaya, 1 cup	CA, CAR, SA
Cherimoya	CA, SA	Passion fruit (granadilla, lilikoi), ¼ cup	A, CA, CAR, PI, SA
Dragonfruit	A	Prickly pear (nopal), 4 cups	CA
Guava (guayaba), ¾ cup	CA, CAR, SA	Rambutan (mamón chino)	A, CA, CAR, PI
Longan (lungan, longyen, dragon eye)	A	Soursop (guanábana, guayabana, graviola), ½ cup nectar	A, CA, CAR, SA
Loquat (nispero)	CA, CAR, SA		
Lychee (Chinese plum), ¼ cup (canned)	A	Star fruit (carambola, Quả Khế), 2 cups	A, PI, SA
Mamey Sapote	CA, CAR, SA		

Region Legend

A = Asia, CA = Central America, CAR = Caribbean, IN = India, PI = Pacific Islands, SA = South America

Note: Fruits in listed serving sizes are raw unless otherwise specified; if no serving size is listed, the author was unable to locate nutrition information.

TABLE 2.7 Serving Sizes for Milk
1 cup fat-free (skim) or low-fat (1%) milk
2/3 cup nonfat or low-fat yogurt, plain or sweetened with artificial sweetener

Note: Other common non-dairy milk or milk substitutes include 1 cup (8 ounces) low-fat, plain soy milk (1 carbohydrate and ½ fat choice); 1 cup (8 ounces) unsweetened almond milk (1 unsaturated fat choice); 1 cup (8 ounces) unsweetened coconut milk beverage (thin) (1 saturated fat choice). Check the Nutrition Facts label for the best fit.

Source: Academy of Nutrition and Dietetics and American Diabetes Association, *Choose Your Foods: Food Lists for Diabetes* (Chicago and Alexandria, Va: Academy of Nutrition and Dietetics and American Diabetes Association, 2014).

TABLE 2.8 Serving Sizes for Greek Yogurt
2/3 cup nonfat Greek yogurt, plain = 1 fat-free milk/carb (about 80–90 calories)
2/3 cup nonfat Greek yogurt, with fruit = 1½ fat-free milk/carb (about 110–140 calories)

Milk Survival Skill

Each serving (choice) of food/beverage from this group contains about **12 g** of carbohydrate. Milk products have vitamins (including vitamin D), calcium, and other minerals, plus protein to help keep your bones strong. Fat-free or low-fat milk products are your best choice. Your individualized meal plan will tell you how many milk servings (choices) are recommended for you. See Table 2.7 for milk serving sizes.

Lactose is a sugar found in milk and some other dairy products. If you are lactose intolerant, consider other sources of calcium such as tofu, soybeans, and orange juice fortified with calcium. You may also choose dairy products that are lactose-free, or you may use over-the-counter medicines that contain lactase enzyme when having lactose-containing dairy products. Natural cheeses, such as cheddar and Swiss, generally are lactose-free, but processed cheeses, such as American, do contain lactose.

Greek yogurt has more protein and less carbohydrate than regular yogurt. Suggested choices for single serve cups are given in Table 2.8. Check the label for grams of carbohydrate for that brand, flavor, and serving size.

For heart health, it's best to choose milk products that are fat-free or low-fat. One way to compare the amount of fat in different types of milk is to visualize the fat as a pat of butter. For every cup of milk, the fat content varies:

- Whole milk: 2 pats of fat (8 g of fat)
- Reduced-fat (2%) milk: 1 pat of fat (5 g of fat)
- Low-fat (1%) milk: ½ pat of fat (3 g of fat)
- Fat-free (skim) milk: 0 pats of fat (0 to 0.5 g of fat)

Adults learn best when they can relate new information to what they already know. Show models of butterfat to simulate the fat in various milk options.

Is whole milk bad for you? That's all I drank as a kid.

Sweets Survival Skill

Many people think that sugar is *off limits* in the diets of those with diabetes, often referred to as the *diabetic diet*. In fact, this used to be the *rule* in years past. Now, however, sugar—like any other carbohydrate—can be fit into the meal plan. Sugary foods usually don't have the same nutrition value as grains or vegetables. Many sweets also have lots of fat in them, so it's best to keep your portions small. Reserve sweets for special occasions. See Table 2.9 for serving sizes for selected sweets.

American Association of Diabetes Educators©

TABLE 2.9 Serving Sizes for Selected Sweets*

Brownie, unfrosted†	1¼-inch square	Gelatin	½ cup
Cake, unfrosted†	2-inch square	Hard candy	3 pieces
Cookies†	2 (2¼ inches across)	Ice cream, regular	½ cup
Frozen yogurt	¼ to ½ cup (check nutrition label, the grams of carb per serving can vary)	Sherbet, sorbet	¼ cup
		Vanilla wafers†	5

*Serving size equals about 15 g of carbohydrate.
†Sweets that also contain fat choices. Check the Nutrition Facts label.
Source: Academy of Nutrition and Dietetics and American Diabetes Association, *Choose your Foods: Food Lists for Diabetes* (Chicago and Alexandria, Va: Academy of Nutrition and Dietetics and American Diabetes Association, 2014).

Do you think people with diabetes can enjoy sweets?
Do you think that sugar is allowed in the diabetes meal plan?

Read labels to see the grams of carbohydrate in sweets, because the amount varies widely. Swap sweets for a carbohydrate serving (choice) in your individualized meal plan. This will help avoid big spikes in your blood glucose level.

Help patients build a positive attitude about diabetes self-care by:
- Confronting erroneous beliefs, expectations, and assumptions about sweets/sugar that might underlie a negative patient attitude.
- Presenting evidence that will help put deprivation fears to rest and promote patient control over his or her situation.

Carbohydrate Problem Solving

If you ran out of milk, what could you substitute for milk?

If you ate an extra serving of oatmeal, what other food could you delete from your breakfast?

If you wanted an extra serving of fruit, could you substitute it for an egg? Why or why not?

Mix and Match

You will notice that starch, fruit, and milk products contain about the same amount of carbohydrate per serving. This gives you flexibility in your meal plan. You can mix and match foods within these groups to fit your situation.

If you don't have any fruit, you can substitute a serving of milk. If you run out of milk, you can substitute a serving of starch. If you take an extra serving of oatmeal, you can skip the toast.

Ideally, you will include foods from all 3 groups for balanced nutrition.

Keep in mind that *serving sizes may vary*, according to the type of food. But serving for serving, starch, fruit, and milk products are about equal in their carbohydrate content. These food groups are all considered carbohydrate choices.

American Association of Diabetes Educators©

Patients using advanced carbohydrate counting to titrate insulin should count *exact grams* of carbohydrates in each serving rather than estimate *about 15 g per serving*.

Nonstarchy Vegetables `Survival Skill`

Nonstarchy vegetables are good sources of fiber, vitamins, and minerals. They also contain carbohydrates, but less per serving than starch, fruit, or milk. Each serving of nonstarchy vegetables contains **about 5 g** of carbohydrates. A balanced meal plan includes at least 2 or more servings (choices) of nonstarchy vegetables per day. Your individualized meal plan will tell you how many nonstarchy vegetable servings (choices) are recommended for you. See Table 2.10.

To get the most nutrition from nonstarchy vegetables, eat them raw, microwaved, or steamed to help preserve the vitamins and minerals.

Can you list some nonstarchy vegetables? What are some of your favorites?

Can you substitute a half cup of cooked broccoli for 1 slice of bread? Why or why not?

Are there other nonstarchy vegetables that are commonly eaten in your culture/family?

TABLE 2.10　Nonstarchy Vegetables

Artichoke	Mixed vegetables (only nonstarchy)
Artichoke hearts	Mushrooms
Asparagus	Okra
Baby corn	Onions
Beans (green, Italian, wax)	Pea pods
Beets	Peppers (all varieties)
Broccoli	Radishes (all varieties)
Brussels sprouts	Rutabaga
Cabbage	Sauerkraut
Carrots	Spinach
Cauliflower	Squash (summer, crookneck, zucchini)
Celery	Swiss chard
Cucumbers	Tomato
Eggplant	Tomato sauce
Greens (collard, mustard, turnip)	Tomato/vegetable juice
Hearts of Palm	Turnips

Note: Foods listed are a half cup cooked or 1 cup raw. Salad greens (eg, chicory, endive, escarole, lettuce, romaine, spinach, arugula, radicchio, kale, watercress) are on the Free Food Choices list.

Sources: Academy of Nutrition and Dietetics and American Diabetes Association, *Choose Your Foods: Food Lists for Diabetes* (Chicago and Alexandria, Va: Academy of Nutrition and Dietetics and American Diabetes Association, 2014); US Department of Agriculture, "What's in the foods you eat search tool, 2011-2012" (cited 2015 July 15), on the Internet at: http://www.ars.usda.gov/News/docs.htm?docid=17032.

> **Advanced Detail**

I've been hearing about the glycemic index. What is it, and should I be using it?

The glycemic index (GI) is a system that ranks carbohydrate foods according to their effect on blood glucose levels. The blood glucose rise from a particular food is compared with the rise caused by pure glucose. The higher the rise in blood glucose, the higher the number on the GI; the lower the rise in blood glucose, the lower the number on the GI.

Glycemic Index Ranking[15]:

High GI = 70 or more   **Medium GI** = 56 to 69   **Low GI** = 55 or less

The glycemic load (GL) combines the GI value with the carbohydrate content of a serving of that food. A GL of 10 or less is low, 11 to 19 is medium, and 20+ is high. To check the GI and GL values of carbohydrate-containing foods, see the University of Sydney site list (http://www.glycemicindex.com).[18]

Should You Use the Glycemic Index?

The American Diabetes Association has concluded that research does not support the GI as a meal planning tool for people with diabetes. Substituting low GL food for higher GL foods may modestly improve blood glucose control.[11] By monitoring your glucose level before a meal and 2 hours later, you can learn how you respond to the carbohydrate in a given meal. This can help you learn how different foods affect your blood glucose levels.[11]

See Table 2.11 for examples of nonstarchy vegetables commonly used in international cuisine.

TABLE 2.11 Nonstarchy Vegetables Commonly Used in International Cuisine

Food Item	Region	Food Item	Region
Amaranth leaves (Chinese spinach)	A	Hot chili peppers	A, CA, CAR, IN, ME, SA
Azuki beans (adzuki, pat, đậu đỏ)	A		
Bamboo shoots (gaz, labong, măng, rebung, take no, tama, sandhna)	A	Jicama (yam bean, singkama)	A, CA, SA
		Kai lam (Japanese kale)	A
Bean sprouts (mung, so)	A	Kohlrabi	EE, IN, NE
Bitter melon	A	Leeks	NE
Bok choy	A	Sauerkraut	EE, NE
Borscht (beet soup)	EE	Snow peas	CA, SA
Burdock root (gobō)	A	Tatuma squash (tatume)	CA, SA
Chayote squash (sayote, mirliton, tayota, choko, chocho)	A, AF, CA, CAR, SA	Tomatillos	A
		Water chestnuts (bíqí, mătí, củ năng)	A, CAR, IN
Choy sum/yu choy	A	Yardlong beans (dangok, thua fak yao, kacang panjang, sitaw, bora, vali, eeril)	A
Daikon (labanos, oriental radish)	A		

Region Legend

A = Asia, AF = Africa, CA = Central America, CAR = Caribbean, EE = Eastern Europe, IN = India, ME = Middle East, NE = Northern Europe, SA = South America

Note: Foods listed are a half cup cooked/canned or 1 cup raw.

Protein `Survival Skill`

Protein is the nutrient in foods that helps tissues grow and repair after injury. Meat and meat substitutes contain protein, vitamins, and minerals. See Table 2.12 and Table 2.13 for examples of meats and meat substitutes.

Your individualized meal plan will tell you how many protein servings (choices) are recommended for you.

Protein does not cause the blood glucose level to rise after a meal in individuals with type 2 diabetes, but it does increase insulin response. Therefore, it is not advised to use protein to treat or prevent hypoglycemia.[11,19]

During pregnancy, your healthcare provider may reduce your carbohydrate intake. If so, to avoid not eating enough calories, your protein intake may be increased.

What sources of protein can you think of?

Do you think a person can get enough protein in his or her diet without eating meat? Why or why not?

Fats `Survival Skill`

Fat is a necessary part of your diet but should be eaten in moderation. Fats provide a concentrated form of energy (calories) and help support the growth of your body's cells. Fats help your body absorb certain nutrients and produce important hormones as well. Each gram of fat contains more than twice the calories of carbohydrates and

TABLE 2.12 Meat and Meat Substitutes and Their Serving Sizes (Weight After Cooking)

Beef, 1 ounce	Fish, 1 ounce; sardines, 2 medium, canned	Pork, 1 ounce
Beef jerky, 1 ounce	Goose, 1 ounce	Rabbit, 1 ounce
Bison, 1 ounce	Hot dog, 1 (low fat)	Ricotta cheese, ¼ cup (2 ounces)
Cheese, 1 ounce; 1 slice (sandwich size)	Lamb, 1 ounce	Scallops, 1 ounce
Chicken, 1 ounce	Lobster, 1 ounce	Shrimp, 1 ounce
Cottage cheese, ¼ cup	Lunch meat, 1 ounce (low fat)	Soy nuts (dry roasted), ¾ ounce
Clams, 1 ounce	Mussels, 1 ounce	Squid, 1 ounce
Duck, 1 ounce	Octopus, 1 ounce	Tofu, 4 ounces; ½ cup
Egg, 1	Oysters, 6 medium	Turkey, 1 ounce
Egg substitute, ¼ cup	Nut butter, 1 tablespoon	Venison, 1 ounce
Egg whites, 2		

Source: Academy of Nutrition and Dietetics and American Diabetes Association, *Choose Your Foods: Food Lists for Diabetes* (Chicago and Alexandria, Va: Academy of Nutrition and Dietetics and American Diabetes Association, 2014).

TABLE 2.13 Meat Substitutes Commonly Used in International Cuisine

Food Item	Region
Baby soybeans (edamame, máodòu), ½ cup cooked	A
Falafel (fava beans and/or chickpeas), 3 patties (2 inches across)	ME, AF
Hummus (chickpea spread), ⅓ cup	ME

Region Legend
A = Asia, AF = Africa, ME = Middle East

proteins. Be aware of portions, as eating too much fat can cause weight gain. Your individualized meal plan will tell you how many fat servings (choices) are recommended for you.

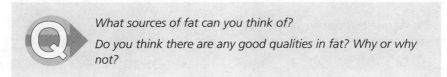

What sources of fat can you think of?

Do you think there are any good qualities in fat? Why or why not?

Fat is naturally found in animal products as well as in some plant products. All fats are not the same.

Unsaturated Fat

Unsaturated fats are found in all foods in differing amounts. Plants and certain fish contain the most unsaturated fats. They can help raise the level of HDL cholesterol in your body. HDL is known as "good" cholesterol because it improves the status of your heart health. Try to choose unsaturated fats over saturated and trans fats. Unsaturated fats are liquid at room temperature but may turn solid if chilled.

Unsaturated fats include *monounsaturated* and *polyunsaturated* fats. Polyunsaturated fats include omega-6 and omega-3 fatty acids. These fats play an important role in your brain function. They also help raise HDL ("good") cholesterol levels and reduce triglycerides and LDL ("bad") cholesterol levels, and so reduce the risk of heart disease. Foods containing monounsaturated fats usually have a good amount of vitamin E, an important antioxidant. Choose monounsaturated fats often to replace saturated fat sources.

Saturated Fat

Saturated fats are found in most foods in differing amounts. Animal products generally contain the most saturated fats, but plants have some also. Saturated fats increase your LDL cholesterol. LDL cholesterol is called "bad" cholesterol because it increases your risk for heart disease. Saturated fats are solid at room temperature.

Trans Fat

Small amounts of trans fats are found naturally in some animal products such as some meats, cheese, butter, milk, and other dairy products. Most trans fats come from a manufacturing process called *hydrogenation*.

Hydrogenation is used to increase the shelf life of baked and processed foods, and it helps maintain the flavor. Since trans fats have been shown to raise LDL levels, their intake should be minimized. On nutrition labels, the words *partially hydrogenated vegetable oil* generally mean trans fat. Check the Nutrition Facts panel for trans-fat content.

Omega-3 Fatty Acids

Omega-3 fatty acids are polyunsaturated fats found in some fatty fish and other foods. Omega-3s can help lower triglycerides and your risk of heart disease. The fish richest in this kind of fat are salmon, sardines, and mackerel. Two servings per week of these fish is recommended (serving size for the meat group is 1 ounce).[20] Sources of omega-3 fatty acids include:

- Albacore tuna
- Herring
- Lake trout
- Mackerel
- Halibut
- Salmon
- Sardines

Advanced Detail

Isn't it true that certain fish are not safe to eat because of mercury levels?

Mercury and other toxic chemicals in the water can build up in fish, posing a health hazard. The heavier fish that swim near the bottom of the ocean contain more mercury, so you should eat them less often. Young children and pregnant or nursing women should avoid shark, swordfish, tilefish, and king mackerel altogether, and limit all other fish to 12 ounces per week.[20-22] When choosing tuna, be aware that albacore tuna contains more mercury than chunk light tuna.

To learn about safety recommendations for eating fish caught or sold in your local area, visit the Food and Drug Administration (FDA) Web site at http://www.fda.gov/NewsEvents/Newsroom/PressAnnouncements/ucm397929.htm.[22] The Environmental Protection Agency issues fish advisories. On its Web site, you can click on your state to learn about current advice on eating fish from freshwater lakes and streams. Also see http://water.epa.gov/scitech/swguidance/fishshellfish/fishadvisories/.

Choose your fat carefully. Eat fat sparingly. Choose unsaturated fats over saturated fats. See Table 2.14 for examples of fats and their serving sizes.

TABLE 2.14 Fats and Their Serving Sizes

Monounsaturated Fats	Polyunsaturated Fats	Saturated Fats
Avocado, 2 tablespoons Nuts • Almonds, 6 • Brazil nuts, 2 • Cashews, 6 • Hazelnuts (Filberts), 5 • Macadamia nuts, 3 • Peanuts, 10 • Pecans, 4 halves • Pistachios, 6 kernels Nut butters, 1½ teaspoons • Almond • Cashew • Peanut Oils, 1 teaspoon • Canola • Olive • Peanut Olives • Green, stuffed, 10 • Black, pitted, 8 Plant stanol esters • Benecol™ • Take Control™ Spreads, 2 teaspoons, regular; 1 tablespoon, light	Dressings, 1 tablespoon, regular; 2 tablespoons, light or reduced-fat Margarine, 1 teaspoon, regular; 1 tablespoon, light or reduced-fat Mayonnaise, 2 teaspoons, regular; 1 tablespoon, light or reduced-fat Nuts • Pine nuts (pignolia), 1 tablespoon • Walnuts, 4 halves Oils, 1 teaspoon • Corn • Flaxseed • Grapeseed • Safflower • Soybean • Sunflower Seeds, 1 tablespoon • Flaxseed, ground • Pumpkin • Sesame	Bacon, 1 slice Butter, 1 teaspoon; whipped, 2 teaspoons Chitterlings, cooked, 2 tablespoons, ½ ounce Coconut, shredded, 2 tablespoons Cream cheese, 1 tablespoon, ½ ounce Half-and-half, 2 tablespoons Heavy whipping cream, 1 tablespoon Lard, 1 teaspoon Oils, 1 teaspoon • Coconut • Palm • Palm kernel Shortening, 1 teaspoon Sour cream, 2 tablespoons, regular; 3 tablespoons, light or reduced-fat Whipped cream, 2 tablespoons

Source: Academy of Nutrition and Dietetics and American Diabetes Association, *Choose Your Foods: Food Lists for Diabetes* (Chicago and Alexandria, Va: Academy of Nutrition and Dietetics and American Diabetes Association, 2014).

Tips for Cutting Fat and Cholesterol[23]

- Trim any obvious fat off meat.
- Remove skin from poultry.
- Grill, roast, bake, or broil rather than frying meat, poultry, or fish.
- Use a rack during cooking so fat will drain off meat.
- Buy tuna packed in water.
- Use a nonstick pan with cooking spray to avoid adding oil or butter.
- When scrambling eggs, use 1 egg yolk; add more egg whites for a larger serving or use an egg substitute.
- When baking, substitute 2 egg whites for 1 whole egg or use one-fourth cup egg substitute.
- Choose fat-free or low-fat dressings, creams, and cheeses.
- Choose fat-free or low-fat milk and yogurt (regular or Greek).
- Consider choosing mustard instead of mayonnaise.
- Steam, boil, grill, or microwave vegetables rather than frying.
- Try lemon juice or flavored vinegar on salads instead of dressing.
- Use herbs and spices to season vegetables instead of butter or sauces.
- Chill soup or broth, then remove the solid fat that rises to the top.
- Dip your fork in gravy or dressing instead of pouring it over the food.

> **Group Learning Activity**
>
> - Copy "Tips for Cutting Fat and Cholesterol."
> - Cut the list into strips of 1 to 4 tips each, depending on group size.
> - Fold each strip and put into a bowl or basket.
> - Pass the bowl around the group.
> - Each participant should take out a strip and read it aloud.
>
> When the material is spoken aloud, learning is enhanced beyond just hearing it or reading it.

I see the words low fat *and* low cholesterol *on the food label. What does this really mean?*

(See Table 2.15 for examples of labeling of food's fat and cholesterol content.)

The FDA sets guidelines for labeling a food's fat and cholesterol content. In order to use certain claims, food manufacturers must follow the rules shown in Table 2.15.[24]

TABLE 2.15 Labeling of Food's Fat and Cholesterol Content

Claim on the Label	Amount of Fat/Cholesterol
Fat-free	Less than 0.5 g per serving
Low-fat	3 g or less per serving than usual product
Reduced or less fat	At least 25% less per serving than usual product
Saturated-fat free	Less than 0.5 g per serving AND less than 0.5 g of trans fats per serving
Low saturated fat	1 g or less per serving AND not more than 15% calories from saturated fats
Reduced or less saturated fat	At least 25% less per serving than usual product
Trans-fat free	Less than 0.5 g per serving, but can be listed on Nutrition Facts label as "0"
Cholesterol-free	Less than 2 mg of cholesterol per serving AND 2 g or less of saturated fat
Low-cholesterol	20 mg of cholesterol or less per serving AND 2 g or less of saturated fat
Reduced or less cholesterol	At least 25% less per serving than usual product
Lean meat	Less than 10 g of fat per serving AND 4.5 g or less saturated fat AND less than 95 mg of cholesterol per serving
Extra lean meat	Less than 5 g of fat per serving AND less than 2 g of saturated fat AND less than 95 mg of cholesterol per serving

Source: US Food and Drug Administration, "Nutrient content claims," last updated 2014 Dec 9 (cited 2015 Sept 22), on the Internet at: http://www.fda.gov/Food/IngredientsPackagingLabeling/LabelingNutrition/ucm2006880.htm.

Sweeteners

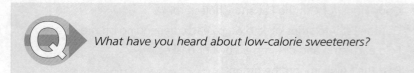

What have you heard about low-calorie sweeteners?

In addition to sugar (sucrose), there are a variety of options for sweetening food. Some sweeteners affect the blood glucose level; others do not.

Safety

There have been some rumors about the dangers of low-calorie, natural as well as artificial sweeteners. None of these claims have been backed up by a reputable scientific study. On the other hand, there have been hundreds of solid studies that prove that high-intensity sweeteners are safe in humans.[25-40]

The FDA approves the use of several low-calorie sweeteners.[41] The FDA sets the safe level of use for each sweetener, called the *acceptable daily intake* (ADI). There is a 100-fold safety factor built into the ADI. This means that even if a person ate 100 times the ADI every day over his or her lifetime, there would be no bad health effects.

In 2001, the FDA *removed* the warning on saccharrin labels that said it could potentially cause cancer. All sweeteners approved by the FDA are also safe for pregnant women and children.[42]

Nutritive Sweeteners[43]

Nutritive sweeteners have calories and can affect the blood glucose level like any carbohydrate source. Nutritive sweeteners include the following:

- Table sugar (sucrose)
- Honey

- Corn syrup
- Molasses
- Dextrose
- Fructose
- Lactose
- Sugar alcohols (includes erythritol, isomalt, lactitol, maltitol, mannitol, sorbitol, xylitol, tagatose, and hydrogenated starch hydrolysates)

Note that many of the sugar alcohol names end in "ol." Sugar alcohols have less of an effect on the blood glucose level than sugar (sucrose). They have about half the carbohydrates and calories of sugar.[43] Sugar alcohols in excess can cause gas, bloating, diarrhea, and a general laxative effect in some individuals.[11] It is suggested that you test sugar alcohols in small amounts to learn their effect on you or avoid completely.

Agave nectar is a highly processed type of sugar from the *Agave tequiliana* (tequila) plant. Agave nectar is about one and a half times sweeter than regular sugar. It has about 60 calories per tablespoon, compared to 40 calories for the same amount of table sugar. Agave nectar is not healthier than honey, sugar, high fructose corn syrup (HFCS), or any other type of sweetener.[43]

High fructose corn syrup and corn syrup are made from corn. Sugar and HFCS have almost the same level of sweetness. High fructose corn syrup is often used in soft drinks, baked goods, and some canned products. There is a lot of scientific debate about the role of HFCS in increasing the risk of type 2 diabetes as well as contributing to escalating rates of obesity.[43]

Help patients build a positive attitude about diabetes self-care by:
- Confronting erroneous beliefs, expectations, and assumptions about low-calorie sweeteners that might underlie a negative patient attitude
- Presenting evidence of the safety of low-calorie sweeteners that will help put fears to rest and promote patient control over his or her situation

Nonnutritive, Low-Calorie Sweeteners and Sugar Substitutes Survival Skill

Nonnutritive, low-calorie sweeteners and sugar substitutes have no effect on the blood glucose level. The FDA has extensively tested and approved many of these products as safe to use.[44] See Table 2.16 for examples of nonnutritive, low-calorie sweeteners and sugar substitutes.

What have you heard about cooking with sugar substitutes or low-calorie sweeteners?

You can cook with several noncaloric sweeteners, substituting them for sugar in the recipe. Saccharin, acesulfame potassium, and sucralose are stable at high temperatures and can be used in cooking. Aspartame breaks down at high temperatures and loses its sweetness, so it is less suitable for baking. Check with the manufacturer (800# or Web site on label) for specific information regarding baking or cooking with the sweetener.

48 Diabetes Education Curriculum

TABLE 2.16 Nonnutritive Low-Calorie Sweeteners and Sugar Substitutes

Chemical Name	Brand Name(s)
Acesulfame potassium (Ace-K)	Sweet One®, Sunett®
Advantame	FDA approved May 2014—no brand name available at press time
Aspartame (blue packet)	NutraSweet®, Equal®
Monk Fruit Extract (orange packet)	PUREFRUIT™, Monk Fruit in the Raw
Neotame	FDA approved 2002—no brand name available at press time
Saccharin (pink packet)	Sweet'N Low®, Sugar Twin®, Sweet Twin®, NectaSweet®
Stevia sweeteners (green packet)	PureVia™ (RebA), Truvia™ (Rebiana), Stevia Extract in the Raw®, Sun Crystals™
Sucralose (yellow packet)	Splenda®

Note: Watch for a brand new category of low-calorie sweeteners, low-calorie sugars, such as allulose (www.dolceprima.com).

Source: National Library of Medicine, NIH, "Sweeteners—sugar substitutes," Medline Plus, updated 2013 Aug 26 (cited 2015 July 15), on the Internet at: http://www.nlm.nih.gov/medlineplus/ency/article/007492.htm.

Advanced Detail

I've heard that Splenda® is made with sugar but that it won't raise blood sugar. How is that possible?

Sucralose (Splenda®) is made with sugar. But it is chemically altered (chlorine molecule added) so that your body cannot absorb it. Therefore, you taste the sugar when you eat it, but it never breaks down into glucose during digestion.[38]

What is stevia, and is it safe?

Stevia is an extract derived from the leaf of a shrub from the Chrysanthemum family—*stevia rebaudiana bertoni*. It has been used as a sweetener for centuries by people in Central and South America. Stevia has no calories and does not affect the blood glucose level.

One safety detail to know about aspartame: People with the rare genetic disease *phenylketonuria* should avoid aspartame. They lack an enzyme in their body that breaks down aspartame correctly.[44]

Free Foods

Free foods are those items that contain 5 g of carbohydrate or less and fewer than 20 calories per serving. The American Diabetes Association recommends limiting free foods to 3 servings per day. Spread those servings out so that the impact on your blood sugar is minimal. Some examples of free foods are listed in Table 2.17.

Is there a particular time of day you tend to get hungry? What do you usually do about it?

American Association of Diabetes Educators©

Module 2 *Healthy Eating* 49

TABLE 2.17 Examples of Free Foods and Their Serving Sizes

Snacks	Beverages*z	Condiments and Flavor Enhancers
Baby carrots and celery sticks, 5 pieces	Bouillon	Barbecue sauce, 2 teaspoons
Blueberries, ¼ cup	Broth	Coffee creamer (liquid, nondairy), 1 tablespoon
Cheese (sliced, fat-free), ½ ounce	Club soda or seltzer	Coffee creamer (powder, nondairy), 2 teaspoons
Crackers	Coffee (black or with sugar substitute)	Dill pickle, 1½ (3¾-inch pickles)
• Goldfish-style crackers, 10	Consommé	Horseradish sauce, 1 tablespoon
• Saltine-style crackers, 2	Drink mixes (sugar-free)	Jelly (low or reduced sugar), 2 teaspoons
Gelatin (sugar-free), 1 cup	Flavored water (sugar-free)	Ketchup, 1 tablespoon
Gum, 1 stick	Soft drink (sugar-free)	Lemon juice, 1 tablespoon
Meat (lean), ½ ounce	Tea (plain or with sugar substitute)	Margarine (fat-free), 1 tablespoon
Popcorn (light), 1 cup	Tonic water (sugar-free)	Mayonnaise (fat-free), 1 tablespoon
Vanilla wafer, 1	Water	Mustard, 1 tablespoon
		Parmesan cheese, 1 tablespoon
		Pickle relish (sweet), 1 tablespoon
		Salad dressing (low-fat or fat-free), 1 tablespoon
		Salad greens (lettuce, spinach, etc), 1 cup
		Salsa, ¼ cup
		Soy sauce, 1 tablespoon
		Sweet & sour sauce, 2 teaspoons
		Taco sauce, 1 tablespoon
		Vinegar, 1 tablespoon

*8 ounces is considered a standard measure for liquids.

Source: Academy of Nutrition and Dietetics and American Diabetes Association, *Choose Your Foods: Food Lists for Diabetes* (Chicago and Alexandria, Va: Academy of Nutrition and Dietetics and American Diabetes Association, 2014).

Snacks

Snacks can be incorporated into your meal plan. Well-timed snacks can help keep your energy up. Snacks can help you avoid becoming overly hungry, so that you are less likely to overeat at mealtimes. If you choose to use part of your day's calories as between-meal snacks, it's best to select foods that also supply positive nutrients.

Snacks containing fiber can help you feel full. Plan ahead so that you aren't tempted to just grab what's available, which may not be as healthful. Healthy snack choices include:

◆ Beef jerky, ½ ounce

◆ Dried fruit and/or nuts, 1 handful

◆ Fresh fruit, 1 piece

◆ Popcorn, plain or reduced fat/sodium, 3 cups popped

◆ Rice cakes, 2

◆ Seeds, 1 handful

Note that a handful is no more than one-fourth cup!

When choosing prepared foods, be sure to check the amount of total carbohydrates on the label, as well as the serving size. Even sugar-free or "no sugar added" foods can still have carbohydrates in them from other ingredient sources.

American Association of Diabetes Educators©

Fiber and Whole Grains

Survival Skill Fiber is an important part of your diet because:

- It provides the bulk that helps move the food along in the intestines. This helps keep your bowel habits more regular.
- It curbs hunger, giving you a feeling of fullness. This helps you avoid overeating.
- Foods containing fiber tend to be rich in vitamins and minerals.
- It may help lower cholesterol.
- It may help lower the risk of colon and rectal cancer and diverticulitis.

One study showed that a very high-fiber diet lowered blood glucose levels by 10%. The diet in this study contained about 50 g of fiber per day.[45] However, most people in the United States consume only about 10 to 20 g of fiber per day, which is not likely to affect the blood glucose level very much.

A very high-fiber diet (50 g per day) would be difficult to attain and can cause a lot of gas, so it may not be tolerated very well. Women should try to get 25 g of fiber per day, and men should try to get 38—the US recommended amount on the Nutrition Facts label. Increase your fiber intake gradually throughout the day, and be sure to drink plenty of water along with other fluids, too.

To get adequate amounts of fiber, certain foods should be included in the meal plan. Sources of fiber include fruit, beans, vegetables, whole grain breads, whole grain pasta, brown or wild rice, and other grains. Check the Nutrition Facts label for grams of dietary fiber per serving.

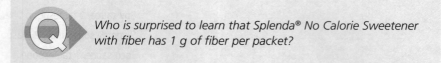

Who is surprised to learn that Splenda® No Calorie Sweetener with fiber has 1 g of fiber per packet?

Whole Grains

People with diabetes should consume at least the amount of fiber (25 g per day) and whole grains (make half your grains whole) recommended for the general population. Whole grains have not been shown to improve blood glucose but may reduce inflammation and heart disease risk.[11] Whole grains include the word "whole" in their name, but also include all oats, quinoa, brown/wild rice, etc. For additional information, check out the Whole Grain Council at: http://wholegrainscouncil.org/.

Other Sources of Fiber

Beans, peas, and lentils are excellent sources of fiber, are naturally low in fat, and also contain plant-based proteins and carbohydrates.[46] Options include:

Beans		Peas	Lentils
Navy	Kidney	Black-eyed	Brown
Black	Lima	Chickpeas	Green
Butter	Pinto	Cowpeas	Red/yellow
Fava	Soy	Green	Specialty varieties
Great Northern	White (Navy)	Split	

Advanced Detail

I see the words high fiber *on the food label. What does this really mean?*

The FDA regulates guidelines for labeling and approved claims of a food's fiber content. In order to use certain claims, food manufacturers must follow the rules listed in Table 2.18.

TABLE 2.18 Labeling of Food's Fiber Content

Claim on the Label	Amount of Fiber
High fiber	20% of the daily value (DV), at least 5 grams per labeled serving
Good source of fiber	10% of the daily value (DV), 3 or more grams per labeled serving

Source: US Food and Drug Administration, "Guidance for industry: a food labeling guide (11. Appendix C: Health Claims)," 2013 Jan (cited 2015 Sept 22), on the Internet at: http://www.fda.gov/Food/GuidanceRegulation/GuidanceDocumentsRegulatoryInformation/LabelingNutrition/ucm064919.htm.

The American Diabetes Association recommends choosing foods with at least 3 g of dietary fiber per serving.[11]

Water

Next to oxygen, water is the most important nutrient for the human body. Your body needs water to carry out all its functions, from supplying oxygen to your cells to removing waste from your system. Adults need at least 6 to 8 glasses of water or other fluids every day (60 to 65 fluid ounces minimum).

By the time you feel thirsty, you are already dehydrated. Also, as people age, they tend to lose their sense of thirst. So you should make an effort to drink water frequently throughout the day. Don't wait until you feel thirsty before you take a drink.

Advanced Detail

Vitamins and Minerals

Should I take vitamins or other supplements?

There is no clear evidence of benefit from vitamin or mineral supplementation in people with diabetes who do not have underlying deficiencies.[11] Individualized meal planning should include optimal food choices so you get all the vitamins and minerals you need for good health. If your diabetes has been out of control for a time, you may have lost water-soluble vitamins (eg, vitamin C, B-complex vitamins) because of excess urination.[15] A healthy, balanced diet will naturally replenish those vitamins.

Some groups of individuals can benefit from multivitamin or mineral supplementation, such as the elderly, women who are pregnant or breastfeeding, strict vegetarians, or those on extreme, medically supervised, calorie-restricted diets.[47] It's important to understand that over-the-counter supplements do not require the strict regulation by the FDA that prescription drugs require. However, any claims that a dietary supplement prevents disease must be backed up by studies and approved by the FDA.

It is advised to choose a multivitamin with no more than 100% to 150% of the recommended dietary allowances (RDA) for all nutrients. Men and postmenopausal women should aim to select a supplement without iron.[15] If you are pregnant, always check with your healthcare provider before taking any type of dietary or herbal supplement. This includes any over-the-counter supplement. Most herbal products are not recommended during pregnancy because they could harm the baby.

For information on specific vitamins and minerals, see Module 4: Taking Medication, and on vitamin and mineral usage during pregnancy, see Module 8: Reducing Risks.

Sodium

Table salt is made up of sodium and chloride. Your body needs sodium to function. It's found naturally in many foods, and it is often added to foods during cooking or at the table. Too much sodium in your diet can cause your body to retain excess fluids. This can raise the blood pressure and put an extra strain on your heart.

Survival Skill People who have high blood pressure can lower it by reducing their sodium intake. Some studies show that lowering sodium intake is a way to help prevent high blood pressure.[45] On the other hand, the DASH eating plan has been useful for lowering blood pressure despite including a sodium intake typical of most Americans. The DASH plan calls for a diet high in fruits, vegetables, and low-fat dairy foods. It is low in overall fat, saturated fat, and cholesterol. People in the DASH study lowered their blood pressure but did not lose weight.[48]

A moderate sodium restriction is defined as 2300 mg per day. One level teaspoon of table salt contains about 2400 mg of sodium. Tips for cutting salt intake include[49]:

- Take the salt shaker off the dinner table.
- Reduce or eliminate added salt or sodium while cooking.
- Rinse and drain canned vegetables before cooking them.
- Choose fresh foods over canned or processed foods.
- Choose low- or no-salt-added canned foods.
- Avoid salty seasonings: bouillon cubes, cooking sherry, meat tenderizer, soy sauce, steak sauce, Worcestershire sauce, salad dressings, packaged seasoning mixes (taco, chili, gravy, rice), and soup mixes or select a reduced- or low-sodium version.
- Cut back on processed meats like ham, bacon, sausage, hot dogs, and lunch meat or select a reduced- or low-sodium version.
- Choose frozen foods with less than 480 mg of sodium and meals or dinners with less than 600 mg of sodium per serving.
- Limit fast food and check the nutrition information onsite or online, if available, for the lowest-sodium choice you prefer.
- Limit salty snacks such as chips, pretzels, olives, cheeses, and pickles or select a reduced- or low-sodium version.
- Season foods with herbs, spices, vinegars, and lemon juice.

Invite participants who have successfully cut their salt intake to share with others in the group how they did it.

If you use salt substitutes that contain potassium, discuss this with your doctor first. **Using a salt supplement that contains potassium may pose a risk for people who have heart disease or who take certain blood pressure drugs called *ACE inhibitors*.**[50-52]

Advanced Detail

The FDA regulates guidelines for labeling and approved claims of a food's sodium content. In order to use certain claims, food manufacturers must follow the rules listed in Table 2.19.[26,53]

TABLE 2.19   Labeling of Food's Sodium Content

Claim on the Label	Amount of Sodium
Sodium-free	Less than 5 mg per serving
Very low sodium	35 mg or less per serving
Low sodium	140 mg or less per serving
Reduced sodium	The usual sodium level has been reduced at least 25%
Unsalted	No salt has been added, but the food may contain naturally occurring sodium. Check Nutrition Facts.
Healthy	No salt has been added, but the food may contain naturally occurring sodium. Food must not exceed 480 mg sodium per serving for individual foods or 600 mg for main dish meals. Check Nutrition Facts.

Alcohol

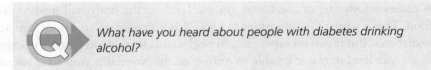

What have you heard about people with diabetes drinking alcohol?

Alcohol is not forbidden for most people with diabetes. If adults with diabetes choose to drink alcohol, they should be advised to do so in moderation (1 drink per day or less for adult women, and 2 drinks per day or less for adult men).[11] Serving sizes for alcohol choices include[54,55]:

- Distilled spirits (scotch, whiskey, rum, vodka, etc): 1½ ounces
- Beer, regular or light: 12 ounces
- Wine, dry red or white: 5 ounces

Keep in mind that some alcoholic drinks typically contain added carbohydrates. Beer contains carbohydrates from the grains in hops, malt, and barley. Wine has carbohydrates from grapes. Cocktails may have carbohydrates from mixers. Even so, you shouldn't eliminate carbohydrate foods from your meal plan in order to have a drink. That action could put you at risk for an episode of low blood sugar later on. Food helps slow the absorption of alcohol in the body, **so always have something to eat if you choose to drink alcohol**.

Each gram of alcohol contributes 7 calories. One serving of alcohol is about 100 calories. Drinking alcohol in moderation will help you avoid too many extra calories and weight gain. Moderation means 1 drink per day (or less) for women and 2 drinks per day (or less) for men.[11]

Certain people should abstain from alcohol: those with a history of alcohol abuse; pregnant women; those with liver disease, pancreatitis, or advanced diabetic nerve disease; and those with very high triglyceride levels (500 mg/dL or above).

Advanced Detail

Some research suggests that drinking moderate amounts of wine may have possible heart health benefits. Since this benefit has not yet been proven in large clinical studies, it is still controversial. The grapes used in making red wine contain flavonoids, which are a type of antioxidant. Antioxidants are substances that can help prevent cell damage. Flavonoids can be found in nonalcoholic sources, too, so don't start drinking just for the possible health benefits. Don't forget wine also adds extra carbohydrates and calories.

Flavonoids can be found in the following foods, which are also rich in vitamins:

- Blueberries
- Red grapes
- Pomegranate juice
- Purple grape juice
- Tea, green and black

Studies show that the antioxidant in pomegranate juice is more powerful than the others listed above. It stimulates the production of nitric oxide, a chemical that helps keep blood vessels open. Include the calories and carbohydrates in your daily plan.[56]

I've heard that alcohol lowers the blood sugar. If that's true, why can't I just drink whenever my blood sugar is too high?

Alcohol *indirectly* causes a lowering of the blood glucose level, as the body will process alcohol first at the expense of digesting food. This is why it's so important to never drink alcohol on an empty stomach, even for those people who don't have diabetes. But if you do experience hypoglycemia (low blood glucose reaction) after drinking too much, your blood glucose level may not be able to recover easily. Normally, your liver releases stored glucose whenever your blood glucose level drops too low. This response helps correct your blood glucose, bringing it to a more normal level. If you are awake, the symptoms of low blood glucose will alert you to take action, and you should eat a snack to raise your blood glucose to normal.

If you have *had too much alcohol* to drink, the liver may not release the amount of glucose it normally would. If you are drunk or asleep when this happens, your symptoms may not alert you to eat a snack. As a result, your blood glucose could continue dropping to dangerously low levels. To avoid this situation, alcohol should *always* be taken with food and in moderation. This is especially true for people who take insulin or diabetes medications that cause insulin production.

Reading Food Labels

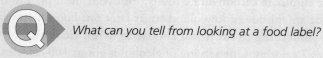

What can you tell from looking at a food label?

By law, the US Department of Agriculture (USDA), along with the FDA, requires that Nutrition Facts labels be placed on packaged foods and beverages for sale. The label has a great deal of information on it. You can use the label to help you make better food choices. Let's look at the Nutrition Facts label in more detail.[57]

Serving Size `Survival Skill`

The amount in the serving size may be more or less than the serving size recommended in your individualized meal plan. In addition to the household serving size measure, the weight of the serving is expressed in grams or milliliters (beverages) within the parentheses. For example, a salad dressing label might state, "Serving size: 2 tablespoons (30 g)" or a fluid milk label might state "Serving size: 1 cup (240 mL)." Do not confuse this information with grams of carbohydrates, protein, fat, or other nutrients.

If the serving size is a half cup, how many servings are there in one and a half cups of the food product?

The serving size listed is 1 cup, but your meal plan calls for a half-cup serving size for this food. Is this a problem?

If you eat double or triple the serving size listed, you are getting double or triple the amount of each aspect of nutrition listed on the label. If you eat half of the serving size listed, you can divide the nutrition information in half to know what you are really getting.

Number of Servings in the Container `Survival Skill`

How many servings are in the *entire* container? Remember, this section is referring to how many servings, based on the serving size, as listed just above on the label.

If the serving size is a half cup and there are 6 servings in the container, how many cups of the food product are there?

Calories per Serving

Calories per serving is the amount of calories in 1 serving. On this line of the label, you can also see how many of the total calories in 1 serving come from fat. Each gram of fat in a serving contributes 9 calories, each gram of protein contributes 4 calories, and each gram of carbohydrate contributes 4 calories. These totals are already calculated for you on the calorie line. The calories are rounded up or down to comply with regulated nutrient rounding rules.

Fat per Serving

Fat per serving tells you the total amount of fat in 1 serving. The amount of fat is expressed in grams. For heart health, choose foods low in saturated fat. Below total fat, the amount of saturated fat in 1 serving is listed as well as the amount of trans fat in 1 serving. Replacing foods that contain trans fats with foods that contain unsaturated fat will help lower cholesterol.

You will notice that the amount of unsaturated fat in 1 serving is not listed. This does not mean that the food product has no unsaturated fat. It's just not required to be on the label. Use the label to help you choose foods that are low in saturated and trans fats.

Cholesterol per Serving

The total amount of cholesterol in 1 serving is listed. Use the label to compare the amount of cholesterol in different foods. Choose those lower in cholesterol. The recommendation is to keep dietary cholesterol less than 300 mg per day.

Sodium per Serving

The total amount of sodium in 1 serving is listed. If you are trying to reduce your sodium/salt intake, choose food items that have less than 480 mg of sodium per serving. If the food item is a meal, then choose meals that have less than 600 mg of sodium.

American Association of Diabetes Educators©

Potassium

The grams of potassium in 1 serving are not required to be listed unless a claim is made or the manufacturer voluntarily provides that information on the label. Potassium is an important element found naturally in many foods. Most people do not get enough potassium in their diet. About 4.7 g (4700 mg) per day is considered an adequate intake of potassium. Potassium can help people maintain a more normal blood pressure. This is especially true if you are "salt or sodium sensitive," which means that your blood pressure goes up when sodium/salt intake is increased.

Taking in enough potassium also helps prevent kidney stones and reduces the risk of bone loss. If you are trying to get more potassium in your diet, choose fruits and vegetables. If your provider has advised you to cut back on potassium, pay attention to this area of the label; follow the guidelines you've been given. If the grams of potassium are not listed, as it's not required by law, contact the manufacturer for that information via its customer service phone line or Web site. This information may be listed on the product label.

Total Carbohydrate Content **Survival Skill**

The total amount of carbohydrate in 1 serving is listed. This is the most important part of the label when figuring out your carbohydrate intake. Consider the number of carbohydrate servings (choices) in your meal plan. Remember that 15 g of carbohydrate is 1 serving (choice) of carbohydrate. Meal plans for women usually call for 3 or 4 carbohydrate servings in a meal; meal plans for men usually call for 4 or 5 carbohydrate servings in a meal.

In this section of the Nutrition Facts label, there is a line for dietary fiber and sugars. Both are types of carbohydrates. What doesn't appear on the label is the amount of starches or other nutrients that also are carbohydrates. This is why it's more important to look at the *total carbohydrates* line.

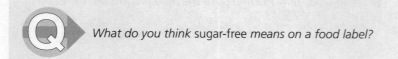

What do you think sugar-free *means on a food label?*

Just because no sugar is in the product does not mean that there are no carbohydrates in it. Other carbohydrates, like starch, may be in the product. The FDA does not require food companies to list the starch content on the label. When sugar is removed from a product, other nutrients (like fat) may be added for consistent texture or flavor. Sugar alcohols contain carbohydrates, but since they do not add to the sugar content of the product, the product can be labeled sugar-free. Sugar alcohols, if present, will be listed separately under carbohydrates in the Nutrition Facts, and you can also check the ingredients list.

Group Learning Activity

- Keep participants actively involved when teaching about the Nutrition Facts label.
- Have them choose from a collection of labels from actual food products.
- Depending on group size, invite participants to pair up in twos.
- Ask each group questions about its product to assess understanding.

    This activity will resonate with those with visual/spatial intelligence, whose learning is enhanced with color-coded charts.

Advanced Detail

Sometimes I see net carbs *on a food package. What does this mean?*

The low-carbohydrate craze of recent years has slowed, but some manufacturers still use this unapproved label claim. You will not see *net carbs* included on the Nutrition Facts label, as it is not approved by the USDA or the FDA.

Some food companies incorrectly subtract the dietary fiber and the sugar alcohols from the total carbohydrate count. These subtractions may appear to lower the total carbohydrate count, but that is not accurate. You may see claims such as *net carbs*, *effective carbs*, *impact carbs*, or *net effective carbs*.

All carbohydrates can affect blood glucose levels and contribute calories. Many people with diabetes figure their insulin dose based on the amount of carbohydrates they eat or drink. A person's insulin dose should be based on the total carbohydrates per serving per the Nutrition Facts panel, unless their diabetes educator has advised differently based on their previous glucose response to a particular food or beverage.

For most people with diabetes, it is no longer advised or necessary to subtract dietary fiber or sugar alcohols from total carbohydrates when carbohydrate counting.[11] However, if you are advised by your healthcare team to do so based on your individual needs, you *may* subtract half the dietary fiber or half the sugar alcohols from the total carbohydrates *if* the serving contains more than 5 g of dietary fiber or more than 5 g of sugar alcohols.

Protein

The total amount of protein in 1 serving is listed. Most people consume adequate protein in their diet. When choosing protein foods, choose those that are lean, low-fat, or fat-free for heart health and calorie control.

Vitamins A and C, Calcium, and Iron

You will notice that the total unit amounts of vitamins A and C, calcium, and iron in 1 serving are not listed but their percent daily value (DV) is listed. Choose foods with a higher percent daily value listed when comparing similar products. The goal is to get 100% of each nutrient's daily value each day.

Percent Daily Value

The percent daily value section of the Nutrition Facts label appears at the bottom. For each nutrient on the label, there is also a percentage shown on the far right side of the label. According to the FDA, "The percent daily value is a general guide to help you link nutrients in a serving of food to their contribution to your total daily diet."[57] The percent daily values are based on a 2000 calorie diet. Your calorie needs may be more or less than 2000 calories per day. Even if your meal plan has a different calorie level, these percentages can be a useful guide.

To see if a food is high or low in a nutrient, look at the percent daily value. If the number is 5% or less, it is low in that nutrient; if the number is 20% or more, it is high in that nutrient.

List of Ingredients Survival Skill

The list of ingredients is below or just to the side of the Nutrition Facts label. Ingredients are listed, by weight, in the order of quantity, from the largest ingredient amount to the smallest.

People with food allergies should always pay close attention to the ingredient list, as it can change!

Eating Out and Reading Restaurant Menus

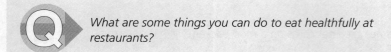
What are some things you can do to eat healthfully at restaurants?

Eating out is part of modern life. There are lots of things you can do to stick to your meal plan while eating out. Here are some suggestions that might work for you:

- Keep snack foods on hand just in case the meal is delayed (long wait times to be seated and/or served).
- If your portion is larger than what your meal plan calls for, ask for half to be served to you and the other half to be placed in a to-go container.
- Consider sharing your entrée.
- Eat a salad first to keep from overeating during the rest of the meal.
- Limit the amount of bread you eat (move the bread basket before the meal comes if it's too tempting to overindulge).
- Ask if fried meat entrées on the menu can be grilled or baked instead.
- Ask if low-calorie or nonfat dressings are available.
- Ask for salad dressing or sauces to be served on the side.
- Be aware of certain words on the menu and what they usually mean. See Table 2.20.

TABLE 2.20   Interpreting Language on a Menu

Words on a Menu	What They Usually Mean
Alfredo	Covered in a white cream sauce
Au gratin	Cooked with breadcrumbs and cheese
Batter-dipped	Breaded and fried
Breaded	Coated with bread crumbs and usually fried
Crispy	Breaded and fried
Creamy or in a cream sauce	Contains or covered in some type of high-fat white sauce
Deluxe, jumbo, giant	Oversized serving, which means more calories, fat, carbohydrates, and sodium
Deep-fried	Breaded and fried
Scalloped	Baked in a sauce with breadcrumbs and sometimes cheese

Group Learning Activity

- Compile menus from as many local restaurants as you can.
- Allow participants to look through your collection and choose a menu from a restaurant they frequent.
- Use the menu as a springboard for discussion about making healthy choices in restaurants.

Identifying Barriers to Healthy Eating

Even though you know that healthy eating is good for you, there may be barriers that prevent you from making healthy food choices. For every barrier there may be many possible solutions.

Group Learning Activity

- Select a reality scenario from the list in the table below.
- Ask for suggestions from participants on possible solutions for overcoming the barrier or have the class work as a group or several small groups to brainstorm possible solutions.

Reality Scenario	Problem Solving Possible Solutions/What Would *You* Do?
Can't afford healthy food *Health food is too expensive.*	• It's not necessary to buy health food. • Everyday foods can be worked into a meal plan. The main things to watch are total calories, total carbohydrates, and portion control.
Guilt *I was taught to eat everything on my plate. I feel guilty when I don't finish my meal.*	• Go with smaller portions. • Use a smaller plate so portions feel bigger. • At restaurants, ask that half be placed in a to-go container before the plate is brought out to you.
Unrealistic expectations about weight *I'll never get to my ideal weight! I haven't been that weight since I was 18 years old.*	• Realize that ideal weight and a realistic healthy weight are not always the same. • Moderate weight loss (5% to 10% of body weight) has lots of health benefits: improves blood pressure, blood glucose level, and blood lipid (fat) levels.
Feelings of hunger and deprivation *I get too hungry whenever I go on a diet. Feeling starved just makes me want to binge later on.*	• Space out your meals and make sure you have enough overall calories. Include snacks so you don't go more than 3 hours without eating. • Eat slowly. Put your fork down between bites. It takes at least 15 minutes for the brain to get the message that you have just eaten. • Include more vegetables so that you feel fuller. Choose raw vegetables or fruits that require more chewing. • Use a smaller plate so that your portions don't look so meager.
Emotional eating when bored or stressed *Stress makes me eat.* *Every night, I just have to have my ice cream when I watch TV.* *When I see those Cheetos® in the pantry, I can't help myself.*	• Consider other ways to deal with stress—talking to someone, going for a walk, relaxation, writing in a journal, imagery, etc. • Consciously try to sever the cue (television) with the behavior (eating ice cream). • Stock your kitchen with healthier snack food choices. Get rid of the ice cream and Cheetos®. These foods are visual cues that prompt you to make poor choices.
Expectations of others (eg, family, friends, coworkers) *I tried to cut out all the fat and add more raw vegetables, but my husband and kids complained.*	• Make changes gradually. Get your family involved in meal planning, one change at a time. Teach them to read labels. Explain why healthy eating is good for the whole family.

American Association of Diabetes Educators©

Reality Scenario	Problem Solving Possible Solutions/What Would *You* Do?
Every day at work, somebody brings doughnuts or some other junk food to the employee lounge. It's so tempting. Whenever there's a coworker's birthday or a holiday, I feel like I have to eat some of the cake they bring to celebrate.	• Bring something healthy to eat. Suggest that employees bring healthier foods. Avoid the employee lounge. Eat a healthy snack before you go to the lounge so you feel full. Then, to join in the celebration, just have a small taste of the junk food.
Lack of time to eat breakfast *I have to be at work by 8:30 in the morning.*	• Fix simple breakfast items before going to bed. Choose breakfast foods or meal replacements that can be eaten on the go.
I have to get the kids ready and off to school. I don't have time to eat breakfast.	• Get up 15 minutes earlier. Eat while the kids are eating breakfast.
Travel a lot/on the road *With my job I travel most of the time, so I have to eat in restaurants. There's nothing healthy on the menu.*	• Learn more about healthy restaurant options. Ask the restaurant waitstaff to make healthy changes to your order. • Carry portable healthy snacks with you so you won't be famished by the time you get to the restaurant. • Consider meal replacements that can be eaten on the go.
Cultural issues about weight *My husband likes me a little on the plump side. He says skinny women are unattractive.*	• You don't have to be skinny to be healthy. Even a moderate weight loss (~10% of body weight) has lots of health benefits: it improves blood pressure, blood glucose level, and cholesterol level. • Tell your husband that your main goal is to be healthy.
Nausea and vomiting during pregnancy *I feel sick especially in the morning and I can't eat my favorite foods.*	• You may not be able to eat your favorite foods right now, but it is important to eat something, especially if you are taking medication to control your blood glucose levels. The registered dietitian will help you find foods that you can keep down. You may have to check your blood glucose more often to make sure your levels aren't going too low.

Identifying Facilitators for Healthy Eating

As important as it is to identify barriers to healthy eating, it's just as important to consider the positives, or facilitators, in your situation. Looking deeper, you may find that there are more positives than you thought.

 What are some things that help you stick with your plan to eat healthy?

Common Facilitators

- Social support—family members, friends, coworkers, etc
- Community resources—free online resources on nutrition and weight, nutrition support groups (see "Resources" section at the end of this module)

♦ Reminders and cues—notes of encouragement (positive affirmations), removing visual stimuli to eat unhealthily

♦ Rewards—incentives to maintain motivation

Setting a SMART Goal for Healthy Eating

S—Specific: identify type of food choices, amount of food eaten, timing of meals, alcohol intake, handling of special situations, etc

M—Measurable: not vague

A—Attainable: challenging but not out of reach

R—Realistic: given person's situation, can it be done?

T—Timeline: short term, for next 2 to 4 weeks?

The participant sets an individual goal for healthy eating. The educator and the participant schedule a date in which to evaluate progress with behavior change.

Follow-up/Outcomes Measurement

Per the Standards for Outcomes Measurement of Diabetes Self-Management Education, the first **follow-up should be conducted within 2 to 4 weeks** after the initial teaching session on healthy eating. At this follow-up, success in implementing healthy eating behavior can be assessed. **Subsequent follow-up is recommended at 3- to 6-month intervals thereafter.** Use the following table as a guide for identifying outcomes measures and how to measure them. Measurement of these outcomes may be objective or subjective.[2]

The exception to this schedule would be during pregnancy. The first follow-up should be conducted within 1 week and subsequent visits at 2 to 4 weeks.

Self-Care Behavior: Healthy Eating Outcomes Measures	Self-Care Behavior: Healthy Eating Methods of Measurement
Immediate outcome: Learning Immediate outcomes of learning can be assessed right away after the educational encounter. Immediate outcomes include: K: Acquiring *knowledge* (*what to do*) S: Acquiring *skills* (*how to do it*) CM: Developing *confidence and motivation* (*want to do it*) PS: Developing *problem-solving/coping skills* to overcome barrier (*can do it*)	Immediate outcomes of learning can be measured by patient knowledge testing (paper-and-pen testing, or questioning to determine that patient understands information taught). Immediate outcomes for acquiring a skill can be measured by patient's demonstration of that skill. The following are various methods of measuring immediate outcomes for the self-care behavior of *healthy eating*.
Effect of food on glucose (K)	<u>Subjective:</u> Patient describes the effect of food on glucose. <u>Objective:</u> Food records and/or logbook data showing effect of food intake on glucose levels.
Sources of carbohydrates (K)	<u>Subjective:</u> Patient lists sources of carbohydrates.
Meal planning (K,S)	<u>Subjective:</u> Patient describes the meal plan (type of food choices, the amount of food, the timing of meals, and responses to special situations, etc) that is appropriate for his or her nutritional goals. <u>Objective:</u> 24-hour recall of food intake, food records, food frequency questionnaires.

American Association of Diabetes Educators©

Self-Care Behavior: Healthy Eating Outcomes Measures	Self-Care Behavior: Healthy Eating Methods of Measurement
Label reading (S)	Objective: Patient correctly interprets food label.
Menu reading (S)	Objective: Patient correctly identifies menu items that are appropriate for his or her meal plan/nutritional goals.
Weighing and measuring food portions (S)	Objective: Patient correctly demonstrates how to measure/weigh food portions.
Carbohydrate counting (S)	Objective: Patient accurately calculates the math in carbohydrate counting; food records and/or logbook data show correct carbohydrate counting calculations.
Food safety in pregnancy (K)	Subjective: Patient lists foods to be avoided during pregnancy.
Potential barriers (environmental triggers: emotional, cultural, financial) and facilitators to healthy eating (PS)	Subjective: Considering his or her individual situation, patient describes anticipated obstacle(s) that may limit the ability to follow the meal plan. Patient describes facilitators which may help him or her to follow the meal plan.
Strategy to overcome potential barriers to healthy eating (PS)	Objective: Patient develops a plan to deal with anticipated obstacle(s) to healthy eating.
Intermediate outcome: Behavior change	Intermediate outcomes measures can be assessed over time, after the educational encounter and once the patient has had adequate time to implement new behavior(s) in a real-life setting. *Behavior change* is an intermediate outcomes measure. It is the ultimate outcome of diabetes self-management and support (DSMES). At follow-up intervals, knowledge and skills (discussed above), as well as behavior change, should be reassessed.
Eating behavior (PS)	Subjective: Patient self-report of eating behavior (eg, type of food choices, amount of food, timing of meals, response to special situations).
	Objective: Review of food records and logbook data.
Barrier identification and resolution (PS)	Subjective: Patient self-report of barriers faced and facilitators and strategies used to implement healthy eating behaviors.
Plan for future behavior change (PS)	Subjective: Patient self-report of healthy eating goals and behavior strategies going forward.

REFERENCES

1. Povey RC, Clark-Carter D. Diabetes and healthy eating: a systematic review of the literature. Diabetes Educ. 2007; 33(6):931-59.

2. Mulcahy K, Maryniuk M, Peeples M, et al. Diabetes self-management education core outcomes measures: technical review. Diabetes Educ. 2003;29(5):768-803.

3. Kittler PG, Sucher KP. Diet counseling in a multicultural society. Diabetes Educ. 1990;16:127-34.

4. Brown TL. Ethnic populations. In: Ross TA, Boucher JL, O'Connell BS, eds. American Dietetic Association Guide to Diabetes Medical Nutrition Therapy and Education. Chicago: American Dietetic Association; 2005:227-38.

5. Brown TL. Meal-planning strategies: ethnic populations. Diabetes Spectr. 2003;16:190-2.

6. Academy of Nutrition and Dietetics (formerly American Dietetic Association). Diabetes type 1 and 2 evidence-based nutrition practice guidelines for adults. 2008 (cited 2015 Jul 19). On the Internet at: http://adaevidencelibrary.com/tmp/pq66.pdf.

7. American Diabetes Association. Standards of medical care in diabetes—2015. Diabetes Care. 2015;38 Suppl 1:S1-59.

8. Pastors JG, Warshaw H, Daly A, Franz M, Kulkarni K. The evidence for the effectiveness of medical nutrition therapy in diabetes management. Diabetes Care. 2002;25:608-13.

9. Kulkarni K, Castle G, Gregory R, et al. Nutrition practice guidelines for type 1 diabetes mellitus positively affect dietitian practices and patient outcomes. J Am Diet Assoc. 1998;98:62-70.

10. Franz MJ, Monk A, Barry B, et al. Effectiveness of medical nutrition therapy provided by dietitians in the management of non-insulin-dependent diabetes mellitus: a randomized, controlled clinical trial. J Am Diet Assoc. 1995; 95:1009-17.

11. Evert AB, Boucher JL, Cypress M, et al; American Diabetes Association. Nutrition therapy recommendations for the management of adults with diabetes. Diabetes Care. 2013;36:3821-42.

12. National Institute of Diabetes and Digestive and Kidney Diseases (NIDDK). Dieting and gallstones. NIH publication no. 02-3677. Last updated 2013 Mar (cited 2015 Jul 15). On the Internet at: http://win.niddk.nih.gov/publications/gallstones.htm.

13. National Heart, Lung, and Blood Institute. Assessing your weight and health risk (cited 2015 Jul 15). On the Internet at: http://www.nhlbi.nih.gov/health/public/heart/obesity/lose_wt/risk.htm.

14. National Institute of Diabetes and Digestive and Kidney Diseases (NIDDK). The practical guide: identification, evaluation, and treatment of overweight and obesity in adults. NIH publication no. 00-4084. October 2000.

15. Campbell AP. Nutrition management for diabetes treatment: clinician's approach to medical nutrition therapy. In: Beaser RS and the staff of Joslin Diabetes Center, eds. Joslin's Diabetes Deskbook. 3rd ed. Boston: Joslin Diabetes Center; 2014:97-153.

16. Franz MJ, Powers MA, Leontos C, et al. The evidence for medical nutrition therapy for type 1 and type 2 diabetes in adults. J Acad Nutr Diet. 2010;110(12):1853-89.

17. US Food and Drug Administration. How to understand and use the nutrition facts label. 2004 Nov (cited 2015 Jul 19). On the Internet at: http://www.fda.gov/Food/IngredientsPackagingLabeling/LabelingNutrition/ucm274593.htm.

18. Glycemic Index Research Service, The University of Sydney. Glycemic index testing & research (cited 2015 Jul 15). On the Internet at: http://www.glycemicindex.com/testing_research.php.

19. Gannon MC, Nuttall JA, Damberg G, Gupta V, Nuttall FQ. Effect of protein ingestion on the glucose appearance rate in people with type 2 diabetes. J Clin Endocrinol Metab. 2001;86:1040-7.

20. Kris-Etherton PM, Harris WS, Appel LJ; American Heart Association Nutrition Committee. Fish consumption, fish oil, omega-3 fatty acids, and cardiovascular disease. Circulation. 2002;106:2747-57.

21. Evans EC. The FDA recommendations on fish intake during pregnancy. J Obstet Gynecol Neonatal Nurs. 2002;31:715-20.

22. US Food and Drug Administration. Fish: what pregnant women and parents should know (cited 2015 Jul 15). On the Internet at: http://www.fda.gov/Food/FoodborneIllnessContaminants/Metals/ucm393070.htm.

23. US Food and Drug Administration. Cardiovascular disease prevention and wellness (cited 2015 Jul 15). On the Internet at: http://www.fda.gov/ForPatients/Illness/Cardiovascular/ucm408484.htm.

24. US Food and Drug Administration. Food labeling guide. Nutrient content claims. Last updated 2014 Dec 9 (cited 2015 Jul 15). On the Internet at: http://www.fda.gov/Food/IngredientsPackagingLabeling/LabelingNutrition/ucm2006880.htm.

25. US Food and Drug Administration. Code of Federal Regulations, Title 21, Volume 3. Food additives permitted for direct addition to food for human consumption: 21CFR172.800. Acesulfame potassium (revised 2014 Apr 1).

26. European Commission, Health and Consumer Protection Directorate-General, Scientific Committee on Food. Opinion. Re-evaluation of acesulfame K with reference to the previous SCF opinion of 1991. SCF/CS/ADD/EDUL/194 Final. Brussels: SCF; 2000 (cited 2015 Jul 15). On the Internet at: http://ec.europa.eu/food/fs/sc/scf/out52_en.pdf.

27. European Food Safety Authority (EFSA), European Commission. Scientific opinion on the re-evaluation of aspartame (E951) as a food additive. EFSA Journal. 2013 Dec 10 (cited 2015 Jul 15);11(12):3496 (263 pp). On the Internet at: http://www.efsa.europa.eu/en/efsajournal/doc/3496.pdf.

American Association of Diabetes Educators©

64   Diabetes Education Curriculum

28. Filer LJ, Baker GL, Stegink LD. Effect of aspartame loading on plasma and erythrocyte free amino acid concentrations in one-year-old infants. J Nutr. 1983;113:1591-9.

29. Stegink LD, Brummel MC, Filer LJ Jr, Baker GL. Blood methanol concentrations in one-year-old infants administered graded doses of aspartame. J Nutr. 1983;113:1600-6.

30. Puthrasingam S, Heybroek WM, Johnston A, et al. Aspartame pharmacokinetics—the effect of ageing. Age Ageing. 1996;25:217-20.

31. Nehrling JK, Kobe P, McLane MP, Olson RE, Kamath S, Horwitz DL. Aspartame use by persons with diabetes. Diabetes Care. 1985;8:415-7.

32. Shaywitz BA, Sullivan CM, Anderson GM, Gillespie SM, Sullivan B, Shaywitz SE. Aspartame, behavior, and cognitive function in children with attention deficit disorder. Pediatrics. 1994b;93:70-5.

33. Lapierre KA, Greenblatt DJ, Goddard JE, Harmatz JS, Shader RI. The neuropsychiatric effects of aspartame in normal volunteers. J Clin Pharmacol. 1990;30:454-60.

34. Morgan RW, Wong O. A review of epidemiological studies on artificial sweeteners and bladder cancer. Food Chem Toxicol. 1985;23:529-33.

35. Elcock M, Morgan RW. Update on artificial sweeteners and bladder cancer. Regul Toxicol Pharmacol. 1993;17:35-43.

36. Armstrong B, Doll R. Bladder cancer mortality in diabetics in relation to saccharin consumption and smoking habits. Br J Prev Soc Med. 1975;29:73-81.

37. Grotz VL, Henry RR, McGill JB, et al. Lack of effect of sucralose on glucose homeostasis in subjects with type 2 diabetes. J Am Diet Assoc. 2003;103:1607-12.

38. Kroger M, Meister K, Kava R. Low-calorie sweeteners and other sugar substitutes: a review of the safety issues. Compr Rev Food Sci Food Saf. 2005;5(2):35-47.

39. PureVia All Natural Zero Calorie Sweetener. What is Reb A? (cited 2015 Jul 15). On the Internet at: www.purevia.com.

40. Truvia. About Truvia (cited 2015 Jul 15). On the Internet at: www.truvia.com.

41. National Library of Medicine, NIH. MedlinePlus. Sweeteners—sugar substitutes. Last updated 2013 Aug 26 (cited 2015 Jul 15). On the Internet at: http://www.nlm.nih.gov/medlineplus/ency/article/007492.htm.

42. International Food Information Council Foundation. Facts about low-calorie sweeteners. Last updated 2014 Sep 17 (cited 2015 Jul 19). On the Internet at: http://www.foodinsight.org/articles/facts-about-low-calorie-sweeteners 2014.

43. National Library of Medicine, NIH. MedlinePlus. Sweeteners—sugars. Updated 2013 Apr 30 (cited 2015 Jul 15). On the Internet at: http://www.nlm.nih.gov/medlineplus/ency/article/002444.htm.

44. Academy of Nutrition and Dietetics. Use of nutritive and nonnutritive sweeteners (position paper). J Acad Nutr Diet. 2012;112(5):739-58.

45. James PA, Opani S, Carter BL, et al. 2014 Evidence-based guideline for the management of high blood pressure in adults. Report from the panel members appointed to the Eighth Joint National Committee (JNC 8). JAMA. 2014;311(5):507-20.

46. US Department of Agriculture, US Department of Health and Human Services. Dietary Guidelines for Americans 2010. Appendix 13: Selected food sources ranked by dietary fiber and calories per standard food portion (cited 2015 Jul 15). On the Internet at: http://www.health.gov/dietaryguidelines/dga2010/DietaryGuidelines2010.pdf.

47. Franz MJ, Bantle JP, Beebe CA, et al. Evidence-based nutrition principles and recommendations for the treatment and prevention of diabetes and related complications. Diabetes Care. 2002;25:148-98.

48. Appel LJ, Moore TJ, Obarzanek E, et al, for the DASH Collaborative Research Group. A clinical trial of the effects of dietary patterns on blood pressure. New Engl J Med. 1997;336:1117-24.

49. American Heart Association. Sodium 411—sodium break up (cited 2015 Jul 15). On the Internet at: http://sodiumbreakup.heart.org/sodium-411/.

50. Burnakis TG. Captopril and increased serum potassium levels (letter). JAMA. 1984;252:1682-3.

51. Ray K, Dorman S, Watson R. Severe hyperkalemia due to the concomitant use of salt substitutes and ACE inhibitors in hypertension: a potentially life threatening interaction. J Hum Hypertens. 1999;13:717-20.

American Association of Diabetes Educators©

Module 2　*Healthy Eating*　65

52. Bicket DP. Using ACE inhibitors appropriately. Am Fam Physician. 2002 Aug 1 (cited 28 Feb 2015);66(3):461-9. On the Internet at: http://www.aafp.org/afp/2002/0801/p461.html.

53. Food and Drug Administration. Food labeling: final rule. Fed Regist. 2005; 70:56828-49.

54. Academy of Nutrition and Dietetics and American Diabetes Association. Choose Your Foods: Food Lists for Diabetes. Chicago and Alexandria, Va: Academy of Nutrition and Dietetics and American Diabetes Association; 2014.

55. US National Library of Medicine and the National Institutes of Health. Medline Plus. Wine and heart health (cited 2015 Jul 15). On the Internet at: http://www.nlm.nih.gov/medlineplus/ency/article/001963.htm.

56. Nigris F. Beneficial effects of pomegranate juice on oxidation-sensitive genes and endothelial nitric oxide synthase activity at sites of perturbed shear stress. Proc Natl Acad Sci USA. 2005;102(13):4896-901.

57. USFDA CFSAN, Office of Nutritional Products, Labeling, and Dietary Supplements. Make your calories count. Use the Nutrition Facts label for healthy weight management. Last updated 2014 Dec 16 (cited 2015 Jul 15). On the Internet at: http://www.fda.gov/Food/IngredientsPackagingLabeling/LabelingNutrition/ucm275438.htm.

HEALTHY EATING: RESOURCES

Measuring Food With Everyday Items as a Guide 65

Free and Reliable Online Food-Related Resources 66

Healthy Eating Handout (English) 67

Healthy Eating Handout (Spanish) 69

MyPlate (English) 71

MyPlate (Spanish) 72

Measuring Food With Everyday Items as a Guide

Hand	About the right size for estimating . . .
Tip of thumb	1 teaspoon
Full thumb	1 ounce
Palm	3 to 5 ounces
Fist	1 to 1½ cups

Household item	About the right size for estimating . . .
Baseball (hard ball)	1 cup food (cereal flakes, yogurt, salad greens, vegetables, chili, or 1 medium fruit)
Cassette tape	3 ounces meat, poultry, 1 slice of bread
Checkbook	3 ounces fish
Child's small toy block	Bagel (1 serving is ¼ to ⅓ bagel)
Compact disc	1 pancake, 1 ounce deli luncheon meat, 6-ounce can of tuna
Computer mouse	1 medium potato
Deck of cards	3 ounces meat, poultry, tofu
Egg	⅓ cup food (rice, quinoa)
Golf ball	Peanut butter or hummus (1 ounce or 2 tablespoons)
Golf ball or ping-pong ball	24 almonds, 29 peanuts, or 49 pistachios, shelled (¼ cup or 1 ounce)
Lightbulb or ice cream scoop	½ cup food (yogurt, pasta, ice cream)
Playing dice, stacked (2)	Cheese (1 ounce)
Poker chip	1 tablespoon salad dressing or mayonnaise
Tennis ball	Medium apple, orange, peach OR ½ cup food

American Association of Diabetes Educators©

66　Diabetes Education Curriculum

Free and Reliable Online Food-Related Resources

WIN—Weight-Control Information Network
http://www.win.niddk.nih.gov/index.htm

Academy of Nutrition and Dietetics
http://www.eatright.org

USDA Choose My Plate
http://www.choosemyplate.gov

Nutrition Support Groups

Weight Watchers
http://www.weightwatchers.com

TOPS: Take Off Pounds Sensibly
http://www.tops.org

Overeaters Anonymous
http://www.oa.org

Patient Assistance Programs

Special Supplemental Nutrition Program for Women, Infants, and Children (WIC)—provides supplemental foods, healthcare referrals, and nutrition education for low-income pregnancy, breastfeeding, and non-breastfeeding postpartum women, and to infants and children up to age 5 who are found to be at nutritional risk
http://www.fns.usda.gov/wic/women-infants-and-children-wic

AADE7™ SELF-CARE BEHAVIORS
HEALTHY EATING

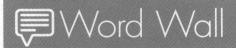

If you've just learned that you have diabetes or prediabetes, you probably have a lot of questions about what you can or can't eat. Do you wonder if you can ever have your favorite food again? What happens when you are eating at a restaurant or a friend's house? Do you have to change your whole diet just because you have diabetes?

The answer is **NO**. There is nothing that you can't eat. You don't have to give up your favorite foods or stop eating at restaurants.

But, it is important to know that everything you eat has an effect on your blood sugar. Learning to eat regular meals, controlling the amount you eat, and making healthy food choices can help you manage your diabetes better and prevent other health problems.

Some skills are more complex, but your diabetes educator or dietitian can help you learn about:

- » Counting carbohydrates
- » Reading food labels
- » Measuring the amount of a serving
- » Developing a practical meal plan
- » Preventing high or low blood sugar
- » Setting goals for healthy eating

Pick one or two of these skills and discuss them with your healthcare provider.

DID YOU KNOW?

There are only 3 main types of nutrients in food: carbohydrates, proteins, and fats. A healthy meal will include all three types.

TRUE OR FALSE:

People with diabetes can't have sugar.

FALSE: Sugar is just another carbohydrate and can fit into a meal plan. Sugary foods, however, do not have the same nutrition as grains or vegetables, and can often be high in fat and calories. It's best to limit sugar-containing foods to small portions, and be sure to count the carbohydrates toward the total recommended in your meal plan.

Word Wall

CARBOHYDRATE (AKA "CARBS"):
One of the three main types of nutrients found in food. Bread, pasta, rice, fruits, vegetables (especially starchy vegetables such as potatoes, corn, peas, dried beans), milk, and sweets are all carbs. Don't forget that carbohydrates can be found in beverages, too.

PORTION:
How much of a food you eat

MEAL PLAN:
A guide for healthy eating developed with your healthcare provider

HYPOGLYCEMIA:
Low blood sugar

HYPERGLYCEMIA:
High blood sugar

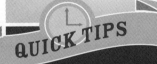

Eat breakfast every day. Breakfast helps begin the calorie-burning process that provides you with energy. Include small snacks between meals as part of your daily intake to help keep your body going.

Space your meals throughout the day. Going too long without eating may result in excessive hunger, which can lead to overeating later on. Try to eat every 4 to 5 hours during waking hours.

AADE American Association of Diabetes Educators

Supported by an educational grant from Eli Lilly and Company.

ACTIVITIES

ASK YOURSELF

When I think about healthy eating, I feel: _____, _____ and
_____. *(Pick 3 words to fill in the blanks)*

What did you eat for dinner last night? _____

Is there anything you could have done to make your meal healthier? _____

For you, what is the hardest part about healthy eating? _____

What is the best part about healthy eating? _____

REMEMBER THAT A HEALTHY MEAL PLAN SHOULD INCLUDE:

» **Complex carbohydrates** such as whole grain bread
» **Fiber,** which is found in beans, whole grains, fruits and vegetables
» **Lean protein,** such as chicken (without skin) or fish
» **Lots of vegetables**—especially the green, leafy ones
» **A limited amount of heart-healthy fats**, such as olive, peanut or canola oil, walnuts, almonds and flax seed

A good first step is to follow the "plate method" of meal planning, which includes a healthy balance of foods and controlled portions.

Visually divide your plate into 4 sections. For lunch or dinner, fill ½ the plate with non-starchy vegetables (such as: greens, green beans, broccoli, cabbage); ¼ should contain meat or other protein (fish, eggs, low-fat cheeses, cottage cheese, beans or legumes); ¼ contains starch (such as a potato or whole grain bread). On the side, include an 8 ounce glass of low fat milk or a small piece of fruit.

PLAN A HEALTHY DINNER THAT YOU WILL ENJOY IN THE SPACE BELOW.

_____
_____
_____
_____
_____
_____
_____

AADE — American Association of Diabetes Educators

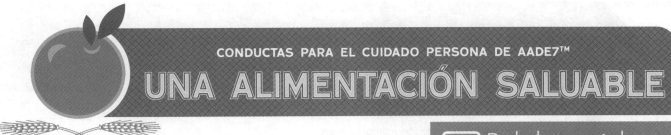

CONDUCTAS PARA EL CUIDADO PERSONA DE AADE7™
UNA ALIMENTACIÓN SALUABLE

Si te acabas de enterar que tienes diabetes o prediabetes, probablemente tengas muchas preguntas sobre qué puedes comer y qué no. ¿Te preguntas si alguna vez podrás volver a comer tu comida favorita? ¿Qué sucede cuando vas a comer a un restaurante o a la casa de un amigo? ¿Tienes que cambiar toda tu dieta sólo porque tienes diabetes?

La respuesta es NO. No hay nada que no puedas comer. No tienes que dejar de comer tus comidas favoritas ni dejar de ir a comer a restaurantes.

Pero es importante que sepas que todo lo que comes afecta tus niveles de azúcar en la sangre. Si aprendes a comer las comidas habituales, controlas la cantidad de alimentos que comes y eliges alimentos saludables, esto puede ayudarte a controlar mejor tu diabetes y prevenir otros problemas de salud.

Algunas técnicas son más complejas, pero tu dietista o educador en diabetes puede ayudarte a aprender cómo:

- » Contar carbohidratos.
- » Leer las etiquetas de los alimentos.
- » Medir el tamaño de una porción.
- » Desarrollar un plan de comidas práctico.
- » Prevenir un nivel alto o bajo de azúcar en la sangre.
- » Fijar objetivos para una alimentación saludable.

Escoge una o dos de estas técnicas y analízalas con tu proveedor de atención médica.

¿LO SABÍAS?

Hay sólo 3 tipos de nutrientes principales en los alimentos: los carbohidratos, las proteínas y las grasas. Una comida saludable incluye los tres tipos de nutrientes.

¿VERDADERO O FALSO?

Las personas con diabetes no pueden comer azúcar.

FALSO: El azúcar es simplemente otro carbohidrato y puede incluirse en un plan de comidas. Sin embargo, los alimentos con azúcar no tienen el mismo valor nutritivo que los granos o las verduras, y a menudo pueden tener un alto contenido de grasas y calorías. Lo mejor es limitar el consumo de alimentos que contienen azúcar a pequeñas porciones; y asegúrate de contar la cantidad de carbohidratos para respetar el total recomendado en tu plan de comidas.

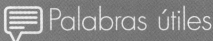 Palabras útiles

CARBOHIDRATOS:
Uno de los tres tipos de nutrientes principales que se encuentran en los alimentos. El pan, las pastas, el arroz, las frutas, las verduras (especialmente las que contienen almidón, como las papas, el maíz, las arvejas, los frijoles secos), la leche y los dulces son todos carbohidratos. No te olvides que los carbohidratos también se pueden encontrar en las bebidas.

PORCIÓN:
La cantidad que comes de un alimento.

PLAN DE COMIDAS:
Una guía para comer sano desarrollada junto con tu proveedor de atención médica.

HIPOGLUCEMIA:
Bajo nivel de azúcar en la sangre.

HIPERGLUCEMIA:
Alto nivel de azúcar en la sangre.

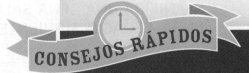

Desayuna todos los días. El desayuno ayuda a comenzar el proceso de quemar calorías que te da energía. Incluye pequeños refrigerios entre las comidas como parte de tu alimentación diaria para ayudar a mantener tu cuerpo en funcionamiento.

Separa tus comidas a lo largo del día. Estar mucho tiempo sin comer puede darte demasiada hambre, y esto puede hacer que más tarde comas en exceso. Trata de comer cada 4 a 5 horas durante las horas que estás despierto.

AADE American Association of Diabetes Educators

Supported by an educational grant from Lilly USA, LLC.

ACTIVIDADES

PREGÚNTATE LO SIGUIENTE

Cuando pienso en una alimentación saludable, siento: _____ y
_____. *(Escoge 3 palabras para completar los espacios en blanco)*

¿Qué cenaste anoche? _____

¿Hay algo que podrías haber hecho para que tu comida fuera más saludable? _____

Para ti, ¿cuál es la parte más difícil de una alimentación saludable? _____

¿Cuál es la mejor parte de una alimentación saludable? _____

RECUERDA QUE UN PLAN DE COMIDAS SALUDABLES DEBE INCLUIR:

- » **Carbohidratos complejos,** como el pan integral.
- » **Fibra,** que se encuentra en los frijoles, los granos integrales, las frutas y las verduras.
- » **Proteínas sin grasa,** como el pollo (sin piel) o el pescado
- » **Muchas verduras,** especialmente las verduras de hoja verde.
- » **Una cantidad limitada de grasas saludables para el corazón,** como el aceite de oliva, maní o canola; las nueces, las almendras y las semillas de lino.

Un buen primer paso es seguir el "método del plato" para planificar las comidas, que incluye un equilibrio saludable de alimentos y porciones controladas.

Divide tu plato visualmente en 4 secciones. Para el almuerzo o la cena, llena medio plato con verduras que no contengan almidón (por ej., verduras verdes, frijoles verdes, brócoli, repollo); ¼ del plato debe contener carne u otra proteína (pescado, huevos, quesos con bajo contenido de grasa, requesón o ricota, frijoles o legumbres); y 1/4 del plato debe contener alimentos con almidón (como una papa o pan integral). A un lado del plato coloca un vaso de 8 onzas de leche con bajo contenido de grasa o una porción pequeña de fruta.

PLANIFICA UNA CENA SALUDABLE QUE DISFRUTES EN EL ESPACIO SIGUIENTE.

_____
_____
_____
_____
_____
_____

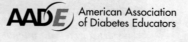

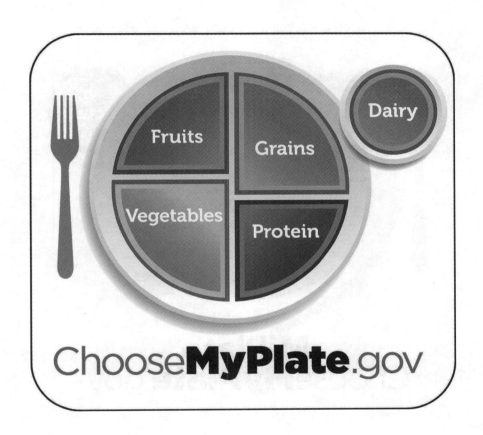

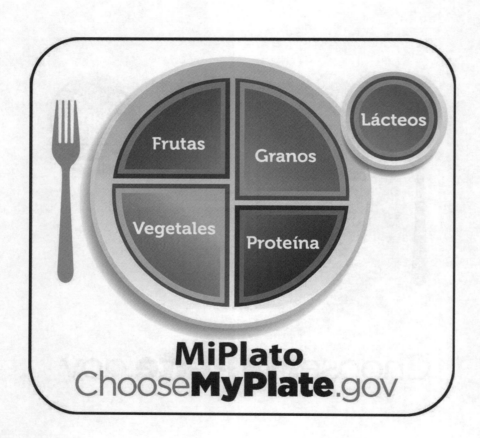

MODULE 3

Being Active

Table of Contents

BEING ACTIVE: AN EDUCATOR'S OVERVIEW 74

    AADE Systematic Review of the Literature. 74

    Background Information and Instructions for the Educator 75

        Exercise Prescription 75

        Progress Comes in Stages 75

        Promoting Physical Activity 76

    Learning Objectives 76

        Knowledge. 76

        Barriers and Facilitators 76

    Behavioral Objectives 76

BEING ACTIVE: INSTRUCTIONAL PLAN 77

    Identifying Participant Understanding of and Interest in Physical Activity 77

    Benefits of Physical Activity 77

        For Those With Prediabetes or Type 2 Diabetes 77

        For Those at Risk for Type 2 Diabetes or Who Already Have Prediabetes. 78

    Lifestyle Approach to Increasing Activity: First Steps for Previously Inactive People 78

    Recommended Types of Physical Activity for People With Diabetes or Prediabetes. 78

        Aerobic Activity. 79

        Resistance Activity 79

        Flexibility and Stretching Exercises. 80

        Balance Exercise 80

    Structured Approach to Moderate Physical Activity 80

        Preparing for Physical Activity 80

        Frequency and Duration of Aerobic Activity 80

        Intensity of Aerobic Activity. 81

        Frequency of Resistance Activity 82

        Intensity of Resistance Activity. 83

74   Diabetes Education Curriculum

Physical Activity and Safety Issues 84

   Medical Clearance 84

   Hydration 84

   Foot Safety... 84

   Medical Identification (ID) 84

   Preventing Hypoglycemia or Hyperglycemia: Balancing Physical Activity
      With Food and Medication... 84

   Physical Activity and Monitoring... 84

   Physical Activity and Insulin 84

   Physical Activity and Diabetes Medication................................. 85

   Timing of Physical Activity 86

Special Considerations/Advanced Detail for Appropriate Participants............... 88

   Obesity/Orthopedic Issues... 88

   Heart Disease/Hypertension 89

   Peripheral Vascular Disease 89

   Moderate to Severe Retinopathy 89

   Visual Impairment/Blindness... 89

   Peripheral Neuropathy/Ulcers 89

   Autonomic Neuropathy 90

   End-Stage Renal Disease 90

Identifying Barriers to Physical Activity 90

Identifying Facilitators for Physical Activity 91

   Common Facilitators 92

Setting a SMART Goal for Physical Activity.................................... 92

Follow-up/Outcomes Measurement 92

REFERENCES 93

BEING ACTIVE: RESOURCES 95

BEING ACTIVE: AN EDUCATOR'S OVERVIEW

AADE Systematic Review of the Literature

A systematic review of the literature was conducted by the American Association of Diabetes Educators (AADE) to assess the existing evidence for the intervention of physical activity among people with diabetes. Overall, the findings suggest that any physical activity is better than none at all. Being active has a positive effect on glucose control and reduces the risk for cardiovascular disease in people with type 2 diabetes. For those with type 1 diabetes, physical activity interventions have not consistently shown an improvement in glycemic control; however, physical activity should be encouraged in this population because of its cardiovascular and other health benefits. Better clinical outcomes tend to be achieved by patients who engage in more intensive, structured physical activity regimens, as compared with regimens that are less intensive in nature and unstructured. To enhance success with physical activity as a self-care behavior, diabetes educators should tailor interventions to meet the patient's individual needs.[1]

American Association of Diabetes Educators©

Background Information and Instructions for the Educator

When interacting with participants, the term *physical activity* or *activity* is preferred over *exercise*. Many people believe that exercise requires certain physical skills or athletic abilities. This perception may cause discouragement and keep them from attempting a physical activity program.[1]

Exercise Prescription

Simply put, the exercise prescription is *the plan one follows to achieve physical fitness.* In an ideal world, each patient would have access to an exercise physiologist (EP) for a well-designed exercise prescription. If your diabetes education team has no EP, then the educator can help the patient design a program that will meet his or her needs. Guide patients in the development of a SMART activity goal that is specific, measurable, attainable, realistic, and that has a timeline. Include the following components—often abbreviated as **FITT**—into patients' written activity plan[2(pp478-9)]:

* **F**requency—How many days per week the activity should take place.
* **I**ntensity—Match it to the patient's capabilities and current fitness level, so it is attainable and realistic. The "talk" test may be used to gauge intensity. For patients requesting more advanced detail, target heart rate may be explained and their range calculated.
* **T**ime—Duration of activity.
* **T**ype of activity—Dependent on patient preference, eg, walking, yoga, swimming, cycling. The educator should ensure that the chosen activity is appropriate, considering the presence of any complications (eg, neuropathy, severe retinopathy, or heart disease).

Progress Comes in Stages[2(pp478-9)]

Unrealistic expectations can derail patients' efforts to become more physically active. Too often, fresh from a diabetes education class and feeling highly motivated, patients will set a behavior change goal for physical activity that is too aggressive, one that may result in either demotivation or physical injury.[2,3] They may truly believe at that moment that they are capable of the goal they have set. One of the most important things the educator can do is to help patients understand the stages of progression they should *realistically expect.*

A sedentary person should progress from the initial stage to the improvement stage to the maintenance stage over a period of about 6 months (see Table 3.1), although allowing extra time for full progression in patients with preexisting comorbidities is perfectly acceptable and recommended to encourage continuation of exercise

TABLE 3.1	Sedentary Person's Rate of Progression Through the 3 Stages of a Physical Activity Program				
Stage of Physical Activity	**Week**	**Key Points**	**Frequency of Activity (per Week)**	**Duration of Activity (Minutes)**	**Intensity (% Heart Rate Reserve)**
Initial	1–4		3–4	15–30	30–59
Improvement	5–24	• Measurable changes begin: ❶ stamina; ❶ endurance • Patient at risk of slacking off • Workload and intensity of activity should increase	3–5	25–40	40–89
Maintenance	25+	• A new goal should be set	3–5	20–60	40–89

Source: Adapted from SR Colberg, "Physical Activity," in C Mensing, ed, *The Art and Science of Diabetes Self-Management Education: A Desk Reference for Healthcare Professionals*, 3rd ed. (Chicago: American Association of Diabetes Educators, 2014), 477.

American Association of Diabetes Educators©

76   Diabetes Education Curriculum

participation. Assist patients with setting a behavior change goal that can be realistically achieved in the first 4 weeks; otherwise, most people will never make it out of this critical stage.[1] At follow-up, assess for the following occurrences:

- Has there been any change in diabetes medication?
- Has any new diagnosis been made?
- Have any diabetes complications occurred/progressed?

If any significant changes have occurred, the physical activity plan should be reevaluated to be certain that it is still safe and effective.

Promoting Physical Activity

Factors that influence patients' decisions to be physically active include self-efficacy, enjoyment level related to activity, support from other people, beliefs about the benefits of activity, and perceived barriers.[3] One of the most consistent predictors of greater levels of activity has been higher levels of self-efficacy, which reflect confidence in the ability to exercise. In individuals with type 2 diabetes in particular, interventions should focus on enhancing self-efficacy, problem solving, and social-environmental support to improve self-management (which includes exercise, dietary, and medication behaviors).[3-6]

To Enhance Self-Efficacy—The educator should help patients pursue activities they feel capable of doing. Help patients set realistic goals, stepped up in small increments. Realistic goals are more likely to be achieved and will consequently promote feelings of mastery. Provide support at regular follow-ups.[3-6]

To Enhance Support—The educator should assess the patient's support system. Help the patient learn to ask for support from others to become and remain physically active. See "Asking for Support From Family" section in Module 7: Healthy Coping for more information.

To Enhance Motivation—The educator should assess conviction and confidence in making a behavior change in the area of physical activity. See "Using Motivational Interviewing Techniques to Enhance Confidence and Conviction" in Module 6: Problem Solving for more information.

Learning Objectives

Knowledge

The participant will:

- state the benefits of physical activity
- describe the elements of an appropriate physical activity plan

Barriers and Facilitators

The participant will:

- identify potential barriers and facilitators that may affect his or her ability to implement a physical activity plan
- develop strategies for reducing barriers and increasing facilitators in order to successfully implement a physical activity plan

Behavioral Objectives

The participant will:

- set realistic, measurable individual goals to increase (or maintain) his or her physical activity level
- continue with his or her physical activity plan through all 3 stages and maintain participation long term

American Association of Diabetes Educators©

BEING ACTIVE: INSTRUCTIONAL PLAN

Identifying Participant Understanding of and Interest in Physical Activity

What information have you been given about physical activity as part of taking care of your diabetes?

What are your thoughts about making physical activity part of your diabetes management plan?

What do you want to learn today about being physically active?

What is your greatest concern about engaging in more physical activity?

Adults learn best when the learning experience is active and not passive. **Keep participants engaged with questions.**

Benefits of Physical Activity

For you, what is the best part about being physically active?

What have you heard about the benefits of being physically active?

For Those With Prediabetes or Type 2 Diabetes

Physical activity can improve blood glucose levels. It helps your body cells use insulin better.[7-10] Blood glucose levels usually improve for anywhere from 2 to 72 hours after physical activity, although the effect varies with the type of activity, intensity, duration, frequency, and other factors.[11]

Physical activity helps strengthen the heart and lowers your risk for heart disease. People with diabetes have at least twice the risk for heart disease compared with people without diabetes, and the risk for coronary death is significantly greater for women with diabetes than for men with diabetes.[12]

Physical activity can lower cholesterol, especially "bad" (small, dense, oxidized) LDL cholesterol, which is thought to lead to plaque formation that can clog the blood vessels. At the same time, physical activity can raise HDL, the "good" type of cholesterol, which may remove cholesterol from the blood and prevent clogging of blood vessels.[13-15]

Sharing of personal experiences has more relevance to patients than passively listening to educational content. Hearing others' accounts of how they successfully and safely integrated physical activity into their lives can encourage patients to do the same.

Blood pressure is also improved with physical activity.[14,15] Physical activity can help with weight loss and can lower the percentage of body fat, especially the fat around your middle, or *belly fat*. Studies show that belly fat is more unhealthy than fat on other areas of the body, as it is highly related to the risk for heart disease.[15-17]

American Association of Diabetes Educators©

Physical activity can have positive effects on your emotional state. It helps lower stress and anxiety and improves feelings of well-being.[18]

Aging is a fact of life. But regular physical activity can delay the usual declines that happen when you get older. Building muscle and endurance helps prevent falls in older people.[19,20]

Studies show that physical activity lowers the risk for certain forms of cancer. It also lowers the risk for osteoporosis by preventing bone loss.[3]

For Those at Risk for Type 2 Diabetes or Who Already Have Prediabetes

Studies have proved that physical activity and weight loss can lower certain people's risk for type 2 diabetes. The participants in these studies had prediabetes. In one study, they did 150 minutes of physical activity per week. They also ate less fat and cut their calorie count. On average, participants lost 10 to 15 lb. This approach lowered their risk for getting type 2 diabetes by almost 60%.[21] Many other studies have shown similar results.[22-24]

Lifestyle Approach to Increasing Activity: First Steps for Previously Inactive People

What do you usually do to add movement into your daily routine?

What can you do to add some extra movement into each day?

Any physical activity is better than none at all. Physical activity as part of your daily lifestyle burns calories even if it's not part of a structured physical activity plan. Standing up counts, as do stretching exercises, taking more daily steps, fidgeting, and moving more any way you can.

Even if you are inactive and out of shape now, you can improve your health by moving just a little more. Take small steps to add more movement into your daily lifestyle.[3,25,26]

Examples of lifestyle activity include the following:

- Doing household chores, yard work, or gardening
- Playing actively with children
- Adding extra "steps" into your routine, eg, walking instead of driving whenever possible
- Taking the stairs instead of the elevator
- Parking farther away from the building when going to work or running errands
- Getting off the bus 1 or 2 stops earlier
- Standing up or pacing when talking on the telephone instead of sitting down

When these activities become easier, it's time to move to the next level, which is a structured activity plan. This includes choosing an activity that you can perform at a moderate-intensity level on most days of the week and for a set amount of time.

Recommended Types of Physical Activity for People With Diabetes or Prediabetes

There are 2 main types of physical activity that can affect the way the body uses glucose: aerobic and resistance. A third type of physical activity is flexibility training or stretching. Flexibility training may not affect the blood glucose level as much, but it does lend to a well-rounded fitness program and helps lower your risk of falling down.[1,19] In addition, frequent balance training is recommended as you get older, and lifestyle exercise should continue to be a daily part of the lifestyle for anyone with diabetes or prediabetes.

Aerobic Activity

Aerobic activity involves moving the large muscles over and over, increasing your body's need for oxygen. Your heart then has to beat faster so it can get enough oxygen to the muscles. The heart continues to beat this fast as long as the activity lasts. Aerobic activity is not a "stop and start" type of activity. Aerobic activity is especially helpful for controlling blood glucose. It is beneficial for circulation and heart health.

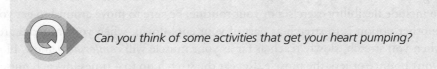

Can you think of some activities that get your heart pumping?

Examples of aerobic activity include the following:

- brisk walking
- jogging or running
- riding a bicycle
- using conditioning machines
- swimming
- tennis or racquetball
- rowing
- dancing

Very vigorous aerobic activity may not be safe if you have heart disease. It may raise your blood pressure too high or cause your heart to work too hard. If you have heart disease, check with your provider to see what kind of activity is safe for you. See the section "Special Considerations" later in this module.

Resistance Activity

Resistance activity strengthens your muscles and keeps you from losing muscle mass as you get older. It helps increase your muscular endurance and helps your body use insulin better, whether it is your own or you have to inject or pump it.[27]

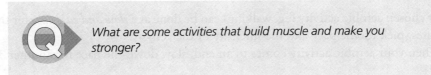

What are some activities that build muscle and make you stronger?

Examples of resistance activity include the following:

- weight lifting with dumbbells or free weights
- weight-lifting machines
- resistance bands or tubing
- certain types of calisthenics—moving your body weight for resistance (abdominal crunches, push-ups, toe raises)

Certain resistance activities may not be safe if you have heart disease, eye disease, or kidney disease. They may raise your blood pressure too high or cause damage to these organs. If you have heart, eye, or kidney disease, check with your provider to see what kind of activity is safe for you. See the section "Special Considerations" later in this module.

American Association of Diabetes Educators©

Flexibility and Stretching Exercises

Stretching the muscles can be done as *part* of your warm-up or cool-down. Recent studies have shown that stretching does not prevent muscle injury as was previously thought.[28] Even so, stretching has other benefits, and exercise programs that include stretching can increase your flexibility.[29] Some studies show that stretching is good for the heart and circulation[30,31]; other studies show that it helps people better use their body's insulin.[32] If you have not been active for a long time, stretching may be a good start for easing into a more active lifestyle.

If you choose to include flexibility exercises in your routine, be sure to move around to get your muscles warm *before* stretching. Another option is to stretch as part of your cool-down, when your muscles are already warmed up. Regardless of when you stretch, slowly reach as far as your muscle will *comfortably* allow. Hold the stretch for 15 to 30 seconds. Don't bounce or jerk the muscle. Repeat the stretch up to 4 times for each muscle.[3,33] Alternately, you can do dynamic stretching, which involves gentle movement during the stretch, and yoga also serves as an excellent stretching and strengthening activity.

Balance Exercise

As you age, it's also critical to do some exercises that help maintain or improve your balance to lower your risk of having a fall.[19] Stretching regularly can help keep you on your feet better by keeping you more flexible.[30] Most lower body and "core" resistance exercises also double as balance training. You can also improve your balance by simply practicing standing on 1 leg as long as you can (alternately with the other one) several times every day.[34]

Structured Approach to Moderate Physical Activity

Preparing for Physical Activity

Have you ever exercised and then were sore later on? What do you think caused the soreness?

Aerobic activity sessions should start with a warm-up and end with a cool-down. The warm-up does just what it says: it warms up your muscles and gets them ready for more intense activity. The warm-up helps prevent injury to your muscles.[15,33] In the cool-down, blood that has built up in your muscles can move back into your general circulation. The cool-down may also limit your stiffness or soreness later on.[33]

Warm-up. Your chosen aerobic activity (eg, walking) can be done at a *slow and easy pace* for the warm-up. After 5 to 10 minutes, pick up the pace and the intensity of the activity.

Cool-down. When your aerobic activity comes to an end, slow down the pace for another 3 to 5 minutes.

Frequency and Duration of Aerobic Activity

How much physical activity do you think you need for good health? Have you been given any specific guidelines?

National guidelines for healthy adults aged 18 to 84 years call for a total of 150 minutes per week of moderate aerobic activity. Preferably, your activity is spread out over the week, for example, 30 minutes 5 days per week.[35] If you have type 2 diabetes, you should aim to get at least 150 minutes per week of moderate to vigorous aerobic activity, allowing no more than 2 consecutive days without any activity.[15] Structured exercise training of more than 150 minutes per week usually leads to greater declines in HbA1c than when you do 150 minutes or less per week, so doing more is recommended for optimal blood glucose control.[36] If you have type 1 diabetes or prediabetes, you should aim for 150 minutes of moderate activity or 75 minutes of vigorous activity weekly, the same that is recommended for all adults.

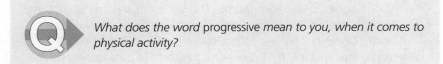
What does the word *progressive* mean to you, when it comes to physical activity?

It's best to start with what you can comfortably do. You may start with 5 to 10 minutes of activity and work up to 30 minutes. This is called *progressive* increases in activity. If you increase the duration of your aerobic activity a little at each session, you lower the chances of getting sore, injured, or discouraged. It gives your body enough time to adapt to the changes in your activity level.

If you push yourself beyond your limits early on, you may become discouraged and want to stop being active. Remember that it may take you a few weeks to progress to 30 minutes *and* feel good while you are doing it.

Which do you think is better: 30 minutes of nonstop activity or three 10-minute sessions?

Studies show that there are still health benefits if you break the activity into three 10-minute sessions.[3,37] Studies have shown that when it comes to controlling blood glucose levels, doing three 10-minute sessions may be just as effective as or even better than doing 30 minutes at once.[37] Even so, health benefits are greater if you do an activity for a longer period of time or at a harder intensity. An analysis of 25 studies showed that the *duration* of an activity session has a greater effect on raising the HDL ("good") cholesterol than increasing the frequency or the intensity of the activity. It showed that 120 minutes of exercise per week was the minimum amount of exercise needed to significantly affect the HDL level.[13] **If weight loss is your goal**, you may need to be active for longer periods. Progressively work up to doing 45 to 60 minutes of continuous activity, 5 to 7 days per week, to help you burn the most calories.[35]

Intensity of Aerobic Activity

The *intensity* of an aerobic activity is determined by how hard it makes your heart work. To get healthier, it is not necessary for your heart to beat as fast as it possibly could, pushed to its full limit.

One easy way to determine a safe and effective intensity is to do the "talk" test. You should be able to talk easily during physical activity. If it is too hard to talk, then the activity is more intense than it needs to be. In this case, you should slow the pace of the activity until you can talk. If you can easily talk during the activity, then it may not be intense enough to optimize your fitness, and you may want to pick up your pace a bit, if possible. Starting out at a lower intensity until your fitness level begins to improve is fine, though, and doing even low-level activity is better than none.

Help patients build a more positive attitude about physical activity by:
- Examining beliefs, expectations, and assumptions about their ability to integrate activity into their lifestyle
- Presenting evidence that breaking activity into multiple short sessions still has merit
- Debunking the idea that one must have special athletic skills or sweat a lot to effectively work out

Pulse-Finding Activity

To find your pulse, press the pads of 2 fingers to the wrist bone close to your thumb. This is the radial pulse. Do not use your thumb to feel for the pulse. (The pulse in your thumb may disrupt your count.) Once your pulse is found, count for 1 minute. Or, count for 15 seconds, then multiply by 4. Exercise equipment (eg, treadmills, stationary bikes) often have sensors in the handles that measure heart rate.

Advanced Detail

Finding Your Target Heart Rate (Based on Heart Rate Reserve)[33]

Aerobic activity should make your heart beat at 40% to 89% of your unique heart rate reserve. There is a formula that can help you find your target heart rate during physical activity.

Target HR = [(Max HR − Resting HR) × Desired percent intensity] + Resting HR

Find the target heart rate for an activity at 50% intensity:

1. Measure your resting heart rate (your pulse rate when you first wake up is best).
2. Subtract your age (eg, 50 years) from 220 to estimate your maximal heart rate (ie, 220 − 50 = 170).
3. Subtract your calculated maximum heart rate (170) from your measured resting value (eg, 70), or in this example, 170 − 70 = 100 beats per minute. This is your "heart rate reserve."
4. Multiply the reserve (100) by your desired intensity level (50%).
5. Add this number (50) back to your resting heart rate to get your target (example: 50 + 70 = 120 beats per minute).

Target heart rate at 50% intensity = 120 beats per minute

In this example, the target heart rate for a 50-year-old person doing an activity at 50% intensity is 120 beats per minute. The same equation can be used to determine the target heart rate for intensity at different levels. Just change the multiplier in step 4 to the desired percentage (within the recommended range of 40% to 89%). For 40% intensity, multiply by 0.40; for 89%, multiply by 0.89.

Learners with strong logical/mathematical intelligence may inquire about the equation for finding target heart rate. They learn best when numbers and math are involved. Share this technique as needed.

Frequency of Resistance Activity

See the section "Special Considerations" for patients who should avoid resistance activities.

Intensity of Resistance Activity

Try lifting hand weights of different loads. Find one that you can lift 8 to 12 times, but no more or less. This is the right weight that you should use for building optimal muscle strength, endurance, and muscle mass.[33] You can also use your own body weight as resistance for many training exercises, such as planks and lunges.

The number of times a weight is lifted is called a *repetition* ("rep"). If you lift a weight 10 times, you have done 10 reps. A *set* is the number of times the reps are done. If you do 10 reps twice, you have done 2 sets of 10 reps. **It is important to rest between sets** to allow your muscles to get ready for the next set. Rest time of **15 seconds to 1 minute** is usually enough.

To build muscle strength and endurance, do 1 to 3 sets of 8 to 12 reps of each resistance activity, and do a minimum of 8 to 10 different exercises. If you are just starting out, you should do only 1 set of each resistance activity for the first 4 weeks, and it is fine to start with a lower resistance that you can lift 12 to 15 times.

Types of hand weight exercises include the following:

- biceps curl
- triceps curl
- fly curl

What kinds of hand weight exercises can you think of?

Tips for proper lifting of hand weights include the following:

- Keep your spine in correct alignment; don't arch your back or hunch over.
- Lift the weight slowly—2 to 3 counts.
- Breathe out when you lift the weight.
- Lower the weight slowly—2 to 3 counts.
- Breathe in when you lower the weight.

If you don't have any hand weights at home, what else can you lift?

Accessible options if no hand weights are available include the following:

- unopened soup can or full water bottle
- plastic jug with handle—partially filled with water, sand, or other substance
- exercises that exclusively use body weight as resistance

Adults learn best when they can relate new information to something they are already familiar with. Show everyday items that can be used as makeshift hand weights, such as full water bottles. This technique is helpful for those with visual/spatial intelligence.

Physical Activity and Safety Issues

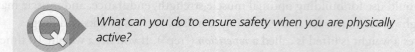
What can you do to ensure safety when you are physically active?

Medical Clearance

You may need to talk with your provider before starting a physical activity program. You may need extra tests to see if physical activity is safe for you, especially if you want to participate in vigorous activities (more vigorous than brisk walking), have not seen your provider within the past year for a checkup, and have developed any diabetes-related health complications.[15]

Hydration

Drink water before, during, and after physical activity. More water will be needed in hot or humid climates because sweating leads to loss of body water.[38]

Foot Safety

Wear the right kind of footwear during physical activity to avoid blisters or other injury. Socks that absorb sweat should be worn. Shoes should provide good support to your foot, with soles that are thick enough to absorb shock.[3,15] Check your feet after activity to see if any injury has occurred.

Medical Identification (ID)

All people with diabetes should carry a medical ID card in case of emergency. Medical ID jewelry is another option, especially if you use insulin.

Preventing Hypoglycemia or Hyperglycemia: Balancing Physical Activity With Food and Medication

You should balance physical activity with food and diabetes medication. This balance is meant to keep your blood glucose level in a safe range.

Physical Activity and Monitoring

Checking your blood glucose with a meter before and after physical activity will show its effect on your blood glucose level. Knowing your blood glucose level before and after will help you make better decisions about physical activity. The timing of monitoring is important if you want to understand cause and effect.

Glucose checks done before and after physical activity *should be done within minutes* before starting and within minutes after ending. In addition, you may need to check your blood glucose an hour or two after the end of your activity, as exercise can have lasting effects on blood glucose.

Physical Activity and Insulin

If you take insulin, you should learn when it lowers your blood glucose level the most. This is called the *peak* of insulin action. Physical activity at the same time the insulin is peaking can cause hypoglycemia (low blood glucose).

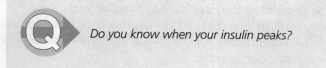
Do you know when your insulin peaks?

American Association of Diabetes Educators©

- You may need to reduce your insulin dose to allow for safe *planned* physical activity. Each person's insulin dose and schedule is unique. A change in insulin should be made *only* after talking with your provider and getting clear instructions.
- If your insulin has already been taken and *unplanned* physical activity occurs during the insulin peak, you should eat a snack to prevent hypoglycemia.
- Insulin should never be injected directly into muscle, as doing so increases its rate of absorption and your risk for hypoglycemia during physical activity. Insulin should always be injected into fat.

Physical Activity and Diabetes Medication

For Participants Who Take Oral Diabetes Agents
Do you know if your diabetes pill(s) can cause you to be at risk for hypoglycemia?

Help participants identify whether they are taking a medication that raises their risk for hypoglycemia during physical activity.

Certain classes of oral diabetes medications (ie, sulfonylureas and meglitinides) raise the risk for hypoglycemia because they cause the pancreas to secrete insulin. This risk is greater if you don't eat on time or you don't eat enough, especially in relation to physical activity.

Examples of Sulfonylureas	Examples of Meglitinides
Glimepiride (Amaryl®)	Repaglinide (Prandin®)
Glipizide (Glucotrol®, Glucotrol XL®); Glipizide in combination with Metformin (Metaglip™)	Nateglinide (Starlix®)
Glyburide (DiaBeta®, Micronase®, Glynase®); Glyburide in combination with Metformin (Glucovance®)	
Chlorpropamide (Diabinese®)	
Tolazamide (Tolinase®)	
Tolbutamide (Orinase®)	
Acetohexamide (Dymelor®)	

Adults learn best when the content is meaningful to their experience and fills a perceived need. Help insulin-using patients understand the relationship between insulin action and physical activity. Ask them to share any experiences they've had when insulin and activity were not in balance.

86   Diabetes Education Curriculum

Timing of Physical Activity

You can be physically active at any time that fits best into your day. Once you know when you are going to be physically active, you need to be aware of how it may affect your blood glucose level.

Advanced Detail

To Snack or Not to Snack Before Activity?

First, you need to know whether your diabetes medication can cause hypoglycemia.

- If you don't take a diabetes medication that can cause hypoglycemia, you may *not* need an extra snack before activity.

- If you take a diabetes medication that may cause you to have hypoglycemia, you may need an extra snack before activity.

    Second, you need to consider when you last ate.

- If your activity is started within 2 hours after a meal or scheduled snack, a pre-activity snack may not be necessary *based on your blood glucose reading*. This is because the meal or snack you just ate is expected to cause the blood glucose level to rise. Activity will help balance out the rise in blood glucose.

- If it has been more than 2 hours since your last meal, a pre-activity snack may or may not be needed, based on your medication regime, type of activity, exercise duration and intensity, and starting blood glucose level. Check your blood glucose beforehand and start activity if it is at the safe level for activity.

    Third, you need to know what a safe pre-activity blood glucose level is for you. Your provider may set blood glucose goals for physical activity. If none has been set, the levels shown in Table 3.2 are a safe place to start.[1]

TABLE 3.2 Blood Glucose Target Levels for Activity Based on Treatment or Situation	
Diabetes Treatment/Situation	**Blood Glucose Level Goal**
If not using diabetes medications or insulin . . .	No specific level
If using diabetes medications that do not cause hypoglycemia . . .	No specific level
If using diabetes medications that may cause hypoglycemia . . .	Keep blood glucose level above 90 mg/dL
If using insulin . . .	Keep blood glucose level above 110 mg/dL
If you have complications that affect your ability to recognize hypoglycemia . . .	Keep blood glucose level above 120 mg/dL

Problem-Solving Example

- Sue has learned that a brisk walk for 30 minutes usually causes her blood glucose level to drop about 30 mg/dL.

- She takes glyburide, so her goal is to keep her blood glucose level above 90 mg/dL during activity.

- To figure out a safe pre-walk blood glucose level, add 30 + 90, which equals 120.

- If Sue's pre-walk blood glucose level is *less than* 120 mg/dL, she needs to consider eating a snack before walking.

- If her walk is just after dinner, she likely will not need the snack.

- If it has been over 2 hours since her last meal, she may need the snack.

American Association of Diabetes Educators©

Fourth, you need to know how many grams of carbohydrate to eat if you need a snack for your physical activity.

- To prevent hypoglycemia in individuals with a relatively high risk for developing it during exercise, a general guideline is that a snack containing 10 to 30 g of carbohydrate should be consumed for every 30 to 45 minutes of moderate physical activity (see Table 3.3).
- The actual carbohydrate need will vary from person to person and even among activities done by one individual, making blood glucose monitoring critical for predicting snack requirements to optimize exercise performance and blood glucose control.

TABLE 3.3 Carbohydrate Requirements During Aerobic Physical Activity

Intensity	Carbohydrate Requirement	Frequency
Mild	0–10 g	Every 30 minutes
Moderate	5–10 g	Every 15 minutes
High	0–15 g	Every 15 minutes

BE AWARE OF THE RISK OF LATE-EVENING ACTIVITY: Late-evening physical activity may cause you to experience hypoglycemia while you are asleep. This risk can be lowered by avoiding late-evening physical activity, eating a bedtime snack, or adjusting your diabetes medication (with your provider's guidance) to lower doses overnight following activity.

Pre-Activity Snacks: What to Eat?

What food items do you usually have available to you for a pre-activity snack?

All snacks are not created equal. Pre-activity snacks are meant to *prevent* your blood glucose level from dropping too low. This kind of snack should contain carbohydrates. It also needs to contain more fiber, protein, and fat than a snack taken to *treat* a low blood glucose (sugar) reaction. For pre-activity snacks, a piece of fresh fruit is a better choice than juice because it contains fiber. Yogurt has protein, so it is also a good option because protein is broken down into glucose more slowly.

To treat low blood glucose, glucose tablets, regular soda, sports drinks, and juice are good choices, but they are not as wise of choices for a pre-activity snack. This is because they are absorbed and used too quickly during activity.

If your activity is going to last less than 30 minutes and be mild to moderate in intensity, you may not need a snack. For moderate activity that lasts 30 minutes to 1 hour, you should consider a pre-activity snack with 15 g of carbohydrate.

American Association of Diabetes Educators©

Advanced Detail

My blood glucose was higher after I exercised than before. Why is that?

Possible explanations include the following:

- If you had a pre-exercise snack, it may have contained too many carbohydrates.
- If you had a hypoglycemic event during activity, it could have prompted your liver to release extra glucose into your blood.
- Your activity may not have used up enough of the stored glucose that was released from your liver or muscles. This commonly happens with power activities like weight lifting or high-intensity activities like sprinting.
- If you were in a competitive situation, you might have had an adrenaline rush that prompted your liver to release extra glucose into your blood.

Engage learners in critical thinking activities. Those with logical/mathematical intelligence will especially benefit from this approach to learning.

Special Considerations/Advanced Detail for Appropriate Participants

Share the following information with patients on an as-needed basis, based on their individual assessment to ensure safety in physical activity.

If you have certain health conditions, your physical activity plan must be adjusted to ensure safety.

Obesity/Orthopedic Issues

- Physical activity *and* a weight-loss meal plan together work better than meal planning alone. This is because physical activity burns up calories. It also helps build muscle, which burns more calories, even at rest. Also, the weight you lose from meal planning alone is often more muscle than fat, and being active helps you retain the muscle while losing more fat.
- Research suggests that for people with type 2 diabetes, combining aerobic activity and resistance training yields better weight loss results than doing one or the other.[35]
- Non-weight-bearing activities such as chair exercises, water activities, and cycling are good activity options for obese people. Walking, running, or jogging may put too much stress on the knees.
- Obese people should aim for activity sessions of 45 to 60 minutes.[35] Start with shorter sessions and increase the time gradually. While it may take months to progress to 45 to 60 minutes, this will burn more calories and lead to more fat loss than shorter sessions.[39]
- The more intense your activity session, the more calories will be burned. Follow the guidelines of the "talk" test to gauge your intensity.

Heart Disease/Hypertension

- Cardiac rehabilitation (rehab) offers a supervised setting for activity if you have heart disease. The staff will help you measure your heart rate and blood pressure during your activity sessions.
- Physical activity can cause blood pressure to rise in people with diabetes and heart disease. For this reason, lower intensity is preferred.
- If you have high blood pressure, you should avoid heavy resistance training or lifting. Activities that cause a "bearing down" or holding of breath should also be avoided.
- Any resistance activities should use lighter weights or less resistance with more repetitions.
- Activities that move the legs are best because they are less likely to raise the blood pressure than upper body activities. Good choices are walking and cycling.

Peripheral Vascular Disease

- People with poor circulation often have leg pain during physical activity. This occurs because the damaged vessels are unable to bring enough oxygen to the muscle cells.
- A walking program that includes frequent rest periods will lessen pain. It may also improve circulation and your ability to exercise.[40,41] The intensity should be low.
- If leg pain occurs during rest or sleep, this means the disease is severe. In this case, a walking program is not recommended and other activity options should be considered.

Moderate to Severe Retinopathy

If you have advanced eye disease, you need to avoid some types of activities, as certain ones may cause the eye blood vessels to bleed inside your eye.[3,15] If you experience a hemorrhage inside your eye while exercising, stop immediately. Additionally, never begin an activity while a hemorrhage is ongoing. Your eye specialist should make the final decision on what kinds of physical activity are safe for you.

In general, avoid movements that:

- place your head below the waist
- cause "bearing down" or holding of your breath (eg, heavy lifting, diving)
- jar your head (eg, jogging, high-impact aerobics, racquet sports, boxing, and competitive sports)

The best options are activities that are low-impact and aerobic. Examples are walking, low-impact aerobics, and stationary cycling.

Visual Impairment/Blindness

Physical activity options should focus on *safety*. Good options are walking on a treadmill with hand rails, stationary cycling, or swimming with lane guides. Dancing with a partner to hold onto is also a safe option, as is tandem biking.

Peripheral Neuropathy/Ulcers

- If you have nerve damage, you may not feel the pain of tight shoes, blisters, or splinters in the feet. Balance may also be affected by nerve damage. Wear appropriate, good-fitting exercise shoes and socks that keep your feet dry.[3,15]
- Special care is needed to prevent injury to the feet. Jogging and other activities that put lots of pressure on your feet should be avoided. Always check your feet after activity.[3,15] Place a mirror on the floor and hold your foot over it to inspect the bottom if it is too hard for you to see it otherwise. Look for areas of redness or potential irritation and treat them appropriately sooner rather than later.
- Do not do weight-bearing or water exercise with an unhealed ulcer on the bottom of your foot. Other activity options include seated exercise, stationary cycling, and non-weight-bearing resistance exercise. Brisk walking is fine as long as all ulcers are fully healed and balance is not affected.[42,43]

American Association of Diabetes Educators©

Autonomic Neuropathy

- This type of nerve damage can affect your ability to keep your blood pressure stable when you change positions. You may want to choose activities like water aerobics or recumbent cycling if you find that you are more prone to falling down with this condition.
- There may be a problem with your ability to keep your body temperature normal. This could cause you to overheat or get too cold.[15] Avoid physical activity in the heat or cold. Wear the right kinds of clothes, depending on the weather.
- "Silent heart attack" is common in people with autonomic neuropathy. Low-intensity aerobic or resistance-training activities are best if you have heart disease.[3,15]
- In autonomic neuropathy, there may be no obvious signs when your blood glucose level drops too low. Frequent monitoring during activity will alert you to dropping glucose levels.[3,15]

End-Stage Renal Disease

The ability to tolerate physical activity will depend on the degree of the disease. The best choices are low-intensity aerobic activities. Examples include walking, swimming, and cycling. You may be able to do low- to moderate-intensity activities during dialysis treatments as well, if you take them.[15]

Identifying Barriers to Physical Activity

Even though you know that physical activity is good for you, there may be barriers that prevent you from making healthy choices. For every barrier there may be many possible solutions.

 What might work to overcome this barrier? Let's brainstorm together and learn from one another's experiences.

Reality Scenario	Problem Solving Possible Solutions/What Would *You* Do?
Too out of shape It's been years since I did any real exercise. I feel flabby and out of shape. At this point, even walking up the stairs makes me tired.	Start with activities you can tolerate. Increase activity slowly over time.
Time constraints I work full time. I have young kids at home. Also, I'm involved with church and the PTA. It seems there is not enough time in the day to add one more thing.	Do an inventory of your time. Prioritize. Consider what else you can reasonably give up. Think of activities that you can do while watching TV. Get up earlier in the morning. Do things with the kids. Add in bits of activity throughout the day that count toward your goals.
Weather (too hot, too cold, rain or snow) I plan to go for a walk after dinner. But then it's too hot.	Do indoor activities. Get an exercise video or DVD. *Ask participants to share the name of any exercise DVDs or videos they use.* Go to the mall or large stores (eg, Wal-Mart) to walk indoors.
Environment/lack of safe place I'd like to walk in my neighborhood, but there are [fill in the blank: mean dogs/gangs/heavy traffic/sidewalks with big cracks and potholes in them]. I'm afraid I might get hurt if I go out there.	Explore options for each barrier. Can you take a safer route to avoid dogs/people? Are there local resources like the YMCA or community centers? Is there a retail center (mall, large store) nearby? Can you consider another choice of activity, perhaps indoors?

Reality Scenario	Problem Solving Possible Solutions/What Would *You* Do?
Fear of low blood glucose *One time I did an aerobics class at the gym after work. Afterward, I had a very low blood glucose level, and I nearly passed out in the locker room. Someone had to run for help. I was so embarrassed! I don't want that to ever happen again.*	Monitor blood glucose levels before and after activity, and occasionally during. Be prepared with a carbohydrate snack, glucose tablets, juice, or regular soda. Plan to do activity after meals when your blood glucose is rising.
Self-conscious about body *I feel like everyone is looking at me. Everybody else at the health club is lean and in great shape. I feel like a fat blob in my workout clothes.*	Do indoor, solo activities. If active in a public area, wear loose clothes that don't emphasize your body shape. Find a gym that caters to people you feel comfortable being with. Try aquatic activities.
Boredom *Exercise is just so boring! After a few days of the same old thing, I just want to quit.*	Choose activities that you enjoy, even dancing. Having fun will help you stay motivated. Do different activities on different days, or do a combination of activities on the same day. Get an exercise buddy, and make activity a social time, too. Listen to music during the activity to distract you.
Lack of motivation *I just don't have any motivation.*	Focus on reasons for living and being more healthy, such as your children, your spouse, or accomplishing your long-term goals in life. Practice *positive affirmations*. These are statements that reflect who you want to be. If you want to be an active, motivated person, repeat to yourself several times a day: *"I am a motivated, active person."* Set small, realistic, and measurable (SMART) goals. Plan for a reward when you meet your goal. Get an activity *accountability partner*. This is someone who is counting on you to be active.
Unrealistic expectations *I've been exercising for a week already, and I don't see any changes in my body. It's discouraging.*	It takes time to see changes in your body. Focus on other positives that activity brings, like more energy, better glucose control, and just the fact that you're taking steps to improve your health. If you're exercising to lose weight, give it a month or more before you expect the scale to change since you may be gaining muscle mass. Use the "clothes test" (ie, do your clothes fit better?) instead of watching your scale weight.
Physical limitations *Balance issues, joint problems, foot problems, obesity, etc. For example: "My bad knee won't let me go out and walk."*	Choose activities that won't aggravate physical ailments. Consider doing stationary cycling, chair or other seated exercises, or water exercise. It is possible to do resistance exercises sitting down as well.

Identifying Facilitators for Physical Activity

 What are some things that help you stick with your plan to stay active?

As important as it is to identify barriers to physical activity, it's just as important to consider the positives in your situation—facilitators. Looking deeper, you may find that there are more positives than you thought.

American Association of Diabetes Educators©

Common Facilitators

- Social support—activity buddy, family members, coworkers, etc
- Community resources—accessible fitness center, local pool, community center, etc
- Reminders and cues—notes, entry on calendar, reminder alarm
- Rewards—incentives to maintain motivation (preferably noncaloric ones)

Setting a SMART Goal for Physical Activity

S—Specific: identify type, frequency, duration, and intensity of activity
M—Measurable: not vague
A—Attainable: challenging but not out of reach
R—Realistic: given person's situation, can it be done?
T—Timeline: short term, for next week or two

The participant sets an individual goal for physical activity. The educator and the participant schedule a date in which to evaluate progress with behavior change.

Using a mnemonic like SMART to help remember an idea can be a useful teaching tool, especially for those with verbal/auditory intelligence.

Follow-up/Outcomes Measurement

Per the Standards for Outcomes Measurement of Diabetes Self-Management Education, the **first follow-up should be conducted within 2 to 4 weeks** after the initial teaching session on physical activity. At this follow-up, success in implementing physical activity behavior can be assessed. **Subsequent follow-up is recommended at 3- to 6-month intervals thereafter**. Use the following table as a guide for identifying outcomes measures and how to measure them. Measurement of these outcomes may be objective or subjective.

The exception to this schedule would be during pregnancy. The first follow-up should be conducted within 1 week and subsequent visits at 2 to 4 weeks.

Self-Care Behavior: Physical Activity Outcomes Measures	Self-Care Behavior: Physical Activity Methods of Measurement
Immediate outcome: Learning Immediate outcomes of learning can be assessed right away after the educational encounter. Immediate outcomes include: K: Acquiring *knowledge* (*what to do*) S: Acquiring *skills* (*how to do it*) CM: Developing *confidence and motivation* (*want to do it*) PS: Developing *problem-solving/coping skills* to overcome barrier (*can do it*)	Immediate outcomes of learning can be measured by patient knowledge testing (paper-and-pen testing, or questioning to determine that patient understands information taught). Immediate outcomes for acquiring a skill can be measured by patient's demonstration of that skill. The following are various methods of measuring immediate outcomes for the self-care behavior of *physical activity*.

Self-Care Behavior: Physical Activity Outcomes Measures	Self-Care Behavior: Physical Activity Methods of Measurement
Benefits of physical activity (K)	Subjective: Patient states expected benefits of physical activity.
Type, duration, and intensity of physical activity (K)	Subjective: Patient describes the types, duration, and intensity levels of physical activities that are appropriate for him/her.
Safety precautions to observe during physical activity (K)	Subjective: Patient explains relevant safety precautions to observe during physical activity.
Physical activity planning (K)	Subjective: Patient develops a specific plan for physical activity within his/her lifestyle.
Potential barriers (physical limitations, time, environment, emotional) to and facilitators of physical activity (PS)	Subjective: Considering his/her individual situation, patient describes anticipated obstacle(s) that may limit the ability to carry out physical activity plan. Patient describes facilitators that may help him/her carry out physical activity plan.
Strategy to overcome potential barriers to physical activity (PS)	Subjective: Patient develops a plan to deal with anticipated obstacle(s) to physical activity.
Intermediate outcome: Behavior change	Intermediate outcomes measures can be assessed over time: after the educational encounter and once the patient has had adequate time to implement new behavior(s) in a real-life setting. *Behavior change* is an intermediate outcomes measure. It is the ultimate outcome of DSME/T. At follow-up intervals, knowledge and skills (discussed above) should be reassessed, as well as behavior change.
Physical activity behavior (S)	Subjective: Patient self-report of adherence to physical activity plan. Objective: Log of pedometer readings; completed physical activity calendar.
Safety precautions during physical activity (K)	Subjective: Patient self-report/description of safety precautions followed during physical activity.
Barriers and strategies for barrier resolution (PS)	Subjective: Patient self-report of barriers faced, facilitators and strategies used, as patient made efforts to implement physical activity behaviors.
Plans for future behavior change (PS)	Subjective: Patient self-report of physical activity goals and behavior strategies going forward.

REFERENCES

1. Colberg SR. Physical activity. In: Mensing C, ed. The Art and Science of Diabetes Self-Management Education: A Desk Reference for Healthcare Professionals. 3rd ed. Chicago: American Association of Diabetes Educators; 2014: 457-90.

2. American College of Sports Medicine. ACSM's Resource Manual for Guidelines for Exercise Testing and Prescription. 7th ed. Baltimore, Md: Lippincott, Williams & Wilkins; 2014.

3. Colberg SR. Being active. In: Mensing C, ed. The Art and Science of Diabetes Self-Management Education: A Desk Reference for Healthcare Professionals. 3rd ed. Chicago: American Association of Diabetes Educators; 2014:143-74.

4. Dutton GR, Tan F, Provost BC, et al. Relationship between self-efficacy and physical activity among patients with type 2 diabetes. J Behav Med. 2009;32(3):270-7.

5. Allen NA. Social cognitive theory in diabetes exercise research: an integrative literature review. Diabetes Educ. 2004;30(5):805-19.

6. Di Loreto C, Fanelli C, Lucidi P, et al. Validation of a counseling strategy to promote the adoption and the maintenance of physical activity by type 2 diabetic subjects. Diabetes Care. 2003;26(2):404-8.

American Association of Diabetes Educators©

94 Diabetes Education Curriculum

7. Kirwan JP, del Aguila LF, Hernandes JM, et al. Regular exercise enhances insulin activation of IRS-1-associated P13K in human skeletal tissue. J Appl Physiol. 2000;88:797-803.

8. Dube JJ, Allison KF, Rousson V, et al. Exercise dose and insulin sensitivity: relevance for diabetes prevention. Med Sci Sports Exerc. 2012;44:793-9.

9. Houmard JA, Tanner CJ, Slentz CA, et al. Effect of the volume and intensity of exercise training on insulin sensitivity. J Appl Physiol. 2004;96:101-6.

10. American Association of Diabetes Educators. Position statement. Diabetes and exercise. Diabetes Educ. 2008;34(1): 37-40.

11. Goulet ED, Melancon MO, Aubertin-Leheudre M, et al. Aerobic training improves insulin sensitivity 72-120 h after the last exercise session in younger but not in older women. Eur J Appl Physiol. 2005;95:146-52.

12. Lee WL, Cheung AM, Cape D, et al. Impact of diabetes on coronary artery disease in women and men: a meta-analysis of prospective studies. Diabetes Care. 2000;23:962-8.

13. Kodama S, Tanaka S, Saito K, et al. Effect of aerobic exercise training on serum levels of high-density lipoprotein cholesterol. Arch Intern Med. 2007;167:999-1008.

14. Buse JB, Ginsberg HN, Bakris GL, et al. Primary prevention of cardiovascular diseases in people with diabetes mellitus: a scientific statement from the American Heart Association and the American Diabetes Association. Circulation. 2007;115:114-26.

15. Colberg SR, Sigal RJ, Fernhall B, et al. Exercise and type 2 diabetes: The American College of Sports Medicine and the American Diabetes Association: joint position statement. Diabetes Care. 2010;33(12):e147-67.

16. Canoy D, Boekholdt SM, Wareham N, et al. Body fat distribution and risk of coronary heart disease in men and women in the European Prospective Investigation into Cancer and Nutrition in Norfolk Cohort: a population-based prospective study. Circulation. 2007;116:2933-43.

17. O'Leary VB, Marchetti CM, Krishnan RK, et al. Exercise-induced reversal of insulin resistance in obese elderly is associated with reduced visceral fat. J Appl Physiol. 2006;100:1584-9.

18. Williamson DA, Rejeski J, Lang W, et al. Impact of a weight management program on health-related quality of life in overweight adults with type 2 diabetes. Arch Intern Med. 2009;169(2):163-71.

19. Morrison S, Colberg SR, Mariano M, et al. Balance training reduces falls risk in older individuals with type 2 diabetes. Diabetes Care. 2010;33:748-50.

20. Willey KA, Flatarone-Singh MA. Battling insulin resistance in elderly obese people with type 2 diabetes: bring on the heavy weights. Diabetes Care. 2003;26:1580-8.

21. Diabetes Prevention Program Research Group. Reduction in the incidence of type 2 diabetes with lifestyle intervention or metformin. N Engl J Med. 2002;346(6):393-403.

22. Tuomilheto J, Lindstrom J, Eriksson JG, et al. Prevention of type 2 diabetes by changes in lifestyle among subjects with impaired glucose tolerance. N Engl J Med. 2001;344(18):1343-50.

23. Ramachandran A, Snehalatha C, Mary S, et al. The Indian Diabetes Prevention Programme shows that lifestyle modification and metformin prevent type 2 diabetes in Asian Indian subjects with impaired glucose tolerance (IDPP-1). Diabetologia. 2006;49:289-97.

24. Kosaka K, Noda M, Kuzuya T. Prevention of type 2 diabetes by lifestyle intervention: a Japanese trial in IGT males. Diabetes Res Clin Pract. 2005;67:152-62.

25. Dunn AL, Marcus BH, Kambert JB, et al. Comparison of lifestyle and structured interventions to increase physical activity and cardiorespiratory fitness. JAMA. 1999;281(4):327-34.

26. Andersen RE, Wadden TA, Bartlett SJ, et al. Effects of lifestyle vs structured aerobic exercise in obese women. JAMA. 1999;281(4):335-40.

27. Dunstan DW, Daly RM, Owen N, et al. High-intensity resistance training improves glycemic control in older patients with type 2 diabetes. Diabetes Care. 2002;25:1729-36.

28. Shier I. Stretching before exercise does not reduce the risk of local muscle injury: a critical review of the clinical and basic science literature. Clin J Sport Med. 1999;9:221-7.

American Association of Diabetes Educators©

29. Herriott MT, Colberg SR, Parson HK, et al. Effects of 8 weeks of flexibility and resistance training in older adults with type 2 diabetes. Diabetes Care. 2004;27:2988-99.

30. Lan C, Lai JS, Chen SY. Tai Chi Chuan: an ancient wisdom on exercise and health promotion. Sports Med. 2002;32(4):217-24.

31. Ray US, Sinha B, Tomer OS, et al. Aerobic capacity and perceived exertion after practice of hatha yoga exercise. Indian J Med Res. 2001;114:215-21.

32. Innes KE, Bourguignon C, Taylor AG. Risk indices associated with the insulin resistance syndrome, cardiovascular disease, and possible protection with yoga: a systematic review. J Am Board Fam Pract. 2005;18:491-519.

33. American College of Sports Medicine. ACSM's Guidelines for Exercise Testing and Prescription. 9th ed. Baltimore, Md: Lippincott, Williams & Wilkins; 2014.

34. Miller KL, Magel JR, Hayes JG. The effects of a home-based exercise program on balance confidence, balance performance, and gait in debilitated, ambulatory community-dwelling older adults: a pilot study. J Geriatr Phys Ther. 2010;33:85-91.

35. US Department of Health and Human Services. 2008 physical activity guidelines for Americans (cited 2015 Jan 12). On the Internet at: http://www.health.gov/PAguidelines.

36. Umpierre D, Ribeiro PA, Kramer CK, et al. Physical activity advice only or structured exercise training and association with HbA1c levels in type 2 diabetes: a systematic review and meta-analysis. JAMA. 2011;305:1790-9.

37. Eriksen L, Dahl-Petersen I, Haugaard SB, et al. Comparison of the effect of multiple short-duration with single long-duration exercise sessions on glucose homeostasis in type 2 diabetes mellitus. Diabetologia. 2007;50:2245-53.

38. Sawka MN, Burke LM, Eichner ER, et al. American College of Sports Medicine position stand. Exercise and fluid replacement. Med Sci Sports Exerc. 2007;39:377-90.

39. Marcus RL, Smith S, Morrell G, et al. Comparison of combined aerobic and high-force eccentric resistance exercise with aerobic exercise only for people with type 2 diabetes mellitus. Phys Ther. 2008;88(11):1345-54.

40. McDermott MM, Ades P, Guralnik JM, et al. Treadmill exercise and resistance training in patients with peripheral arterial disease with and without intermittent claudication: a randomized controlled trial. JAMA. 2009;301:165-74.

41. Hiatt WR, Regensteiner JG, Hargarten ME, et al. Benefit of exercise conditioning for patients with peripheral arterial disease. Circulation. 1990;81:602-9.

42. Lemaster JW, Reiber GE, Smith DG, et al. Daily weight-bearing activity does not increase the risk of diabetic foot ulcers. Med Sci Sports Exerc. 2003;35:1093-9.

43. Lemaster JW, Mueller MJ, Reiber GE, et al. Effect of weight-bearing activity on foot ulcer incidence in people with diabetic peripheral neuropathy: feet first randomized controlled trial. Phys Ther. 2008;88:1385-98.

BEING ACTIVE: RESOURCES

Being Active Handout (English) 96

Being Active Handout (Spanish) 98

Physical Activity Calendar 100

AADE7™ SELF-CARE BEHAVIORS
BEING ACTIVE

Being active is not just about losing weight. It has many health benefits like lowering cholesterol, improving blood pressure, lowering stress and anxiety, and improving your mood. If you have diabetes, physical activity can also help keep your blood sugar levels closer to normal and help you keep your diabetes in control.

It can be difficult to find the time or the motivation to start an exercise program. Everyone's physical abilities and schedules are different; choose the best ways to fit physical activity into your daily life—whether it's walking to work, doing chair exercises or working out at the gym.

The important thing to remember is to choose activities that you enjoy doing and to set goals that are realistic.

Your healthcare provider can help you design an activity plan that works for you.

DID YOU KNOW?

Breaking activity into three 10 minute sessions throughout the day is as good as one 30 minute session. This can help you fit exercise into your schedule.

TRUE OR FALSE?

You are not working out hard enough if you can carry on a conversation.

FALSE. You should be able to talk when doing an activity. If you can't, then your body is working too hard and you need to slow your pace.

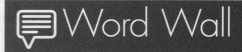

Word Wall

EXERCISE (OR PHYSICAL ACTIVITY):
Activities that get your body moving and help you stay healthy

CARDIO:
Exercise that raises your heart rate

RESISTANCE TRAINING:
Activities that help you build muscle and strength

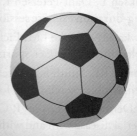

QUICK TIPS

Any amount of physical activity is better than none at all. Making physical activity part of your daily lifestyle burns calories even if it's not part of a structured plan.

Even if you are inactive and out of shape now, you can improve your health by moving just a little more. Take small steps to add more movement into your daily lifestyle. In time, you will find that you are stronger and will be able to move even more!

*Check your glucose before and after physical activity to learn how **your** body responds.*

AADE American Association of Diabetes Educators

Supported by an educational grant from Eli Lilly and Company.

ACTIVITIES

ASK YOURSELF

What's your all-time favorite activity that gets you moving? _____

What stops you from doing it? *(Circle as many as you want)*

- » Not enough time
- » Too out of shape
- » Too tired
- » Not motivated
- » Can't afford it
- » My _____ hurts too much

What can you do to get started doing this activity or working up to it? _____
_____

Pick some other activities that you enjoy doing:

_____
_____
_____
_____
_____

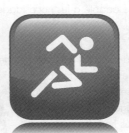

MAKE A FITT PLAN FOR YOUR PHYSICAL ACTIVITY:

- » **Frequency**—How often will you do this activity? Work up to 5 or more days a week.
- » **Intensity**—How hard should you be working? Remember, you should be able to talk, but not sing during an activity.
- » **Time**—How long will you do it? Be realistic. Start with 5 or 10 minutes, and work up to 30 minutes.
- » **Type of Activity**—What will you be doing? Do something you enjoy!

GET CREATIVE!

- » Partner with a friend to find creative ways to be more physically active.
- » Take your dog for a walk or play fetch at the park.
- » Call a friend to go dancing or put on your favorite song and make the living room your personal dance floor.
- » Find a gym buddy to motivate you to stay active.
- » Take the stairs instead of the elevator.
- » If you eat lunch with a co-worker, ask him/her to join you for a short walk after you eat.

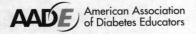

CONDUCTAS PARA EL CUIDADO PERSONA DE AADE7™

MANTENERSE ACTIVO

Mantenerse activo no sólo está relacionado con perder peso. También tiene muchos beneficios para la salud: ayuda a bajar el colesterol, mejora la presión arterial, baja el estrés y la ansiedad, y mejora tu estado de ánimo. Si tienes diabetes, la actividad física también puede ayudar a mantener tus niveles de azúcar en la sangre más cerca de los valores normales y mantener tu diabetes bajo control.

Puede ser difícil encontrar el momento o la motivación para comenzar un programa de ejercicios. Las capacidades físicas y los horarios de todas las personas son diferentes. Escoge las mejores maneras de incluir la actividad física en tu vida diaria; puedes ir al trabajo caminando, hacer ejercicios en una silla o ir a un gimnasio.

Lo importante que tienes que recordar es que debes elegir actividades que disfrutes y fijar metas que sean realistas.

Tu proveedor de atención médica puede ayudarte a diseñar un plan de actividades que se adapte a tus necesidades.

¿LO SABÍAS?

Dividir la actividad física en tres sesiones de 10 minutos durante el día es tan bueno como hacer una sesión de 30 minutos. Esto puede ayudarte a adaptar el ejercicio físico a tus horarios.

¿VERDADERO O FALSO?

Si puedes mantener una conversación, no estás haciendo los ejercicios con la intensidad suficiente.

FALSO. Debes poder hablar mientras realizas una actividad física. Si no puedes, tu cuerpo está trabajando con demasiada intensidad y debes bajar el ritmo.

Palabras útiles

EJERCICIO (O ACTIVIDAD FÍSICA): Actividades que ponen tu cuerpo en movimiento y te ayudan a mantenerte saludable.

EJERCICIO CARDIOVASCULAR: Ejercicio que eleva tu frecuencia cardíaca.

ENTRENAMIENTO DE RESISTENCIA: Actividades que te ayudan a formar músculo y tener fuerza.

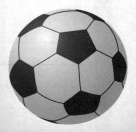

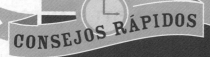

Una mínima cantidad de actividad física es mejor que nada. Al incorporar la actividad física a tu vida diaria, quemas calorías aunque la actividad no forme parte de un plan estructurado.

Aunque estés inactivo y fuera de forma ahora, puedes mejorar tu salud moviéndote un poco más. Avanza de a poco y agrega más movimiento a tu estilo de vida diaria. Con el tiempo, verás que eres más fuerte y podrás moverte aun más. Controla tu nivel de glucosa antes y después de realizar actividad física para aprender cómo responde tu cuerpo.

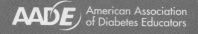

Supported by an educational grant from Lilly USA, LLC.

ACTIVIDADES

PREGÚNTATE LO SIGUIENTE

¿Cuál es tu actividad favorita que te pone en movimiento? _____

¿Qué te impide hacerla? *(Encierra todas las respuestas que desees)*

- » No tengo suficiente tiempo.
- » Estoy muy fuera de forma.
- » Estoy demasiado cansado.
- » No estoy motivado.
- » No tengo suficiente dinero.
- » Mi _____ me duele demasiado.

¿Qué puedes hacer para comenzar con esta actividad o prepararte para ella? _____
_____

Escoge otras actividades que disfrutes hacer:

_____
_____
_____
_____
_____

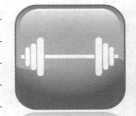
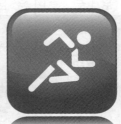

ELABORA UN PLAN FITT PARA TU ACTIVIDAD FÍSICA

- » **Frecuencia:** ¿Con qué frecuencia harás esta actividad? Debes hacer ejercicio 5 días o más a la semana.
- » **Intensidad:** ¿Con qué intensidad trabajarás? Recuerda que debes poder hablar pero no cantar durante
- » una actividad.
- » **Tiempo:** ¿Por cuánto tiempo la harás? Sé realista. Comienza con 5 o 10 minutos y ejercita hasta 30 minutos.
- » **Tipo de actividad:** ¿Qué harás? ¡Haz algo que disfrutes!

SÉ CREATIVO

- » Reúnete con un amigo para buscar maneras creativas de estar físicamente más activo.
- » Saca a pasear a tu perro o juega con él en el parque.
- » Llama a un amigo para ir a bailar o pon tu canción favorita y convierte tu sala en una pista de baile personal.
- » Busca un compañero de gimnasio que te motive para mantenerte activo.
- » Usa las escaleras en lugar del ascensor.
- » Si almuerzas con un compañero de trabajo, pídele que te acompañe a dar un paseo corto después de comer.

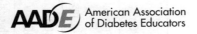

Physical Activity Calendar

Sunday	Monday	Tuesday	Wednesday	Thursday	Friday	Saturday
BGB: BGA:	BGB: BGA:	BGB: BGA:	BGB: BGA:	BGB: BGA:	BGB: BGA:	BGB: BGA:
Physical Activity ___ Yes ___ No	Physical Activity ___ Yes ___ No	Physical Activity ___ Yes ___ No	Physical Activity ___ Yes ___ No	Physical Activity ___ Yes ___ No	Physical Activity ___ Yes ___ No	Physical Activity ___ Yes ___ No
BGB: BGA:	BGB: BGA:	BGB: BGA:	BGB: BGA:	BGB: BGA:	BGB: BGA:	BGB: BGA:
Physical Activity ___ Yes ___ No	Physical Activity ___ Yes ___ No	Physical Activity ___ Yes ___ No	Physical Activity ___ Yes ___ No	Physical Activity ___ Yes ___ No	Physical Activity ___ Yes ___ No	Physical Activity ___ Yes ___ No
BGB: BGA:	BGB: BGA:	BGB: BGA:	BGB: BGA:	BGB: BGA:	BGB: BGA:	BGB: BGA:
Physical Activity ___ Yes ___ No	Physical Activity ___ Yes ___ No	Physical Activity ___ Yes ___ No	Physical Activity ___ Yes ___ No	Physical Activity ___ Yes ___ No	Physical Activity ___ Yes ___ No	Physical Activity ___ Yes ___ No
BGB: BGA:	BGB: BGA:	BGB: BGA:	BGB: BGA:	BGB: BGA:	BGB: BGA:	BGB: BGA:
Physical Activity ___ Yes ___ No	Physical Activity ___ Yes ___ No	Physical Activity ___ Yes ___ No	Physical Activity ___ Yes ___ No	Physical Activity ___ Yes ___ No	Physical Activity ___ Yes ___ No	Physical Activity ___ Yes ___ No
BGB: BGA:	BGB: BGA:	BGB: BGA:	BGB: BGA:	BGB: BGA:	BGB: BGA:	BGB: BGA:
Physical Activity ___ Yes ___ No	Physical Activity ___ Yes ___ No	Physical Activity ___ Yes ___ No	Physical Activity ___ Yes ___ No	Physical Activity ___ Yes ___ No	Physical Activity ___ Yes ___ No	Physical Activity ___ Yes ___ No

BGB: Blood glucose before   BGA: Blood glucose after   Physical activity: Activities you agree to do.   Yes or No: Whether or not you did the physical activities.

MODULE 4

Taking Medication

Table of Contents

TAKING MEDICATION: AN EDUCATOR'S OVERVIEW 102

AADE Systematic Review of the Literature 102

Background Information and Instructions for the Educator 102

Assessing Barriers 103

Learning Objectives 104

Knowledge 104

Skills 104

Barriers and Facilitators 104

Behavioral Objective 104

TAKING MEDICATION: INSTRUCTIONAL PLAN 104

Identifying Participant Thoughts and Feelings About Taking Medication 104

Why Is Medication Necessary? 105

Oral Diabetes Medications 105

Insulin Sensitizers 106

DPP-IV Inhibitors 108

Insulin Secretagogues 110

Alpha-Glucosidase Inhibitors 111

Sodium-Glucose Co-Transporter 2 Inhibitors 112

Combination Oral Diabetes Medications 113

Bile Acid Sequestrants 113

Injected Diabetes Medications 114

Insulin 114

GLP-1 Agonists 123

Amylin Analogs 126

Injecting Diabetes Medication 127

102   Diabetes Education Curriculum

Complementary and Alternative Medications. 133

What Is Complementary and Alternative Medicine? 133

Who Uses CAM? 133

Common CAM Usage. 133

Is CAM Safe? 133

Side Effects and Drug Interactions. 133

Identifying Barriers to Taking Medication 136

Identifying Facilitators for Taking Medication 140

Common Facilitators 140

Setting a SMART Goal for Taking Medication. 140

Follow-up/Outcomes Measurement 140

REFERENCES 142

TAKING MEDICATION: RESOURCES 147

TAKING MEDICATION: AN EDUCATOR'S OVERVIEW

AADE Systematic Review of the Literature

A systematic review of the literature was conducted by the American Association of Diabetes Educators (AADE) to "evaluate the evidence of the challenges and barriers to medication taking (adherence) and to summarize the interventions that improve medication taking in type 1 and type 2 diabetes mellitus." The literature lists several barriers to taking medication. These barriers include a complex medication regimen, depression, lack of understanding about the medication regimen, and forgetting to take meds or refill prescriptions. Barriers encountered by those on insulin include fear of needles, fear of side effects like hypoglycemia, sense of personal failure, belief that disease is worsening, weight gain, and lack of confidence in the ability to manage self-care using insulin. Diabetes educators can promote medication-taking behavior by (1) screening patients to identify barriers, (2) helping patients develop strategies to address barriers, and (3) assessing medication-taking behaviors at follow-up encounters.[1]

Background Information and Instructions for the Educator

The evidence that diabetes complications are reduced by improved glycemic control is overwhelming.[2-6] Today, the pharmacologic armamentarium abounds with options that effectively target the different physiologic problems in diabetes. Data from the latest National Health and Nutrition Examination Survey (NHANES) are encouraging in that the percentage of those with diabetes who had an A1C <7% is now above 50%. However, diabetes control in the United States is far from optimal and recent data suggest a slight decline in control rates from 2003 to 2006 (57%), to 2007 to 2010 (52.5%).[7] The percentage of those with an A1C *above* the American Diabetes Association (ADA) target of 7% remains high at over 47%. Effective drugs are useless if not taken or taken incorrectly. The educator can intervene by facilitating patients' behavior change to help them achieve better metabolic control.

Taking medication is a key behavior in the self-management of diabetes. Insulin therapy is imperative for survival as well as for glycemic control in those with type 1 diabetes. In type 2 diabetes, the natural progression of the disease will eventually require medication therapy.[3] Medication therapy is now being considered at the onset of type 2 diabetes, following the 2006 consensus algorithm jointly published by the ADA and the European Association for the Study of Diabetes, which recommends initiating metformin along with lifestyle intervention

American Association of Diabetes Educators©

(unless there are clear contraindications).[8] Since people with diabetes are also at high risk for other comorbidities such as hypertension and hyperlipidemia, additional medications are typically needed beyond those for glucose control. This module focuses on the medications for glucose control, vitamins and minerals, and complementary and alternative medication use. See Module 8: Reducing Risks for important information for the safe and effective use of medications for blood pressure and lipid control. The diabetes educator plays a critical role in promoting medication-taking behavior. The educator's obvious role is explaining the medications' purpose as well as when and how to take them properly. But just as importantly, the educator should identify barriers that impact this self-care behavior.

Assessing Barriers

Depression is twice as common in people with diabetes as it is in the general population.[9] Depression has been cited as a significant factor affecting medication adherence.[10,11] Including a depression screen in the patient assessment is useful for diabetes education programs.[1] See "Psychological Assessment and Screening Tools" in Module 7: Healthy Coping for a listing of validated screening tools for depression.

Educators should consider incorporating questions into their assessment that would help identify patients at risk for medication adherence problems.[12] Two such questions are derived from the *Brief Medication Questionnaire*, a validated tool for identifying and diagnosing problems with adherence.[13] They are:

1. "Taking medications on a regular basis can be difficult. Do you ever find it difficult to remember to take [*insert medication name*]?" If yes, then,

2. "How many times over the last two weeks have you missed a dose?"

Cue-dose training (eg, linking medication taking with a daily activity like brushing teeth) initially improved adherence in a study by Rosen et al, although improvement declined after the intervention period.[14] This technique, however, may prove useful for some patients who frequently forget to take their medication.

Additionally, educators can ask patients to read aloud what is written on the prescription label. This task may reveal if the patient has difficulty with reading. Often, adherence problems arise because the font on the prescription label is too small. Solutions for visual acuity or health literacy problems include getting the pharmacy to print the label in a larger font and/or using a medication instruction calendar. The medication instruction calendar should use a large font easily read by the patient, and color-coding of prescription vials that correspond to the instructions.[12] Pictograms on the instruction calendar are helpful for those with low literacy or those who use English as a second language.[15] The use of pictograms should always be accompanied by a verbal explanation and then patients' understanding ascertained, as their interpretation may be different from that intended.[16] The USP Pictogram Library may be downloaded free of charge by professionals and used in patient information instructions: http://www.usp.org/usp-healthcare-professionals/related-topics-resources/usp-pictograms.[17]

The complexity of a medication regimen influences adherence, specifically the following factors: the medication is required more than twice a day, tablets must be split, or products must be mixed.[18] Many oral diabetes agents are now available in combination form, which can simplify the medication regimen by reducing the overall number of pills that must be taken. Whenever it is possible to simplify the regimen, the educator can advocate for the patient by communicating with the prescribing provider to see if such a change is feasible. The educator can help selected patients with the barrier of cost by informing them of pharmaceutical patient assistance programs. See Diabetes Resources Appendix at the end of the book for contact information for assistance programs.

People with type 2 diabetes often feel a sense of personal failure or believe that their condition is worsening when they are transitioned from lifestyle to oral medication therapy or from oral therapy to insulin therapy. Educators should emphasize the natural progression of the disease and the importance of addressing all of the multiple defects in the disease process—insulin resistance, declining insulin production, excess hepatic glucose production, etc. Focused training on timing medications with regard to meals and activity, and how to minimize side effects can help address common barriers to adherence.

American Association of Diabetes Educators©

Learning Objectives

Knowledge

The participant will:

- name his or her prescribed diabetes medication and state its proper dose and frequency
- state the purpose of his or her medication
- explain relevant side effects to watch for
- describe actions to minimize side effects and what to do if side effects occur
- demonstrate awareness of relevant precautions about his or her medication
- describe proper storage and transport of medication

Skills

Participants who are taking injected medications will:

- demonstrate proper preparation and self-administration of injection
- demonstrate proper disposal of used needles

Barriers and Facilitators

The participant will:

- identify potential barriers/facilitators which may impact his or her ability to appropriately take medication
- develop strategies for reducing barriers and increasing facilitators in order to successfully take medication

Behavioral Objective

- The participant will set realistic and measurable individual goals for taking medication.

TAKING MEDICATION: INSTRUCTIONAL PLAN

Identifying Participant Thoughts and Feelings About Taking Medication

How do you feel about having to take diabetes medicine?
What do you want to learn today about your medicine?
What is your greatest concern/frustration about taking medicine?
What is the hardest part about taking your medicine?
What do you think would help you take your medicine the way it's prescribed?
What kind of effect do you think the medication will have on you and your baby?

Adults learn best when they feel valued and respected for the experiences and perspectives they bring. **Use probing questions to elicit learners' experiences and perspectives.**

Why Is Medication Necessary? `Survival Skill`

In type 1 diabetes, insulin is always needed to replace what the pancreas no longer produces. Type 2 diabetes is a progressive condition. It starts with insulin resistance. This means that the body is unable to respond properly to its own insulin. Physical activity and healthy eating, combined with weight loss, can help reverse insulin resistance, but only to a point. There comes a time when medicine is needed to help your body cells be more sensitive—and less resistant—to insulin.

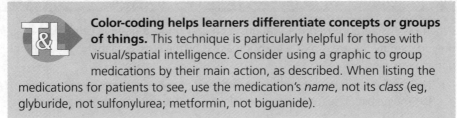

Color-coding helps learners differentiate concepts or groups of things. This technique is particularly helpful for those with visual/spatial intelligence. Consider using a graphic to group medications by their main action, as described. When listing the medications for patients to see, use the medication's *name*, not its *class* (eg, glyburide, not sulfonylurea; metformin, not biguanide).

The next thing that happens in type 2 diabetes is a decline in production of insulin. This decline continues for as long as you live. When your pancreas cannot make enough insulin, medicine is needed to help you control your blood glucose level. In the earliest stages of type 2 diabetes, pills can often help you make more insulin. If your body doesn't respond to the pills, insulin can be taken.

Medication use in pregnancy may be necessary to achieve good blood glucose control. If blood glucose control cannot be achieved by medical nutrition therapy alone, medication will be necessary.

Many people feel that taking medicine is proof that they didn't do a good enough job with their efforts to change their lifestyle. This is not entirely true. Your efforts to eat properly and be active are indeed important. You should continue to do your best with meal planning and activity to control your weight and help prevent other health problems. But even your best efforts at lifestyle change are eventually not enough to overcome the problems caused by type 2 diabetes. It's just the natural progression of the disease.

It's not your fault, so you don't need to feel guilty. You wouldn't blame your car if it ran out of gas or oil, would you? You just replace the needed fluids and move on. Try to see medication taking the same way. Taking medicines is just part of the process of managing your diabetes.

Adults learn best when they can relate new information to what they already know. Consider using the car analogy provided. This technique is particularly helpful for those with visual/spatial intelligence.

Oral Diabetes Medications

For each main problem in diabetes, there is a medicine which can help. Usually, it takes more than one medicine to control the blood glucose level. Your provider won't know which medicine is effective until you try it. The exception is in pregnancy—most diabetes medications are not recommended because of their possible harm to the fetus. It takes time to learn how your body responds to each medicine. That means your provider may try one medicine first, adjust the dose after a while, then perhaps switch to another medicine, or add another one. It's important to be patient while your provider discovers the right combination of medicines for you.

`Survival Skill` You should learn the name, dose, and when to take each of your medicines. Knowing what side effects to watch for is crucial.

American Association of Diabetes Educators©

The following sections are an extensive list of currently approved medications for the treatment of diabetes. Share with participants only the amount of information that is relevant to their prescribed medications to facilitate safe and effective medication-taking behavior.

Group Learning Activity

When discussing approved medications, consider using a graphic of human anatomy to identify the areas of the body impacted by the various diabetes medications participants take.

- Next to the pancreas, list the *names* of the medications in these classes: insulin, DPP-IV inhibitors, sulfonylureas, meglitinides, GLP-1 agonists, and amylin analogs.
- Next to the liver, list the *names* of the medications in these classes: biguanides, DPP-IV inhibitors, GLP-1 agonists, and amylin analogs.
- Next to the intestines, list the *names* of the medications in these classes: alpha-glucosidase inhibitors, GLP-1 agonists, and amylin analogs.
- Next to the muscle, list the *names* of the medications in these classes: thiazolidinediones and biguanides.
- Next to the brain, list the *names* of the medications in these classes: GLP-1 agonists and amylin analogs.
- Next to the kidney, list the *names* of the medications in the class of SGLT inhibitors.

Insulin Sensitizers
Metformin

Metformin is the generic name for Glucophage®, Glucophage XR®, Riomet®, Glumetza®, and Fortamet®.

How It Works

Metformin works in 2 ways. The main effect is to reduce the amount of glucose your liver produces. This is especially important in the early morning hours, when the liver tends to release the most glucose. The provider will review your fasting (upon waking) glucose to see if the metformin is effective.

Metformin also helps your body cells (fat and muscle) use insulin better. It does not cause you to make more insulin. If you take metformin in combination with certain other diabetes medicines, there may be a risk for hypoglycemia (low blood glucose). But used by itself, metformin usually does not cause hypoglycemia. As lifestyle efforts become more effective at controlling glucose levels, any symptoms of hypoglycemia are a sign that the metformin dose may need to be lowered.[19]

How to Take It `Survival Skill`

Typically, your provider will start you at a low dose and increase it gradually until the desired effect is seen. Once the maximum daily dose of 2000 mg is reached, your provider will decide if additional diabetes medicines are needed.[19] The lowest usual starting dose is 500 mg (adults)/250 mg (children); the maximum daily dose is 2550 mg. It comes in pill or liquid form. If taking the extended release (XR) form of metformin, do not crush the pill. Metformin is prescribed once or twice a day. It should be taken with the first bite of a meal.

Precautions

◆ You should have a blood test to check your kidneys before starting metformin therapy. People over age 80 should have a 24-hour urine test done in addition to the blood test.[19]

◆ **Survival Skill** Metformin should be temporarily stopped if you are seriously ill (eg, heart attack, surgery, worsening of heart failure)[20]

◆ **Survival Skill** Metformin should not be taken the day of having an X-Ray that uses injected dye containing iodine. Wait 2 days to restart metformin.[20]

◆ Make sure all of your healthcare providers know that you take metformin. This information is important in case you need surgery, are seriously ill, or need to have an X-Ray with iodine contrast dye.

◆ Women who have been unable to ovulate due to insulin resistance may begin ovulating after taking metformin. If not planning pregnancy, contraception should be used.

◆ Randomized controlled trials support the short-term use of glyburide, which is classified in pregnancy by the US Food and Drug Administration (FDA) as Category B, although long-term safety data are not available.[21,22]

Who Should Not Take Metformin[23(pp508-9)]

◆ Metformin should not be taken by people with type 1 diabetes.

◆ Metformin use in certain rare instances can lead to a serious (sometimes fatal) condition called lactic acidosis. For this reason, certain people should not take metformin. This includes those who have:

—Kidney problems (blood creatinine level >1.5 mg/dL in males or >1.4 mg/dL in females)

—Liver problems

—History of alcoholism, or those who binge drink

—Chronic obstructive pulmonary disease (COPD)

—Congestive heart failure that requires medication

Side Effects

Some of the side effects of metformin may be beneficial for those with diabetes:

◆ Slight weight loss (up to about 10 lb) may occur

◆ Improvement in lipids: triglycerides (~16% reduction), LDL cholesterol (~8% reduction), total cholesterol (~5% reduction), and HDL cholesterol (~2% increase).[4]

Survival Skill Side effects that can cause some discomfort include:

◆ Gastrointestinal (GI) effects: metallic taste, abdominal bloating, nausea, diarrhea, cramping, and feeling full. Gastrointestinal effects are the most common problems with metformin, and they usually go away on their own within a week or two. Taking metformin with food will help limit GI effects. The extended-release (XR) formulation of metformin is associated with fewer GI effects than the immediate-release (IR) metformin.

Pioglitazone and Rosiglitazone

Pioglitazone is the generic name for Actos®. Rosiglitazone is the generic name for Avandia®. Together, these medications belong to a class of drugs referred to as TZDs (thiazolidinediones).

How It Works

Pioglitazone and rosiglitazone work by helping your body cells (fat, muscle, and liver) use insulin better. It does not cause you to make more insulin. If you take it in combination with certain other diabetes medicines, there

American Association of Diabetes Educators©

108   Diabetes Education Curriculum

may be a risk for hypoglycemia (low blood glucose). But used by itself, neither pioglitazone nor rosiglitazone causes hypoglycemia. It takes several weeks (8 to 12) to see the full effect of pioglitazone or rosiglitazone. So do not be discouraged if you don't see immediate improvements in your blood glucose level.

How to Take It [23(p502)]

Typically, your provider will start you at a low dose and increase it gradually until the desired effect is seen. Once the maximum daily dose is reached, your provider will decide if additional diabetes medicines are needed.

- Pioglitazone: lowest usual starting dose is 15 mg; maximum daily dose is 45 mg
- Rosiglitazone: lowest usual starting dose is 2 mg; maximum daily dose is 8 mg

Survival Skill It comes in pill form only. It is prescribed once or twice a day. It doesn't matter whether you take this pill with or without food. But if you take it with your main meal(s), it will help you remember to take it.

Precautions

You should have a blood test to check your liver before starting pioglitazone or rosiglitazone therapy. Your provider should repeat the liver function tests (transaminase) periodically while you are taking this medicine.[24] Pioglitazone and rosiglitazone should not be taken by pregnant or breastfeeding women or by children.

Women who have been unable to ovulate due to insulin resistance may begin ovulating after taking pioglitazone or rosiglitazone. If not planning pregnancy, contraception should be used.

Who Should Not Take Pioglitazone or Rosiglitazone

- People with type 1 diabetes should not take pioglitazone or rosiglitazone.
- Pioglitazone and rosiglitazone can be dangerous in people with certain other conditions, including moderate to severe heart failure (New York Heart Association [NYHA] class III or IV) or liver disease.[25]

Side Effects

- Small changes in lipids may occur with either pioglitazone or rosiglitazone.
- **Survival Skill** Weight gain, probably due to fluid retention (edema). Edema tends to be worse in those who take insulin along with either pioglitazone or rosiglitazone. If you notice an increase of weight of over 7 lb (3.3 kg), notify your provider.[26]
- **Survival Skill** Any swelling in the feet or lower legs, shortness of breath, trouble breathing at night, or unexplained cough should be reported promptly to your provider.[26]
- **Survival Skill** Muscle aches, abdominal pain, or flank pain should be reported to your provider.

DPP-IV Inhibitors (Sitagliptin, Alogliptin, Linagliptin, Saxagliptin)

Sitagliptin is the generic name for Januvia®. Alogliptin is the generic name for Nesina®. Linagliptin is the generic name for Tradjenta®. Saxagliptin is the generic name for Onglyza®.

How It Works[27]

Sitagliptin, alogliptin, linagliptin, and saxagliptin work by blocking the action of an enzyme so that it cannot destroy GLP-1. GLP-1 is a hormone produced by your intestine. It stimulates your pancreas to produce insulin after a meal. GLP-1 also helps lower the amount of glucose released by your liver after a meal. These 2 actions of GLP-1 work to blunt the rise in blood glucose after eating. Because these medications cause insulin to be released only in response to a rise in blood glucose, they usually do not cause hypoglycemia when used alone. But if you take these medications along with certain other diabetes medicines (eg, insulin secretagogues), you may be at risk

American Association of Diabetes Educators©

Advanced Detail

I heard in the news that Avandia® (rosiglitazone) causes heart attacks. Shouldn't my doctor take me off Avandia®?

Information drawn from a group of studies focusing on rosiglitazone was analyzed. The data called into question the safety of rosiglitazone, mainly about an increased risk of heart attacks.[28-31] This increased risk was based on information that is not considered by many experts to be definitive.[32] In 2013, results from a large clinical trial found no elevated cardiovascular risk with rosiglitazone (RECORD).[33] As a result, the FDA lifted restrictions on rosiglitazone but did report in a statement: "Some scientific uncertainty about the cardiovascular safety of rosiglitazone still remains."[33] Of note, pioglitazone may have a protective effect on the cardiovascular system.[34]

The FDA still requires a *black box* warning to be placed on the product label for rosiglitazone and pioglitazone regarding risk of congestive heart failure in certain patients.[35,36]

Lessons to be learned regarding news reports about the safety of medication are as follows:

- The risks of taking a medication are not necessarily the same for every person.
- Providers should consider each person's individual health status when they prescribe a medication.
- Always talk to your provider if you are concerned about a news report about a medication you are taking.
- Do not stop taking your medication until you have discussed your situation and treatment options with your provider. Stopping a medication abruptly can sometimes be dangerous.

---

for hypoglycemia. Studies show that this class of medications is *weight neutral*; that is, it does not cause you to gain or lose weight. Checking your glucose levels just before meals and 2 hours later may help show you whether sitagliptin is effective.

How to Take It[27] Survival Skill

All of these medications come in pill form and can be taken with or without food.

- Sitagliptin: The usual starting dose is 100 mg once daily. If kidney function is reduced, the dose may be reduced to 25 to 50 mg daily.
- Alogliptin: The usual starting dose is 25 mg once daily. If kidney function is reduced, the dose may be reduced to 6.25 to 12.5 mg daily.
- Linagliptin: Only a 5-mg once-daily dose is available. No dose adjustment is needed in patients with kidney or liver disease.
- Saxagliptin: The usual starting dose is 5 mg once daily. If kidney function is reduced, the dose may be reduced to 2.5 mg daily.

Who Should Not Take It

- People with type 1 diabetes
- Nursing mothers
- Pregnant women

Side Effects

Gastrointestinal effects like diarrhea or abdominal pain, headache, and runny nose are rare but may occur. In short, these medicines have very few side effects, so any unusual problems that occur after starting them should be reported to your healthcare provider.

Insulin Secretagogues

Glyburide, Glipizide, and Glimepiride

Glyburide is the generic name for Micronase® and Glynase® (micronized form). Glipizide is the generic name for Glucotrol® and Glucotrol XL®. Glimepiride is the generic name for Amaryl®.

How It Works

Glyburide, glipizide, and glimepiride work by increasing the amount of insulin your pancreas releases. In some people, they work well at first but then stop working later on. If your pancreas can no longer produce enough insulin, these medicines will not be effective. When taking these medicines, there is a risk for hypoglycemia (low blood glucose) because of the increase in insulin. Glyburide is also used in the treatment of gestational diabetes. It is classified as Category B in pregnancy by the FDA.

How to Take It

Typically, your provider will start you at a low dose and increase it gradually until the desired effect is seen. Once the maximum daily dose is reached, your provider will decide if different diabetes medicines are needed.

- Glyburide: lowest usual starting dose is 2.5 mg (1.5 mg if micronized); maximum daily dose is 20 mg (12 mg if micronized)
- Glipizide: lowest usual starting dose is 2.5 mg; maximum effective daily dose is 20 mg
- Glimepiride: lowest usual starting dose is 1 mg; maximum daily dose is 8 mg

Survival Skill These medicines are taken every day. Do not skip doses, because your blood glucose will be affected for the next 24 hours. It comes in pill form only. It is prescribed once or twice a day. Take just before or with meal(s) to prevent hypoglycemia.

Precautions

- Your provider should have lab results in your file that prove you have good kidney and liver function to safely take these medicines.
- **Survival Skill** The main precaution to watch for is hypoglycemia. Older people and those with impaired kidney function are most at risk for hypoglycemia while using these medicines. You should take steps to prevent hypoglycemia, for example, eating meals on a regular schedule.
- Do not split or crush a Glucotrol XL® pill. Splitting or crushing it will increase the risk of hypoglycemia.
- Hypersensitivity rash after sun exposure is possible. Use a sunscreen to limit skin problems with sun exposure.

Who Should Not Take It

People with type 1 diabetes should not take glyburide, glipizide, or glimepiride.

Side Effects

- **Survival Skill** Hypoglycemia
- Weight gain, probably related to increased insulin (which promotes the storage of fat)

American Association of Diabetes Educators©

Repaglinide and Nateglinide

Repaglinide is the generic name for Prandin®. Nateglinide is the generic name for Starlix®.

How It Works

Repaglinide and nateglinide work by increasing the amount of insulin released from your pancreas. If your pancreas can no longer produce enough insulin, these medicines will not be effective. When taking these medicines, there is a lower risk for hypoglycemia (low blood glucose) than with similar medicines that affect insulin release. Checking your pre- and postmeal glucose levels will show you whether repaglinide or nateglinide is effective.

How to Take It

Typically, your provider will start you at a low dose and increase it gradually until the desired effect is seen. Once the maximum dose is reached, your provider will decide whether additional or different diabetes medicines are needed.

- ◆ Repaglinide: usual starting dose is 0.5 mg; maximum daily dose is 16 mg.
- ◆ Nateglinide: usual starting dose is 60 to 120 mg; maximum daily dose is 360 mg.

Survival Skill Both repaglinide and nateglinide come in pill form only. Take within 30 minutes of eating a meal. If you skip the meal, don't take the medicine.

Precautions

- ◆ Repaglinide and nateglinide should not be taken by pregnant or breastfeeding women or by children.
- ◆ They should be used with caution in those with liver disease.

Who Should Not Take It

People with type 1 diabetes should not take repaglinide or nateglinide.

Side Effects **Survival Skill**

Hypoglycemia is possible.

Alpha-Glucosidase Inhibitors (Miglitol and Acarbose)

Miglitol is the generic name for Glyset®. Acarbose is the generic name for Precose®.

How It Works

Miglitol and acarbose work by limiting the absorption of carbohydrate in your intestine during digestion. This blunts the rise in blood glucose after meals. Checking the blood glucose 2 hours after meals will show whether miglitol or acarbose is effective. Because they do not cause an increase in insulin, neither miglitol nor acarbose causes hypoglycemia. But if you take either of these medicines in combination with certain other diabetes medicines (eg, insulin secretagogues), you may be at risk for hypoglycemia.

Survival Skill If hypoglycemia occurs while taking miglitol or acarbose, treatment should be with glucose tablets or glucose gel. Because of how miglitol and acarbose work, hypoglycemia treatment with other types of carbohydrates (like table sugar, juice, or soda) will not be effective.

How to Take It **Survival Skill**

The usual starting dose is 25 mg at each meal or large snack. Typically, your provider will increase it gradually until the desired effect is seen. Take with the first bite of each meal. Once the maximum dose is reached, your provider will decide whether additional diabetes medicines are needed.

American Association of Diabetes Educators©

112   Diabetes Education Curriculum

Who Should Not Take It

- ◆ Miglitol and acarbose should not be taken by pregnant or breastfeeding women or by children.
- ◆ People with major intestinal problems should not take miglitol or acarbose.
- ◆ Those with cirrhosis of the liver should not take acarbose.
- ◆ People with kidney disease (creatinine >2 mg/mL) should not take acarbose; neither miglitol nor acarbose should be taken if creatinine clearance is <25 mL per minute.

Side Effects `Survival Skill`

Gastrointestinal effects like flatulence, diarrhea, and abdominal pain are the main side effects of miglitol and acarbose. They are generally worse when the medicine is first started and when the dosage is increased. Side effects usually subside after several weeks of taking miglitol or acarbose. Being active after a meal will help limit the buildup of gas.

Sodium-Glucose Co-Transporter 2 Inhibitors (Canagliflozin, Dapagliflozin, Empagliflozin)

Canagliflozin is the generic name for Invokana®. Dapagliflozin is the generic name for Farxiga®. Empagliflozin is the generic name for Jardiance®.

How It Works[37]

Canagliflozin, dapagliflozin, and empagliflozin work by blocking the reabsorption of glucose in the kidney. This increases the excretion of glucose in the urine and decreases blood glucose levels. These medicines can cause hypoglycemia, but the risk of hypoglycemia is increased if taken with sulfonylureas or insulin.

How to Take It[37]

Typically, your provider will start you at a low dose and increase it gradually until the desired effect is seen. Once the maximum daily dose is reached, your provider will decide whether different diabetes medicines are needed.

- ◆ Canagliflozin: lowest usual starting dose is 100 mg once daily; the maximum dose is 300 mg daily in patients with good kidney function
- ◆ Dapagliflozin: lowest usual starting dose is 5 mg once daily; the maximum dose is 10 mg daily in patients with good kidney function
- ◆ Empagliflozin: lowest usual starting dose is 10 mg once daily; the maximum dose is 25 mg daily in patients with good kidney function

`Survival Skill` These medicines only come in pill form and should be taken first thing in the morning before the first meal of the day. This is because the medicines can increase urination frequency.

Precautions

- ◆ Dehydration may occur in people who have low blood pressure, take blood pressure medications, have kidney problems, or are ≥65 years old.
- ◆ Women and men may experience yeast infections and urinary tract infections. Those prone to these infections are more susceptible.
- ◆ Increases in LDL ("bad") cholesterol have been observed, yet the clinical relevance of this has yet to be understood.

Who Should Not Take It

- ◆ People with severe kidney impairment or end-stage kidney disease or people who are on dialysis.
- ◆ At this time, it is unknown whether these medicines will harm an unborn fetus or pass into breast milk.
- ◆ Women who are pregnant or are breastfeeding.

American Association of Diabetes Educators©

Side Effects

Side effects include an increased risk of infection, particularly of the urinary tract, genitals, and upper respiratory tract. These are more likely to occur in those prone to such infections. Increased urination frequency is also common, so patients should avoid taking these medications during daytime activities or at night.

Combination Oral Diabetes Medications

There are a number of combination diabetes medicines today. Combinations may simplify your diabetes therapy. If you take one of these medicines, you should be aware of how each part works, as well as possible side effects. The available combination medicines (as of early 2015) include (* indicates the combination is available as a generic medication):

- *ACTOplus met®: pioglitazone and metformin
- ACTOplus met XR®: pioglitazone and metformin ER
- Avandaryl®: rosiglitazone and glimepiride
- Avandamet®: rosiglitazone and metformin
- *Duetact®: pioglitazone and glimepiride
- *Glucovance®: glyburide and metformin
- Invokamet®: canagliflozin and metformin
- Janumet®: sitagliptin and metformin
- Janumet XR®: sitagliptin and metformin ER
- Jentadueto®: linagliptin and metformin
- Kazano®: alogliptin and metformin
- Kombiglyze XR®: saxagliptin and metformin ER
- *Metaglip®: glipizide and metformin
- Oseni®: alogliptin and pioglitazone
- PrandiMet®: repaglinide and metformin
- Xigduo XR®: dapagliflozin and metformin ER

Bile Acid Sequestrants (Colesevelam)

Colesevelam is the generic name for WelChol®.

Colesevelam is a medication that is well established in the treatment of abnormal lipids. It has not traditionally been used as a treatment for diabetes. Research, however, shows that colesevelam also has a favorable effect on glucose levels. It lowers fasting blood glucose by 12%. A1C, as well as postprandial blood glucose, is significantly lowered as well. It is weight-neutral, and studies report no serious adverse effects. The most common side effect is constipation.[38] How colesevelam lowers glucose is unclear, but it is thought that it may slow the absorption of carbohydrates and fat in food. It may also increase the release of GLP-1 and GIP, thereby stimulating insulin release.[38-40] However, cholesterol-lowering medications are not used in pregnancy.

Antihypertensive Drugs and Pregnancy

Pregnant women with chronic hypertension or pregnancy-induced hypertension may need medication or a change in medication to bring their blood pressure under control. ACE inhibitors and angiotensin receptor blockers are contraindicated because they may cause fetal damage. There are antihypertensive drugs, however, that are effective and safe for use in pregnancy. These include methyldopa, labetalol, diltiazem, clonidine, and prazosin.[41]

Tocolytic Agents

Tocolytic agents are medications that are used in pregnancy to treat premature labor. These agents can raise blood glucose levels and cause ketosis. If these agents must be used, the blood glucose levels must be carefully monitored.

Injected Diabetes Medications (Insulin, GLP-1 Agonists, Pramlintide)

For Participants for Whom Insulin Is Prescribed

What have you heard about insulin?

How do you feel about having to take insulin?

What do you want to learn today about insulin?

What is your greatest concern/frustration about taking insulin?

What's the hardest part about taking your insulin?

What do you think would help you to take your insulin the way it's prescribed?

If patient is new to injection therapy, instruct on the injection technique *before* instructing on how to draw up the medication or how it works. Allow the patient to first deal with any anxiety he or she may have about the injection itself. Then, the information that follows is more likely to be retained.

Help patients new to injection therapy to minimize negativity that gets in the way of learning by:

- Examining beliefs, expectations, and assumptions about taking medications by injection (particularly insulin).
- Presenting evidence that will help put fears to rest and promote the notion that by taking the medication they are exerting control over their situation.

Insulin

Normally, the pancreas releases a small amount of insulin in a slow, steady stream throughout the day that is commonly referred to as basal insulin. When a meal is eaten, the food breaks down into glucose, which is fuel for the body. The glucose gets into the bloodstream as the food is digested. When you begin to eat, a burst of insulin, also known as bolus insulin, is released from the pancreas into the bloodstream. Insulin moves the glucose from the bloodstream into the body cells. Once glucose is inside the cells, energy is released. This is how the body gets the energy it needs.

When a person has diabetes, there is a problem with insulin production. In type 1 diabetes, insulin production stops completely. Insulin therapy is always needed to maintain life and regulate the blood glucose level. In type 2 diabetes, there is a continual decline in the amount of insulin produced. **In most people with type 2 diabetes, the** time will come when their pancreas can no longer make enough insulin to meet their needs. At that point, insulin therapy is needed to regulate the blood glucose level.

Insulin is available by injection or by way of an insulin pump. Insulin cannot be taken in pill form, because the digestive juices will destroy it.

More recently, inhaled insulin was approved by the FDA and is on the market.[42] (Note: this product is different from the inhaled insulin Exubera® that was withdrawn from the market by manufacturer Pfizer due to poor sales in 2007.)

> *Once you start insulin, do you have to take it forever?*

The answer to that question depends on the situation. In type 1 diabetes, the need for insulin will last throughout a person's lifetime. As discussed above, insulin is often needed as an ongoing therapy in those with type 2 diabetes. Short-term insulin therapy for those with type 2 diabetes is usually needed during the following situations:

- **Extreme Hyperglycemia at Diagnosis**—Sometimes, a person's blood glucose level is dangerously high at the time of diagnosis. In this case, insulin is the only medication that will adequately treat the hyperglycemia. Once the glucose levels are controlled, the provider may change from insulin to oral diabetes medication.

- **Hospitalization**—During a hospital stay, a person's meals are often interrupted for tests, procedures, or surgery. Or, the illness that prompted the hospital admission affects one's ability to eat. If the kidney or liver function is affected, then oral diabetes medicines can be toxic. Insulin therapy is a safe and accurate way to control the blood glucose level during a hospital stay. In many cases, a person's oral diabetes medicines are resumed after discharge.

- **Severe Illness**—During a severe physical illness, especially infection, many *stress hormones* are released into the bloodstream. These stress hormones make it hard for the pancreas to release insulin. They also cause the body's cells to be even more resistant to insulin. The result is hyperglycemia, or a very high blood glucose level. Sometimes this situation is referred to as *glucose toxicity*.

    Short-term insulin therapy can help to "rest the pancreas" for a while. When the illness resolves, and the glucose level begins to lower, then the pancreas can produce insulin again. The body cells become more sensitive to insulin again. In this case, a person's oral diabetes medicines may be resumed. If the blood glucose remains high, though, insulin may need to be continued.

- **Pregnancy**—If meal planning does not adequately control the blood glucose, pregnant women with type 2 or gestational diabetes will need insulin therapy. It's very important to control blood glucose levels during pregnancy in order to avoid birth defects or delivery problems. If the blood glucose levels normalize after delivery, then the prepregnancy therapy may be resumed.

 Invite any participants who have successfully integrated injection therapy into their life to share with others in the group how they managed it and how it improved their metabolic control. Adults with social/interpersonal intelligence learn by telling their story; hearing and telling stories helps those with verbal/auditory intelligence learn.

Source of Insulin

What is "human" insulin? Is it taken from humans?

Human insulin is made in a laboratory using special gene technology. It is *not* made from the pancreases of humans. Its chemical structure is the same as human insulin. In the past, insulin was made from the pancreases of pigs and cows. This form of insulin is no longer available in the United States. For people who follow strict religious rules against beef or pork consumption, human insulin is permitted. Insulin is obtained at a pharmacy. A prescription is required for certain formulations of insulin called *analogs*. This group includes glargine, detemir, lispro, aspart, and glulisine. Other insulin types generally do not require a prescription.

Concentration of Insulin

Insulin is measured in *units*. In the United States, insulin is made in two strengths: U-100 and U-500. U-100 means that there are 100 units of insulin in each milliliter of liquid. It is the most common strength of insulin prescribed in the United States.

U-500 means that there are 500 units of insulin in each milliliter of liquid; this is five times more concentrated than U-100 insulin. U-500 is needed for those people who require unusually large doses of insulin.

If you travel outside the United States, be aware that insulin may only be available in U-40 strength. U-40 means that there are only 40 units of insulin in each milliliter of liquid; this is less than half the concentration of U-100. U-40 insulin also requires a special syringe. Always discuss any international travel with your provider so that you can safely plan for your insulin needs.

Types of Insulin and How They Work

There are many types of insulin, and they work in different ways after they are injected. When the insulin first starts to lower the glucose level is called the *onset of action* (see Table 4.1). When it lowers the glucose the most it is called the *peak*. The period of time the insulin is lowering the glucose is called the *duration of action*. Insulin types

TABLE 4.1 Insulin and Its Action

Classification	Generic Name	Brand Name	Onset	Peak	Duration	Color
Rapid-acting	Aspart Glulisine Lispro	Novolog® Apidra® Humalog®	5–15 minutes	1–2 hours	4–6 hours	Clear
	Inhaled insulin	Afrezza®	12–15 minutes	1 hour	3 hours	N/A
Short-acting	Regular, human	Humulin® R Novolin® R Relion®/Novolin® R	30–60 minutes	2–4 hours	6–10 hours	Clear
Intermediate-acting	Isophane, human (NPH)	Humulin® N Novolin® N Relion®/Novolin® N	1–2 hours	4–8 hours	10–18 hours	Cloudy
Long-acting	Detemir Glargine	Levemir® Lantus®	1–2 hours	No peak	Up to 24 hours	Clear

Source: EM Sisson, DL Dixon, "Pharmacotherapy for Glucose Management," in C Mensing, ed, *The Art and Science of Diabetes Self-Management Education: A Desk Reference for Healthcare Professionals*, 3rd ed. (Chicago: American Association of Diabetes Educators, 2014), 522.

are classified according to their onset, peak, and duration. For safety reasons, it's important to know when your dose of insulin is working to lower your blood glucose.

For Participants Who Take Insulin
Do you know when your prescribed insulin starts to work?
Do you know when it lowers glucose the most?
Do you know how long it lasts (when it wears off)?

Side Effects Survival Skill

Because insulin lowers glucose, there is always a possibility the glucose level could drop *too low*. This is called hypoglycemia. To keep hypoglycemia from occurring, you should balance your food and activity with insulin's action. You should also monitor glucose to see how you respond to insulin.

If you take insulin that "peaks," you should eat a meal during the peak time. As food raises the glucose, the insulin works to lower the glucose. With the right dose of insulin and the right amount of food, the glucose is kept at a controlled level. If you take insulin that "peaks" and you fail to eat during the peak time, hypoglycemia may occur.

If you take insulin that "peaks," it is best not to exercise during the peak time. Physical activity lowers the glucose level. If both insulin and activity are lowering glucose at the same time, hypoglycemia may occur. Time your activity for when the insulin is not peaking.

Adults learn best when the content is meaningful to their own experience and fills a perceived need. Relating meal times to the time of insulin action helps patients connect the two. Use of charts that plot meals and insulin action times resonates with learners, especially those with visual/spatial intelligence.

For Participants Who Take Insulin That "Peaks"
What time do you normally eat your first meal of the day?
What time do you eat your second meal? third meal?
When do you plan for physical activity?

Work with each patient to customize timing for meals, activity, and insulin. Use take-home diagrams or charts to help the patient understand, and to promote safe and effective medication-taking.

Storage[23(pp528-9)43,44]

- **Survival Skill** **Unopened,** unused vials of insulin should be kept **refrigerated** (36°F to 46°F [2°C to 8°C]) and protected from light. Refrigerated, unopened vials of insulin can be used until the printed **expiration date.**
- If the **unopened,** unused vial of insulin is kept at **room temperature** (not to exceed 86°F (30°C)), it must be discarded after **1 month.**
- Opened vial or pen device of insulin that is **in use** at home or while traveling: store at **room temperature**, not to exceed 86°F (30°C).

American Association of Diabetes Educators©

- Most brands of insulin are good for 1 month at room temperature after opening the vial or pen device. Throw away after 30 days, even if some insulin is left in the vial.
- It is OK to keep the vial or pen device you are using in the refrigerator. If injection with cold insulin is uncomfortable, you can roll the syringe with insulin between your palms to warm it up before injecting. Never warm insulin in the microwave or by floating it in hot water, as this will harm the insulin.
- Never freeze insulin. If it has been frozen, do not use.

Rapid-Acting Insulin

There are currently 3 rapid-acting insulin brands (also known as analogs) on the market:

- Insulin aspart is the generic name for Novolog® brand insulin.
- Insulin glulisine is the generic name for Apidra® brand insulin.
- Insulin lispro is the generic name for Humalog® brand insulin.

Rapid-acting insulin is clear. If you see a colored tint to the solution, or if a colored ring has formed at the top, do not use.

Survival Skill Rapid-acting insulin is intended to control the blood glucose rise that happens after a meal. Once injected, the insulin starts to enter the bloodstream quickly, within 5 to 15 minutes. **You should begin to eat within 15 minutes of injecting rapid-acting insulin.** After you eat, the food is actively raising your glucose level for the next 1 to 2 hours. Rapid-acting insulin is actively moving this glucose into your body cells during this same time. The insulin continues to lower blood glucose somewhat until it wears off, in about 4 to 6 hours.

Properly prescribed and taken, rapid-acting insulin most closely mimics the action of insulin at mealtime in a person without diabetes. Rapid-acting insulin is typically prescribed to be taken before meals. Take as directed.

- If you take rapid-acting insulin before your breakfast, it will peak about the same time that breakfast raises your glucose level.
- If you take rapid-acting insulin before your lunch, it will peak about the same time that lunch raises your glucose level.
- If you take rapid-acting insulin before your dinner, it will peak about the same time that dinner raises your glucose level.

If you plan to eat a snack that contains more than 15 g of carbohydrate, an injection of rapid-acting insulin may be needed. This should be discussed with the prescribing provider.[23] Eating within 15 minutes of taking rapid-acting insulin is very important. If you don't eat within 15 minutes, your glucose can drop to a dangerously low level. If you are concerned that eating is likely to be delayed after your injection, consider taking it at the time you sit down to eat instead.

For Participants for Whom Rapid-Acting Insulin Is Prescribed
What do you think might happen if you take your rapid-acting insulin and then eat 30 minutes later?

Short-Acting Insulin

Regular insulin is the generic name for short-acting insulin. The brand names for regular insulin are Humulin® R, Novolin® R, and Relion®/Novolin R. Regular insulin is clear. If you see a colored tint to the solution, or if a colored ring has formed at the top, do not use.

Survival Skill Regular insulin is intended to impact the blood glucose rise that happens after a meal, but there is a lag in its action. For this reason, you should **take regular insulin 30 to 45 minutes before eating**. This gives the insulin a head start. It takes 30 to 60 minutes for regular insulin to enter the bloodstream. After you eat, the food is actively raising your glucose level for the next 1 to 2 hours. Regular insulin moves this glucose into your body cells the most (it peaks) in 2 to 4 hours. The insulin continues to lower blood glucose somewhat until it wears off, in about 6 to 10 hours. *The larger the dose of regular insulin, the longer it stays in your system.* Regular insulin is typically prescribed before meals. Take as directed.

- If you take regular insulin before your breakfast, it will peak about 1 hour after breakfast raises your glucose level.
- If you take regular insulin before your lunch, it will peak about 1 hour after lunch raises your glucose level.
- If you take regular insulin before your dinner, it will peak about 1 hour after dinner raises your glucose level.

Engage learners in critical thinking activities. Those with logical/mathematical intelligence will especially benefit from this approach to learning.

For Participants for Whom Regular Insulin Is Prescribed
If you took your regular insulin after eating, do you think it would control the glucose rise from the meal? Explain why or why not.

Important point: If regular insulin is taken **after** you eat, it is impossible for that dose to control the glucose rise from your meal. Remember, glucose rises quickly after a meal, reaching a high point about 1 to 2 hours after you eat. By the time the regular insulin is peaking, the glucose level has long since passed its high point. Insulin cannot work backward.

Intermediate-Acting Insulin

Insulin isophane is the generic name for intermediate-acting insulin. It is commonly referred to as NPH. Some brand names for NPH insulin are Humulin® N, Novolin® N, and Relion®/Novolin® N.

NPH insulin has a cloudy white color. It is cloudy because a substance has been added to the insulin to slow down its action. If NPH insulin has spoiled, it will look different. If you see any white clumps floating in the solution after mixing, or if the bottle has a frosted look to it, do not use.

Survival Skill *You must gently and thoroughly mix this solution before you prepare your injection.* To mix, roll the container (vial, pen, or prefilled syringe) between your palms several times. Do not vigorously shake the container, as this can cause bubbles to form.

Survival Skill NPH insulin is intended to impact the blood glucose rise that occurs many hours after injection. Once injected, NPH begins to enter the bloodstream in 1 to 2 hours. It has a long, drawn-out peak time, 4 to 8 hours after injection. During this time, it is actively moving glucose into your body cells. It stays in the system for 10 to 18 hours before it wears off. NPH is typically prescribed once or twice a day. Take as directed.

For Participants for Whom NPH Insulin Is Prescribed Pre-breakfast
If you took NPH before breakfast, the blood glucose rise from which meal is most affected? Explain.

If you take NPH before your breakfast, it will peak about the same time that lunch raises your glucose level. The pre-breakfast dose is intended to control the lunchtime glucose rise the most.

American Association of Diabetes Educators©

For Participants for Whom NPH Insulin Is Prescribed Pre-dinner

Would it be a problem if you took NPH in the evening but then ate a very light dinner? Explain why or why not.

If you took NPH before dinner, what could you do to prevent hypoglycemia from occurring during the night?

If you take NPH before dinner, it will peak in the middle of the night. If you haven't had enough to eat the evening before, this could cause your blood glucose to go too low. Eating enough at dinner and having a snack before going to bed can help prevent low blood glucose from happening in the night. Keep in mind that the bedtime snack is included as part of your overall daily calories—it's not extra.

If you take NPH at bedtime, it will peak during the early morning hours. For people with diabetes, the liver releases too much glucose during the early morning hours. NPH will help control the glucose rise at this time.

Long-Acting Insulin

There are 2 long-acting insulin products currently on the market. Insulin detemir is the generic name for Levemir®. Insulin glargine is the generic name for Lantus®. Both of these are clear solutions. If you see a colored tint to the solution, or if a colored ring has formed at the top, do not use.

Survival Skill Long-acting insulin is intended to mimic the constant, steady release of insulin that occurs in people without diabetes. Once injected, long-acting insulin begins to enter the bloodstream in 1 to 2 hours. It has no peak. Instead, a little insulin at a time enters the bloodstream. Long-acting insulin continues to work for up to 24 hours after injection.

Long-acting insulin is typically prescribed once a day, often at bedtime. This timing is meant for convenience more than anything else. It can be taken at any time of day or night, just as long as the timing is consistent day to day.[45] In some people, long-acting insulin wears off earlier than 24 hours, so twice-daily injection is needed. Take as directed.

Be aware that Lantus® (insulin glargine) may cause a mild burning sensation when injected. This is because the pH level is slightly on the acidic side. It is usually not a big problem for people who use Lantus®.

Premixed Insulin

Premixed insulin is generally prescribed for people who may have problems mixing 2 separate types of insulin into 1 syringe (see Figure 4.1).

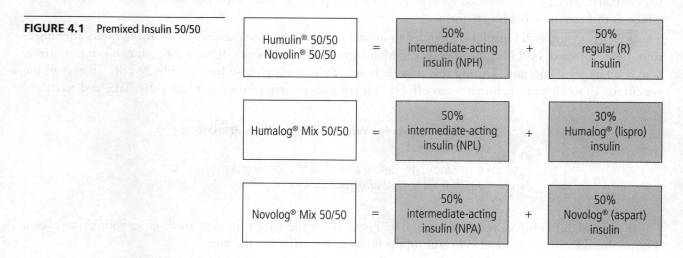

FIGURE 4.1 Premixed Insulin 50/50

Inhaled Insulin

Inhaled insulin is the generic name for Afrezza®. It is the only orally inhaled insulin product currently available and is available in single-use cartridges. Inhaled insulin is suitable for those with type 1 or type 2 diabetes, especially individuals who are afraid of needles.[42]

Survival Skill Inhaled insulin is rapid-acting, so it must be used at the beginning of a meal. Inhaled insulin is NOT a substitute for long-acting insulin.

How to Use It[42]

- The starting dose for insulin-naive patients is 4 units (or 1 blue cartridge) at each meal initially.
- The cartridges come in 2 doses: 4 units per cartridge and 8 units per cartridge.
- Dose adjustment may be necessary when switching from injectable to inhaled insulin.
- For doses greater than 24 units, combinations of different cartridges may be used (see Table 4.2).

    Step 1: ALWAYS make sure to have the correct number of cartridges out before you start.

    Step 2: Remove a blister card from the foil package and remove a cartridge from the strip by pressing the clear side.

    Step 3: Load the cartridge by opening the inhaler (lift the white mouthpiece) and placing the cartridge into the inhaler so that the pointed end lines up with the pointed end of the inhaler. Close the inhaler and remove the purple mouthpiece cover while keeping the inhaler level.

    Step 4: While keeping the inhaler level, fully exhale. Place the mouthpiece in the mouth and tilt the inhaler toward your chin. Form a tight seal with your lips and inhale deeply while holding your breath as long as you are comfortable. Then remove the inhaler, exhale, and breathe normally.

    Step 5: Remove the used cartridge by placing the purple mouthpiece cover back on the inhaler to lift up the mouthpiece. The cartridge may be disposed of in your regular household trash.

    *Repeat steps 2 through 5 if necessary to get the full, prescribed dose.

Storage and Inhaler Care[43,44]

- Cartridges should be at room temperature for 10 minutes prior to use.
- Cartridges NOT in use should be refrigerated and may be used until the expiration date.
- Cartridges in use can be stored at room temperature but must be used within 10 days.

TABLE 4.2 Inhaled Insulin Dose Conversion Chart

Injected Mealtime Insulin Dose	Inhaled Insulin Dose	Number of 4-Unit Cartridges (Blue)		Number of 8-Unit Cartridges (Green)
Up to 4 units	4 units	1		–
5–8 units	8 units	–		1
9–12 units	12 units	1	PLUS	1
13–16 units	16 units	–		2
17–20 units	20 units	1	PLUS	2
21–24 units	24 units	–		3

American Association of Diabetes Educators©

122   Diabetes Education Curriculum

- ◆ An open strip of 3 cartridges must be used within 3 days.
- ◆ The inhaler should be kept at room temperature in a clean, dry place.
- ◆ Use 1 inhaler at a time and replace the inhaler every 15 days.

Precautions

- ◆ Lung function should be assessed before starting inhaled insulin, 6 months after starting it, and annually, regardless of whether the person develops symptoms (eg, shortness of breath, cough).
- ◆ **Survival Skill** Inhaled insulin might cause acute bronchospasm in those with asthma or chronic obstructive pulmonary disease (COPD).

Who Should Not Use It

- ◆ People with chronic lung diseases (eg, asthma, COPD)
- ◆ Those with a history of, or at risk for, lung cancer (eg, smokers)

Side Effects

- ◆ Similar to injectable insulin, inhaled insulin can cause the blood sugar to go too low. The same precautions regarding the need to self-monitor blood glucose and an understanding of how to manage low blood glucose are warranted.
- ◆ Throat pain or irritation and cough may develop from exposure to the inhaled drug powder.
- ◆ A decrease in lung function and cough may develop.

Insulin Pump Therapy[45]

Survival Skill Disposable insulin delivery systems have entered the market in recent years and are intended for those patients who are unable to inject insulin and are on multiple daily injections. These systems are essentially "pump-like" devices that deliver basal-bolus insulin through a small needle that is part of the device without any tubes. After 24 hours, the patient must remove the device and apply a new one. Limitations of these devices are that they are only available in specific preset basal rates that may not work for all patients and that there are no programmable features. Furthermore, disposable insulin delivery systems are only approved for use in type 2 diabetes.

Advanced Detail

An insulin pump can deliver a steady amount of insulin constantly throughout the day and night. The constant flow is the *basal* insulin. At mealtime, it can deliver a larger burst of insulin, which is called a *bolus* of insulin. In this way, it mimics the normal action of the pancreas.

An insulin pump consists of:

- ◆ a reservoir of rapid-acting insulin.
- ◆ pump casing, which is about the size of a cell phone. The casing houses the insulin reservoir. Within the casing is a computer chip that allows programming of the insulin doses.
- ◆ plastic tubing which connects the insulin pump. This tubing is referred to as an infusion set.
- ◆ a thin, flexible needle, called a cannula, that is attached to the end of the tubing. The cannula is inserted into the layer of fat beneath the skin. It is taped into place and can stay for up to 3 days, after which it should be replaced.

American Association of Diabetes Educators©

Advantages of Insulin Pump Therapy

◆ Insulin pump therapy can help users achieve blood glucose levels that are normal or very near to normal. Fasting high blood glucose, often referred to as the *dawn phenomenon*, is reduced with insulin therapy.[46]

◆ Users' lifestyles can be spontaneous in terms of mealtimes, timing of activity, and the ability to sleep in. This is because the pump can allow insulin dosage adjustment during these times to match the user's needs.

◆ Insulin doses given with a pump are very precise. Absorption of the insulin is predictable.

◆ With a pump, users can respond very quickly to any changes in their blood glucose level.

◆ The risk of severe hypoglycemia (low blood glucose) is about 75% less with pump therapy as compared with other ways of taking insulin.[47]

Realities of Insulin Pump Therapy

◆ It takes a lot of initial training to learn how to use a pump. The person must be willing and motivated to accept the extra responsibility.

◆ Not all healthcare providers are familiar with pump therapy. Ideally, training should be done by a skilled diabetes care team that is familiar with pump therapy. This team should be available at all times for immediate consultation.[48]

◆ About half of all people who start using a pump quit within 2 years' time.[49,50] A person who has first mastered multiple daily insulin injections and related problem solving may be more likely to be successful with pump therapy. Also, trying the pump out for a while using saline instead of insulin increases the odds a person will be successful with a pump. It gives the person a chance to see what it's like to do usual daily activities while connected to a pump.[50,51]

◆ Using a pump requires ongoing trial-and-error experiments to learn to match insulin to food and activity. An advanced approach to meal planning, called *carbohydrate counting*, allows for more flexibility and freedom in terms of eating schedule and food choices when using a pump.[52]

◆ Pump users must be willing to monitor and record their blood glucose levels frequently each day.[53(p549)]

◆ Pump therapy is expensive. The pump may cost over $6000. Supplies can exceed $200 per month. Insurance plans vary in coverage of the pump, supplies, and training.[53(p549)]

◆ Infection at the cannula insertion site is possible, although proper skin care and insertion technique lower this risk.

◆ Although insulin pumps are generally very reliable, there is always the possibility that insulin delivery could be interrupted. The pump itself could fail, there could be an error in programming, the insulin in the reservoir could go bad, or there could be a problem with the tubing or cannula. Pump failure can lead to a diabetes crisis (diabetic ketoacidosis) within just a few hours in those with type 1 diabetes.

◆ Having a pump constantly attached to the body is a reminder of the disease. This can cause an emotional burden for some people.

◆ The ongoing demands of pump therapy may lead to burnout in some people. A temporary holiday from the pump can help, in which case the person switches to insulin injections.

Survival Skill **GLP-1 Agonists (Exenatide, Exenatide LAR, Liraglutide, Albiglutide, Dulaglutide)**

Exenatide is the generic name for Byetta®. Extended-release exenatide is the generic name for Bydureon®. Once-weekly (Bydureon) formulation is suspension, not a solution. Liraglutide is the generic name for Victoza®. Albiglutide is the generic name for Tanzeum®. Dulaglutide is the generic name for Trulicity®. Together, these medications belong to a class of drugs known as GLP-1 agonists.

American Association of Diabetes Educators©

Weight loss is common with GLP-1 agonists. In fact, liraglutide is also the generic for Saxenda®. This is the ONLY GLP-1 agonist that has been approved by the FDA for chronic weight management. It is for those with a BMI of at least 30 kg/m² or a BMI of 27 kg/m² PLUS one weight-related condition (eg, diabetes, high blood pressure). It should NOT be used with any of the GLP-1 agonists for diabetes.[54]

How It Works[54-57]

Exenatide, extended-release exenatide, liraglutide, albiglutide, and dulaglutide are intended for people with type 2 diabetes who take 1 or more oral diabetes medicines, but whose glucose levels remain above target. While these medications may be used along with other diabetes medicines—insulin, or those from the sulfonylurea, thiazolidinediones, or biguanide class—these agents are NOT a replacement for insulin. These medications give you a feeling of fullness after eating, which may lead to less eating and weight loss. Also, your sugar levels will not increase as much after meals since these medications slow down the time it takes food to leave the stomach. Weight loss is common with these medications and can be a favorable effect in people with diabetes who are overweight or obese. Used alone, the agents usually do not cause hypoglycemia (low blood glucose). But if taken along with certain other diabetes medicines (eg, insulin, sulfonylureas), hypoglycemia is possible.

How to Take It[58-62]

Survival Skill Each of the GLP-1 agonists has specific dosing intervals, and careful consideration must be given to ensure the patient follows the appropriate dosing interval. These injectable agents are subcutaneous injections and can be administered in the thigh, upper arm, or abdomen.

- Exenatide is injected twice a day. The starting dose is 5 mcg twice daily, and the dose can be increased to 10 mcg twice daily after 1 month. The pens come in a fixed dose (5 mcg or 10 mcg). To ensure exenatide works and to minimize nausea, exenatide should be administered within 1 hour of eating breakfast (first meal of the day) and dinner (last meal of the day). Skip your dose if you skip a meal. Your 2 doses should be at least 6 hours apart.

Advanced Detail

I heard that Byetta® is made from lizard spit. Is that really true?

No, exenatide and the other drugs in this class are not made from lizard spit. You may have heard about this strange connection on the TV news or in the newspaper. It is true, though, that this medicine has an interesting connection to a lizard. The Gila monster is a large lizard that is native to the southwestern United States and Mexico. Researchers discovered that this lizard eats only a few times a year.

Whenever it eats, a substance is released from its spit glands. This substance helps the lizard digest the meal very slowly. It helps the lizard's pancreas make just the right amount of insulin to process the glucose from the meal. This substance causes its liver to release the right amount of stored glucose into the bloodstream, as needed, to provide energy to the lizard during the months between meals. It causes the lizard to not feel hungry for months at a time.

Scientists discovered that the human body releases a similar substance—called GLP-1—after eating. The intestines release the GLP-1, which works like the substance from the lizard, but on a different time frame, of course.

Studies have shown that people with type 2 diabetes don't produce enough GLP-1. Researchers then developed a synthetic (manufactured) version of GLP-1 to help correct some of the problems that occur in type 2 diabetes.

Module 4   *Taking Medication*   125

- Extended-release exenatide is a very long-acting form of exenatide and is only available in 1 dose, 2 mg ONCE weekly. The long-acting exenatide suspension can be given at any time of day, with or without food.

- The starting dose for liraglutide is 0.6 mg for 1 week, THEN increase to 1.2 mg daily. If glucose levels remain elevated, the dose can be increased to 1.8 mg daily. Take at any time of day, with or without food.

- The starting dose for albiglutide is 30 mg ONCE weekly, but can be increased to 50 mg ONCE weekly if glucose control is inadequate.

- The starting dose for dulaglutide is 0.75 mg ONCE weekly, but can be increased to 1.5 mg ONCE weekly if glucose control is inadequate.

Survival Skill Albiglutide and extended-release exenatide must be reconstituted prior to use. After reconstitution, the albiglutide dose must be injected within 8 hours. Extended-release exenatide must be administered immediately after reconstitution.[63]

Precautions

Since GLP-1 agonists slow down the emptying of your stomach, the action of certain oral medicines may be affected. This is especially true for pain pills, birth control pills, and antibiotics. Take any oral medicines 1 hour before your injection. Pain pills, however, should be taken 2 hours before or 2 hours after your injection.[58]

Side Effects

The most common side effect is nausea. It is more likely to occur when first beginning therapy. In most cases, nausea decreases over time. To lower the risk and severity of nausea, eat slowly and stop eating when you feel the least bit full. Nausea is less likely with the longer acting GLP-1 agonists, such as exenatide LAR, liraglutide, albiglutide, and dulaglutide.

Survival Skill If nausea is severe, or if you develop vomiting or abdominal pain, notify your provider right away.

Who Should Not Take It

- Children—at this time, effectiveness and safety studies have not been published

- Pregnant or nursing women

- People with a personal or family history of medullary thyroid cancer or multiple endocrine neoplasia syndrome type 2

- People with gastroparesis, a condition in which the movement of the intestines is abnormal

- People with a personal history of pancreatitis

- People with severe kidney disease[64]

Storage[61-65]

- Unopened, unused packages of all GLP-1 agonists: keep refrigerated (36°F to 46°F [2°C to 8°C]) and protected from light. Good until expiration date.

- Prior to first use, extended-release exenatide and albiglutide may be kept at room temperature, not to exceed 77°F (25°C), for up to 4 weeks, while dulaglutide may be keep at room temperature for up to 14 days.

- Opened pen device of exenatide and liraglutide that is in use at home or while traveling: store at room temperature, not to exceed 77°F (25°C), for up to 30 days. Throw away after 30 days, even if some medicine is left in the pen device.

- Remove needle from pen device in between injections. If the needle stays on the pen device, medicine may leak out and/or air may leak in.

- Never freeze ANY of the GLP-1 agonists. If frozen, do not use.

American Association of Diabetes Educators©

126   Diabetes Education Curriculum

Amylin Analogs (Pramlintide)

Pramlintide is the generic name for Symlin®. It is intended for people with type 1 or type 2 diabetes who take mealtime insulin, but whose blood glucose levels are still not at target level. Pramlintide does not replace insulin therapy. The usual amount of insulin you take before meals will need to be adjusted. While taking pramlintide, you will need less insulin before meals. Your provider will make the necessary insulin adjustments. Pramlintide is available in a pen device. It is a clear solution. If you see a colored tint to the solution, or if a colored ring has formed at the top of the vial or in the pen cartridge, do not use.

How It Works[66-68]

Normally, the pancreas releases a hormone called amylin along with insulin. People with type 1 diabetes make no amylin; people with type 2 diabetes make too little amylin and eventually none at all. Pramlintide is the synthetic (manufactured) version of amylin. It works in 3 ways:

- Through its action on the brain, it gives you a feeling of fullness after eating. This may cause you to eat less, and weight loss may occur.
- It slows down how quickly food leaves the stomach. This helps to blunt the rise of glucose after meals.
- It limits the amount of glucose that is released by the liver, especially after meals when you do not need any extra glucose.

How to Take It `Survival Skill`

- Pramlintide is injected just before your *major meals*. A major meal is defined as at least 250 calories or 30 g of carbohydrate. After injecting, don't delay eating for long, or pramlintide won't work as it should. Never take pramlintide after eating. The starting dose is 15 mcg. Your provider will tell you when to increase your dose.
- Pramlintide is dosed in micrograms. In order to use a standard U-100 syringe, you need to first convert the micrograms to units. Table 4.3 is the dosing chart and is found in the product packaging for your convenience.

If you are using the pramlintide pen device, you can select the dose in micrograms—15, 30, 45, 60, or 120—depending on which pen size is prescribed.

Precautions `Survival Skill`

- Never mix pramlintide with insulin in the same syringe.
- Space the injections with pramlintide and insulin at least 2 inches apart.[69]

TABLE 4.3   Pramlintide Dose Conversion Chart

Ordered Dose in Micrograms (mcg)	Units to Draw Up in U-100 Syringe
15 mcg	2.5 units
30 mcg	5 units
45 mcg	7.5 units
60 mcg	10 units
120 mcg	20 units

American Association of Diabetes Educators©

- Use the abdomen or thigh for injection.[69]
- If you skip a meal, do not take pramlintide.
- When you are ill and cannot eat as usual, do not take pramlintide.
- If you are having surgery, do not take pramlintide until directed (probably once you are eating again as usual).
- If you are having lab tests or procedures that require you to fast, do not take the pramlintide until you can eat again.

Side Effects

The most common side effect of pramlintide is nausea, and it is most likely to occur in the first few weeks of therapy. In most people, the nausea goes away after a few weeks. Because pramlintide lowers glucose, there is always a possibility the blood glucose level could drop **too low** (hypoglycemia). To keep hypoglycemia from occurring, you should balance your food and activity with the action of your pramlintide and insulin. If pramlintide does cause hypoglycemia, it will occur within 3 hours of injection. You should monitor your glucose level to see how you respond to pramlintide therapy. The best monitoring schedule to see your response is before and after each meal and at bedtime. Share these results with your provider.

Storage[69]

- Unopened, unused packages of pramlintide: keep refrigerated (36°F to 46°F [2°C to 8°C]) and protected from light. Good until expiration date.
- Opened vial or pen device of pramlintide that is in use at home or while traveling: store at room temperature, not to exceed 86°F (30°C).
- Never freeze pramlintide. If it has been frozen, do not use.
- Pramlintide (unexpired) is good for 30 days at room temperature after opening the vial or pen device. Throw away after 30 days, even if some pramlintide is left in the vial or pen device.
- Remove needle from pen device in between injections. If the needle stays on the device, medicine may leak out and/or air may leak in.

Injecting Diabetes Medication (Insulin, GLP-1 agonists, and Pramlintide)

Where to Inject   Survival Skill

Insulin, GLP-1 agonists, and pramlintide should be injected into the fat layer between the skin and the muscle. This is called a subcutaneous injection. There are many places on the body that can be used for a subcutaneous injection:

- back of the upper arm
- tops and outer part of the thigh
- hips/outer part of the buttock
- abdomen

Have a diagram of injection sites available to show participants. Use of graphics helps learners, particularly those with visual/spatial intelligence.

Some exceptions apply to pramlintide and GLP-1 agonist injections:

- Pramlintide users should inject this medicine only in the abdomen or thighs.[66,67]
- GLP-1 agonist users should inject this medicine only in the thighs, upper arms, or abdomen.[57-61]

Never inject into the muscle, as it can cause the medication to be absorbed much too quickly. Avoid injecting into any scars. Don't inject within 2 inches of the belly button.[69] To make sure you don't inject into the muscle, pinch up the fat between your fingers and insert the needle at a 90° angle. Extremely thin people may need to angle the needle more in order to avoid injecting into the muscle.[68] Never inject into a vein, as this is very dangerous. Sometimes the needle will strike a tiny blood vessel (capillary) in the fat layer. You may see a small blood drop on the skin just after the injection, or you may bruise later on. This is common and nothing to worry about. You did not do anything wrong, and it does not mean that the medicine went directly into the vein.

Rotating Injection Sites[69] `Survival Skill`

Injecting into the same area for too long can cause scar tissue to develop. Medicine injected into scar tissue will not be absorbed and used properly.

Different areas of the body absorb medicine differently. It is not recommended to change randomly from area to area for injection every day. If you do this, you may get a different response from your medication each time. This makes controlling your blood glucose levels more difficult.

Try to inject into a slightly different spot within an area for no more than 2 weeks. For example, inject into the arms in slightly different spots each time for up to 2 weeks. Then rotate to the thighs, using slightly different spots for the next 2 weeks. If you choose to inject into the abdomen, you do not need to rotate to other areas of the body. The abdomen is large enough to simply rotate your injection sites within this area.

Needles for Injection

Standard injection needles come attached to a disposable syringe. Pen needles are separate disposable needles that are screwed onto a pen device. The needles used to inject insulin and other medicines into the subcutaneous space are very fine.

The thickness of a needle is called its *gauge*. The smaller the gauge number, the thicker the needle; the larger the gauge number, the thinner the needle. For example, a 31-gauge needle is thinner than a 28-gauge needle.

Needles come in a variety of lengths. The standard length is ½ inch (12.7 mm). A "short" needle is 5/16 of an inch (8 mm). A "mini" needle is 3/16 of an inch (5 mm).

Use of short- or mini-length needles by people who are overweight or obese may affect glucose control. Glucose monitoring needs to be done to see if the needle length is affecting glucose control.

Is it okay to use the needle more than once?

Manufacturers don't recommend reuse of needles or syringes. Using a needle more than once may increase the risk of infection for some people. In reality, though, needles and syringes can be safely reused.[69] If you choose to reuse needles and syringes, follow these guidelines to reduce your risk of problems:

- Be sure to clean your skin before each injection.
- Recap the needle after use. Store the used needle at room temperature.
- Prior to each reuse, inspect your syringe and needle, as the number markings on the syringe may rub off after repeated use. After repeated injections, the needle becomes dull and may hurt more.
- Do not clean the needle with alcohol after use, as this rubs off the silicone coating, making future injections more uncomfortable.

Be mindful of adult learners' numeracy when teaching injection technique. Ask them to identify their dose on the syringe and/or calculate the total dosage when mixing 2 insulins. Comments like "I forgot my glasses" may indicate low literacy/numeracy. Involve family members as needed to ensure success.

Preparing and Taking an Injection Using a Syringe and Vial

Break down complicated tasks into smaller units. Demonstrate and then ask for return demonstration. Provide positive feedback as the learner successfully completes each step.

1. Wash your hands.
2. Make sure the skin where you plan to inject is clean.
3. Using alcohol, clean the rubber top of the vial.
4. Draw air into the syringe. *The amount of air you draw up is the same as the dose of medicine you need from the vial* (eg, if your medicine dose is 10 units, draw 10 units of air into the syringe).
5. With the vial upright, stick the needle into the rubber top of the vial. Inject the air into the vial, but don't take the needle out yet. Adding air into the vial is a very important step. It makes it easier to draw out the medicine from the vial.
6. Hold the vial and syringe firmly together as a unit, and turn it upside down.
7. Slowly draw the medicine into the syringe.
8. If you see air bubbles, slowly inject back into the vial and redraw. Tapping sharply on the syringe helps the bubbles rise to the top. Repeat until no bubbles are seen and your dose is correct.

    Air bubbles are not dangerous if they are accidentally injected into the fat layer. The reason to rid the syringe of air is to ensure that the entire dose injected is all medicine.

    Make sure the top of the black rubber stopper is aligned with the measuring line on the syringe for the dose you want.
9. Remove needle from vial.
10. Gently pinch up a layer of fat. Quickly insert the needle into the skin. Inject.
11. After waiting a few seconds, remove the needle. This allows the medicine to begin to absorb. If you remove the needle too quickly, sometimes a bit of the medicine leaks out. Do not massage the skin after injection.

Mixing 2 Kinds of Insulin in the Syringe

Some insulin types may be manually mixed together in the same syringe. Others come premixed in a vial or pen device. If you mix insulin types, they should be of the same brand (eg, Humulin® or Novolin® or Relion®/Novolin®). Be sure that the time delay between mixing and injecting is about the same each time. Otherwise, the action of the mixed insulin may vary from injection to injection.

There are some insulin types that should *never* be mixed together. Never mix long-acting insulin detemir or glargine with another type of insulin in the same syringe. When taking detemir or glargine, don't use a syringe that was previously used for another type of insulin.

If mixing NPH and regular insulin, always draw up the regular (clear) insulin into the syringe first. This prevents accidentally injecting NPH into the vial of regular insulin, which will slow down the action of the regular insulin.

American Association of Diabetes Educators©

Steps for Mixing Clear and Cloudy Insulin (Regular + NPH; Lispro + NPL; Aspart + NPA)

1. Wash your hands.
2. Clean the skin where you plan to inject.
3. Using alcohol, clean the rubber top of BOTH vials.
4. Draw air into the syringe. The amount of air you draw up is the same as your dose of CLOUDY insulin.
5. With the vial upright, stick the needle into the rubber top of the vial of CLOUDY insulin. Inject the air into the vial and remove the needle.
6. Draw air into the syringe a second time. The amount of air you draw up is the same as your dose of CLEAR insulin.
7. With the vial upright, stick the needle into the rubber top of the vial of CLEAR insulin. Inject the air into the vial, but don't remove the needle.
8. Hold the vial and syringe firmly together as a unit, and turn it upside down.
9. Slowly draw the CLEAR insulin into the syringe.
10. If you see air bubbles, slowly inject back into the vial and redraw. Tapping sharply on the syringe helps the bubbles rise to the top. Repeat until no bubbles are seen and your dose is correct.
11. Remove needle from the vial.
12. Now, stick the needle into the rubber top of the vial of CLOUDY insulin.
13. Slowly draw the CLOUDY insulin into the syringe until you reach your total insulin dose.
14. Gently pinch up a layer of fat. Quickly insert the needle into the skin. Inject.
15. After waiting a few seconds, remove the needle. This allows the medicine to begin to absorb. If you remove the needle too quickly, sometimes the medicine leaks out a bit. Do not massage the skin after injection.

Your total dose equals the units of CLEAR insulin *plus* the units of the CLOUDY insulin.

Preparing and Taking an Injection Using a Pen Device

There are many brands of injection pens. Follow the manufacturer's directions for setting your dose and injecting using a pen device. Disposable needles are purchased separately and may require a prescription. Always remove the needle from the pen device in between injections. If the needle stays on the device, medicine may leak out and/or air may leak in.

Before a pen device may be used, a procedure called an *air shot* is done. Sometimes this is called *priming the pen*. To perform an air shot, dial the device as directed to expel any air that may be in the cartridge. Follow the manufacturer's directions for when to perform an air shot and how far to dial the device.

Can I fix all of my insulin syringes for the week all at once?

Prefilled Syringes

Single formulations or mixed insulin can be safely prefilled in syringes and used later on. Follow these guidelines[66,67]:

- Prefilled syringes must be kept in the refrigerator.
- Use prefilled syringes of insulin within 21 to 30 days.

- Store syringes containing a mix of insulin upright or at an angle, with the needle pointing up. This will help avoid problems with the needle becoming plugged with dried insulin particles.
- Cloudy insulin (NPH, or a mixture of intermediate-acting insulin with another insulin) must be rolled several times between the palms to properly mix the 2 insulin types before injecting. Also, slightly pull back and forth on the plunger to help agitate the insulin before injecting.

Disposal of Used Needles

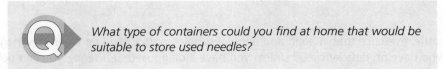

What type of containers could you find at home that would be suitable to store used needles?

Used needles are a health hazard. They should be stored in a container that is shatterproof and has a lid that holds firm if the container is dropped.

Heavy plastic containers like detergent or bleach jugs are ideal. When the needles are ready for disposal, the top of the container should be tightly closed and the words *medical sharps* written on the container. Another option is to use a store-bought sharps disposal unit. Follow your local sanitation department rules for disposal of either type of container. Some areas allow marked sharps containers to be placed in the regular trash. **Sharps containers should never be placed in the recycle bin.**

Never break the needle off the syringe. This practice allows very tiny shards of metal to scatter when the needle is broken. These tiny metal pieces could penetrate your skin and cause an infection. Place the entire syringe into the sharps container. Another alternative is to use a needle clipper, which safely breaks off the tip of the needle and stores it inside the unit.

Advanced Detail

Traveling with Injectable Medicines[70]

When you travel, take extra care to keep your injectable medicines safe from harm. The cargo compartments of buses, airplanes, or trains, as well as the trunk of a car, may be too hot or too cold for your medicines. Carry all injectable medicines on board with you when traveling by these modes of transportation.

Be aware of the current Transportation Safety Administration (TSA) regulations that apply to most modes of public transportation. Notify the TSA officer that you have diabetes and have the supplies with you. The following diabetes-related supplies and equipment are allowed through the TSA checkpoint after screening:

- Injectable medication in vials, injector devices, and pen devices. Insulin and other injectable medication must be clearly identified.
- Unused syringes, when accompanied by injectable medication.
- Used syringes, carried inside a sharps disposal unit or similar hard-surface container.
- Insulin pump and supplies, when accompanied by insulin.

If you wear an insulin pump, you can ask the TSA officer for a full-body pat-down and a visual inspection of the pump OR you may go through the metal detector. You should tell the officer that the pump cannot be removed, since it is connected to your body.

Advanced Detail

Vitamins and Minerals

Should I take vitamins or mineral supplements?

There is no scientific evidence that vitamin and mineral supplements should be taken *routinely* by people with diabetes who have no deficiencies.[71] Unless you have a diagnosed deficiency, you can get all the vitamins and minerals you need for good health from a balanced diet. If your diabetes has been out of control for a time, you may have lost water-soluble vitamins (eg, vitamin C, B-complex vitamins) due to excess urination.[72]

Some people can benefit from multivitamins, however: the elderly, women who are pregnant or breastfeeding, strict vegetarians, or those on calorie-restricted diets.[73] It's important to understand that over-the-counter (OTC) supplements do not require the strict regulation by the FDA that prescription drugs do. However, any health claims that a supplement prevents disease must be backed up by studies and approved by the FDA.

Vitamins E, C, and Beta Carotene

Health claims that antioxidants such as vitamins E, C, and beta carotene prevent cancer and heart disease have not been proven in clinical studies. In fact, megadoses of vitamin E, vitamin C, and beta carotene can cause diarrhea, bleeding, and toxic reactions.[74,75]

Chromium

Chromium is a trace mineral that has a role in insulin action and glucose tolerance. There is no scientific evidence that people with diabetes are chromium deficient, though. Research has not yet shown a clear benefit from supplementing with chromium, so its use is not recommended at this time.[74] In 2005, the FDA rejected health claims that chromium picolinate reduced the risk of diabetes complications caused by insulin resistance, high blood sugar, or type 2 diabetes.[76]

Vanadium

Vanadium is a trace element that occurs naturally in foods such as black pepper, parsley, dill seeds, mushrooms, spinach, and shellfish.[76] Very small, short-term studies have been done in humans that showed that high doses of vanadium lowered glucose levels and A1C in those with diabetes. Other studies have shown that there is a potential for toxic accumulation. At this time, there is a lack of solid scientific evidence that vanadium is safe or effective for use as a supplement.[77-80]

Alpha Lipoic Acid (ALA)

Alpha lipoic acid is a vitamin-like substance, also known as thioctic acid. It is naturally produced in the liver and also found in many foods (including spinach, broccoli, tomatoes, garden peas, Brussels sprouts, and rice bran).[81] Strong studies show that using oral ALA supplements for up to 2 years improves the symptoms of diabetic peripheral neuropathy. Because there was a lack of side effects shown in the studies, ALA can be considered a valid treatment option for those with diabetic neuropathy.[82]

Complementary and Alternative Medications

What Is Complementary and Alternative Medicine?[83]

Complementary and alternative medicine (CAM) is defined as healthcare practices and treatments that are not generally considered part of mainstream Western medicine. The National Center for Complementary and Alternative Medicine (NCCAM) is a federal agency (part of the National Institutes of Health) whose purpose is to conduct rigorous CAM research. NCCAM helps the public and healthcare professionals understand which CAM therapies have been proven to be safe and effective. Complementary therapies are those that are *used along with* conventional medicine; alternative therapies are *used in place of* conventional medicine. *Integrative medicine* refers to therapy that *combines* conventional medicine with CAM for which there is proven safety and efficacy.

Who Uses CAM?[84]

According to the NCCAM, women with higher levels of education and income make up the largest group of CAM users. In the United States, CAM is used by 50% of American Indians and Alaska Natives, 43% of Caucasians, 40% of Asians, 26% of blacks, and 24% of Latinos.

Common CAM Usage[85]

The type of CAM products that are most used are the non-vitamin, non-mineral natural products. The top 10 CAM products used in 2007 in the United States were (starting with most used): fish oil/omega-3, glucosamine, echinacea, flaxseed oil, ginseng, combination herb pills, ginkgo biloba, chondroitin, garlic supplements, and coenzyme Q-10.

Is CAM Safe?

It's important to understand that OTC supplements do not require the same strict regulation by the FDA that prescription drugs do. However, any health claims that a supplement prevents disease must be backed up by studies and approved by the FDA. Most CAM products are not recommended during pregnancy, so if you are a woman considering having a baby you should consult your healthcare provider before taking any herbal or dietary supplements.

Side Effects and Drug Interactions

Side effects and drug interactions are 2 primary concerns with CAM therapies.[86-97] CAM therapies can interact with prescription drugs as well as with other CAM therapies. CAM therapies can exaggerate the effects of prescribed medications. Conversely, they can diminish the action of prescribed medications, so that their effects are subtherapeutic. Fewer than 40% of patients inform their healthcare provider about CAM use.[89] The provider, unaware of the CAM usage, may attribute side effects to a prescribed medication, and subsequently discontinue it.

Educators should assess for the use of CAM products. Since so many patients use CAM, it is advisable that the educator have at least a basic knowledge of the most common CAM products used for the treatment of diabetes.

For more detail about CAM safety concerns, refer to Chapter 20, Biologically Based Practices: A Focus on Dietary Supplements for Diabetes, in *The Art and Science of Diabetes Self-Management Education Desk Reference*, 3rd edition. The following instructional content is included for 2 reasons: (1) to respond to patients' queries about specific supplements that are marketed for diabetes control or the prevention of complications, and (2) to facilitate effective decision making for those patients who currently use CAM.

American Association of Diabetes Educators©

Advanced Detail

I read in a natural health magazine that certain herbs are good for lowering blood glucose. Is this true?

There are a number of supplements on the market—some are plant-based, others are not—that claim to improve diabetes control or help treat diabetes complications (see Table 4.4). They may be labeled as an *herbal supplement* or a *nutraceutical*. Even though these products are *natural*, it does not necessarily mean that they are safe. Like prescription medications, some supplements can have dangerous side effects. They can also interact with other supplements as well as with prescribed medicines. They may cause your prescribed medicines to have an exaggerated effect, much like taking an overdose. Or, supplements can cause your prescribed medicines to lose their effectiveness.

Always inform your provider of all the OTC products or natural remedies that you take. If your provider does not know about everything you take, it's hard for him or her to make informed decisions about your care. Here's an example:

- The patient goes to the doctor complaining of fast heart rate and swelling in the feet. Her blood pressure is also higher than usual. These symptoms are common side effects and drug interactions of a supplement that she has recently started taking (ginseng).
- The doctor doesn't know about the supplement. He decides to lower the dosage of her heart medicine to slow the heart rate down to normal. He increases the dose of her diuretic (water pill) to lower the blood pressure and ease the swelling in her feet.
- Days later, the patient becomes very sick with heart problems caused by changing the prescription medicines. She is hospitalized.
- If the doctor had known about the supplement, he could have advised her to stop taking it because of its known side effects and drug interaction with her diuretic.

Supplements vary in their ability to carry out their advertised claims. It's important to understand that OTC supplements do not require the same strict regulation by the FDA that prescription drugs do. However, any health claims that a supplement prevents disease must be backed up by studies and approved by the FDA.

TABLE 4.4 Common Supplements Used to Lower Blood Glucose

Name of Supplement	Possible Side Effects	Possible Drug Interactions	Summary
Aloe gel (Desert plant, *Liliaceae*. Spanish name: *savila*)	• Cathartic effects, which may cause fluid and electrolyte imbalance	• Hypoglycemia possible, if taking with insulin secretagogues • Blood loss during surgery if the anesthetic sevoflurane is used*	• Not enough evidence to support its use • Not recommended as an oral supplement
Banaba (tea made from leaves of crepe myrtle tree grown in Southeast Asia and Australia, *Lagerstroemia speciosa L*)	• None reported	• Hypoglycemia possible, if taking with insulin secretagogues	• Only very small studies have been done • No long-term safety information available
Bilberry (dried fruit extract of berry from *Vaccinium myrtillus* plant)	• Mild gastrointestinal distress • Skin rashes	• None known	• No studies have been done in humans to show effectiveness in lowering glucose.

American Association of Diabetes Educators©

Module 4 *Taking Medication* 135

TABLE 4.4 Common Supplements Used to Lower Blood Glucose *(continued)*

Name of Supplement	Possible Side Effects	Possible Drug Interactions	Summary
Bitter melon (*Mamordica charantia*, grown in tropical areas)	• Gastrointestinal discomfort and vomiting • Hypoglycemic coma • Serious onset of anemia from destruction of red blood cells (favism) • Can cause miscarriage	• Hypoglycemia possible, if taking with insulin secretagogues	• Safe to be used as a food • May be unsafe in persons of Mediterranean descent (higher risk of favism)[†] • May be unsafe in women of childbearing age[†]
Caiapo (a white sweet potato grown in Japan, *Ipomoea batatas*)	• Constipation • Gastrointestinal pain • Gas accumulation with distention	• Hypoglycemia possible, if taking with insulin secretagogues	• Promising research shows that it significantly reduces fasting and postmeal glucose, lowers weight, and reduces cholesterol[‡] • No long-term safety information available
Cinnamon (from the bark of a tropical evergreen tree, *Cinnamomum cassia*)	• None reported	• Hypoglycemia possible, if taking with insulin secretagogues	• Studies show that it significantly improves fasting glucose and lipids[§]
Fenugreek (a legume related to peanuts and chickpeas, *Trigonella foenum-graecum*)	• Diarrhea, gas • Uterine contractions • Allergic reactions	• May increase anticoagulant effect of warfarin • May increase anticoagulant effect of herbs such as garlic, boldo, and ginger	
Ginseng (a root of ginseng plant, *Panax ginseng CA Meyer* or *Panax quinquefolius L*)	• Insomnia • Headache • Restlessness • Increased blood pressure • Increased heart rate • Breast pain • Mood changes, nervousness	• Decreases the effectiveness of warfarin • Decreases the effectiveness of diuretics • Increases effect of estrogen • Possibly increases the effects of certain analgesics and antidepressants • Hypoglycemia possible, if taking with insulin secretagogues	• Studies show that it may lower glucose in those with type 2 diabetes[¶] • Safety questionable due to effects on blood pressure and central nervous system
Gymnema (plant from milkweed family found in India and Africa, *Gymnena sylvestre R.Br.*)	• May cause hypoglycemia	• Hypoglycemia possible, if taking with insulin secretagogues	• Limited evidence of effectiveness in humans
Milk thistle (plant from the aster family, *Silybum marianum*)	• Gastrointestinal upset and diarrhea • Allergic reactions possible if allergic to ragweed, daisies, marigolds, and chrysanthemums	• Beneficial interactions in those with liver disease. May attenuate liver toxicity from acetaminophen, antipsychotic, halothane and alcohol.[#]	• Long-term safety and exact doses are unknown

American Association of Diabetes Educators©

TABLE 4.4 Common Supplements Used to Lower Blood Glucose *(continued)*

Name of Supplement	Possible Side Effects	Possible Drug Interactions	Summary
Nopal (prickly pear cactus leaf, *Opuntia streptacantha*)	• Diarrhea, nausea, abdominal fullness • Increased volume of stool	• Improved blood glucose with sulfonylurea use	• Safe as a food • Small studies show it decreases postmeal glucose • May help lower glucose when cooked or taken as a supplement • No long-term studies done on oral supplement form

*B Ludvik, B Neuffer, G Pacini, "Efficacy of *Ipomoea batatas* (Caiapo) on diabetes control in type 2 diabetes subjects treated with diet," *Diabetes Care* 27 (2004): 436-40.

†A Khan, M Safdar, MM Ali Khan, et al, "Cinnamon improves glucose and lipids of people with type 2 diabetes," *Diabetes Care* 26 (2003): 3215-8.

‡V Vuksan, JL Sievenpiper, VY Koo, et al, "American ginseng (*Panax quinquefolius* L) reduces postprandial glycemia in nondiabetic subjects and subjects with type 2 diabetes mellitus," *Arch Intern Med* 160 (2000): 1009-13.

§EA Sotaniemi, E Haapakoski, A Rautio, "Ginseng therapy in non-insulin dependent diabetic patients," *Diabetes Care* 18 (1995): 1373-5.

¶V Vuksan, MP Stavro, Sievenpiper JL, et al, "Similar postprandial glycemic reductions with escalation of dose and administration time of American ginseng in type 2 diabetes," *Diabetes Care* 23 (2000): 1221-6; J Pepping, "Alternative therapies—milk thistle: *Silybum marianum*," *Am J Health Syst Pharm* 56 (1999): 1195-7; MS Knowles, EF Holton, RA Swanson, eds, *The Adult Learner: The Definitive Classic in Adult Education and Human Resource Development* (Houston: Gulf Professional Publishing, 1998).

#JM Jellin, PJ Gregory, et al, *Pharmacist's Letter/Prescriber's Letter Natural Medicines Comprehensive Database*, 13th ed (Stockton, Calif: Therapeutic Research Faculty; 2013); J Pepping, "Alternative therapies: milk thistle (*Silybum marianum*) for the therapy of liver disease," *Am J Gastroenterol* 93 (1998): 139-43.

Source: Table adapted from L Shane-McWhorter, "Biologically Based Practices: A Focus on Dietary Supplements for Diabetes," in C Mensing, ed, *The Art and Science of Diabetes Self-Management Education: Desk Reference*, 3rd ed (Chicago: American Association of Diabetes Educators, 2014), 586-7.

Identifying Barriers to Taking Medication

Even though you know that taking prescribed medication is good for you, there may be barriers that prevent you from making healthy choices about taking medication. For every barrier there may be many possible solutions.

What might work to overcome this barrier? Let's brainstorm together and learn from one another's experiences.

From Malcolm Knowles, the father of adult learning theory:

"Lessons that make the most sense are those that deal with authentic responses of learners to a particular problem:

- The kinds of questions they will face
- The obstacles they will face
- Their attitudes
- The possible solutions they will offer"[98]

Reality Scenario	Problem Solving Possible Solutions/What Would *You* Do?
Emotional: perception that need for meds = failure *I just want another chance at diet and exercise. I know I can do it. I don't want to go on meds.*	• Understand that type 2 diabetes is naturally progressive. Needing medicine, even insulin, is not a sign that you have failed. • Prolonging medicine therapy will allow your blood glucose to stay too high for too long. This can lead to complications, which would require treatment with even more medications.
Emotional: perception that need for meds = worsening diabetes *Being on meds means my diabetes is getting worse.*	• Understand that type 2 diabetes is naturally progressive. Needing medicine, even insulin, is not a sign that you have failed. • Putting off medicine therapy will allow your blood glucose to stay too high for too long. This can lead to complications. • Taking a "little bit" of medicine now might keep you from taking more medicine later (eg, slowing progression and avoiding or reducing severity of potential complications).
Insulin causes blindness.	Validate that the belief about insulin causing blindness is common in certain populations. Explore the patient's health beliefs. Ascertain in what context the patient heard about insulin and blindness being linked. Explain what causes complications like blindness, and how glycemic control (often by using insulin) can help to prevent them.
Health beliefs: lack of confidence in effectiveness of therapy *Why should I take these meds? I'm going to end up with complications like my mother anyway. It's inevitable.*	Discuss the patient's actual risk of complications with adherence to medicine plan. The patient may be surprised that the risk for complications is much lower than he or she actually believed. Give examples of patients who felt the same way and who have had success managing their diabetes with medications when they initially thought they would not. • Try to look at it as an experiment. Try it for a while and see if it works.
Concern about side effects *The doctor said this medicine might cause weight gain. I'm supposed to be losing weight, not gaining it.*	• Think about the positives of the medicine: blood glucose control, lowering risk for complications. • Consider other parts of your self-care plan that affect weight, like your meal plan and your activity level. Are you taking in too many calories? Are you regularly active? Making needed adjustments in these areas may help you avoid, or at least limit, weight gain.
I feel bad when I take it, so I stopped.	• Be sure you are taking the medicine correctly: right dose and right time (in relation to food, etc). • Talk to your provider about side effects that persist despite taking your medication properly. There may be an alternative medication with fewer side effects.
Sometimes I take less medicine than I should. I don't want my blood sugar to go too low. I had a bad experience with hypoglycemia when I first started my medication.	• Monitor blood glucose more often. • Time medication with meals to avoid lows. • Be prepared if hypoglycemia occurs, and treat right away.

Reality Scenario	Problem Solving Possible Solutions/What Would You Do?
Financial I can't afford my medication.	• Ask your provider for samples to tide you over until you can afford to buy your prescription. • Ask your provider or pharmacist if a "therapeutic equivalent" or less expensive generic form of the medication could be used. Ask your pharmacist how he or she can save you money. • Patient assistance programs may be able to help if you qualify for assistance. See the "Resources" section at the end of this module for contact information for pharmaceutical assistance programs. It can be used as a patient handout. • Consider any other sources of support besides insurance that may be able to assist. • Consider safe reuse of needles/syringes if you can't afford to use a new syringe or needle with each injection.
Complex regimen I've got so many medicines to keep up with.	• Ask provider if any of your medications can be combined. • Ask if a simpler dosing regimen is possible. • Use a daily pill-case to simplify pill-taking each day.
Lack of organization Gets distracted, and often misses insulin dose or diabetes medication. Takes diabetes medication(s) at the wrong time, due to poor organization. I keep forgetting to take my medicine.	• Build in some reminders to take your meds (alarm on your watch, cell phone, or PDA). • Until you get a firm habit in place, post little reminder notes to help you remember when your medication is due. Remind yourself that your needs are important, that you are worth the effort to take your medicine. • Use a daily pill-case system. Put your medication where you will see it before the first dose is due every day. • Organize all your diabetes supplies in one central place so you have everything you need when it's time to take your medication. Include the following supplies (as applicable): medication, insulin or insulin pen, syringes or pen needles, alcohol wipes, meter, lancets, strips, and logbook. • If your medication is due during work hours, keep a small kit with supplies at your workplace. If you don't have a safe, temperature-controlled area to keep your supplies at work, carry a portable kit with you. A variety of insulin cooling cases are available through the Internet. Your local pharmacy may also carry such kits.
Before I know it, I'm out of medicine. Then, it takes several days to get the prescription refilled.	• Set up a routine: Mark your calendar to remind you to refill your pill case on the same day every week. When you have less than 10 days' medication remaining in the pill bottle, call for a refill.
Physical limitations I have trouble drawing up insulin because of arthritis/neuropathy in my hands.	• Consider alternative ways of loading syringe using an adaptive device. • Consider using an insulin pen. • Have someone else draw up syringes ahead of time.
I have trouble drawing up insulin because of my vision.	• Consider using a syringe magnifier. • Consider using insulin pen (with magnifier, if available). • Ask a reliable person to help fill syringe.
I have poor vision, so managing my medication is difficult.	• Use a magnifier to see pill bottle labels. • Consider adaptive devices such as the Timex Weekly Medication Manager, which is a talking pill organizer widely available through catalogs. • Ask a reliable person for help to fill your pill-case system once a week.

Reality Scenario	Problem Solving Possible Solutions/What Would *You* Do?
Cognitive limitations Limited cognitive skills to calculate amount of medication to take or when to take it.	Get patient's family involved if possible. • Ask provider to simplify regimen. • Use aids like pill boxes. • Use prefilled insulin syringes, if applicable.

For Those Prescribed Injected Medication

Reality Scenario	Problem Solving Possible Solutions/What Would *You* Do?
Emotional: fear of needles/pain *I don't want to stick myself. I'm afraid of needles. Shots hurt!*	• Use the thinnest gauge needle possible. • Use sites with fewer nerve endings, like the abdomen, for injection. Consider having the patient try a saline self-injection to help allay fear. Consider first demonstrating an injection on yourself.
Emotional: perception of stigma *I don't want to be on the needle. It makes me feel like an addict.*	Discuss and validate patient's feelings. Help the patient to weigh positives against the negatives, and align desire for good health outcomes with taking insulin.
Emotional/social *It's embarrassing to have to take my insulin when I'm out with other people, so I just skip it sometimes.* *Insulin makes me gain weight.*	Discuss patient's agenda.* • If you use a syringe and vial, consider switching to an insulin pen, which is more discreet to use in public places. Discuss patient's agenda.* It's true that insulin can cause weight gain. But also realize that there is a strong link between DKA and omitted insulin if you have type 1 diabetes.† This is a big risk to take. Consider other parts of your self-care plan that affect weight, like your meal plan and your activity level. Are you taking in too many calories? Are you regularly active? Making needed adjustments in these areas may help you avoid, or at least limit, weight gain.

*The patient's problem-solving efforts for the scenarios *involving intentional omission of insulin* may uncover his/her attitudes and beliefs about having diabetes, as well as potential emotional problems, such as depression, anxiety, or alcohol and drug abuse. These must be investigated and addressed first in order to successfully resolve the secondary problem of omitting insulin (G Boden, X Chen, J Ruiz, et al, "Effects of vanadyl sulfate on carbohydrate and lipid metabolism in patients with non-insulin dependent diabetes mellitus," *Metabolism* 45 [1996]: 1130-5).

†AB Goldfine, DC Simonson, F Folli, et al, "Metabolic effects of sodium meta-vanadate in humans with insulin-dependent and non-insulin-dependent diabetes mellitus: in vivo and in vitro studies," *J Clin Endocrinol Metab* 80 (1995): 3311-20; L Packer, EH Witt, HJ Tritschler, "Alpha-lipoic acid as a biological antioxidant," *Free Rad Biol Med* 19 (1995): 227-50; TS Foster, "Efficacy and safety of α-lipoic acid supplementation in the treatment of symptomatic diabetic neuropathy," *Diabetes Educ* 33, no. 1 (2007): 111-7.

Identifying Facilitators for Taking Medication

As important as it is to identify barriers to taking medication, it's just as important to consider the positives in our situation—facilitators. Looking deeper, you may find that there are more positives than you thought.

What are some things that help you take medications as prescribed?

Common Facilitators

- Social support—family members, coworkers, work environment, etc.
- Community resources—medication assistance programs such as Partnership for Prescription Assistance, NeedyMeds, health departments, and free clinics.

See the "Resources" section at the end of this module for more information on these assistance programs, and the Diabetes Resources Appendix for a listing of state health departments. Use these as patient handouts.

- Reminders and cues—reminder notes, reminder alarm, visual reminders, notes of encouragement (positive affirmations).
- Rewards—incentives to maintain motivation.

Setting a SMART Goal for Taking Medication

S—Specific: not vague
M—Measurable: you can measure it (how much, how often, etc)
A—Attainable: challenging, but not out of reach
R—Realistic: given person's situation, can it be done?
T—Timeline: short term, for next week or two

The participant sets an individual goal for taking medication. The educator and the participant schedule a date in which to evaluate progress with behavior change.

Using a mnemonic like SMART to help remember an idea can be a useful teaching tool, especially for those with verbal/auditory intelligence.

Follow-up/Outcomes Measurement

Per the Standards for Outcomes Measurement of Diabetes Self-Management Education, the **first follow-up should be conducted within 2 to 4 weeks** after the initial teaching session on taking oral medication. **Patients new to injection therapy** (insulin, GLP-1 agonists, pramlintide) should have a **follow-up earlier** than 2 weeks after the initial teaching session. At this follow-up, success in implementing medication-taking behavior can be assessed. **Subsequent follow-up is recommended at 3- to 6-month intervals thereafter.** Use the following table as a guide for identifying outcomes measures and how to measure them. Measurement of these outcomes may be objective or subjective.

The exception to this schedule would be during pregnancy. The first follow-up should be conducted within 1 week and subsequent visits at 2 to 4 weeks.

Self-Care Behavior: Taking Medication Outcomes Measures	Self-Care Behavior: Taking Medication Methods of Measurement
Immediate outcome: Learning Immediate outcomes of learning can be assessed right away after the educational encounter. Immediate outcomes include: K: Acquiring *knowledge* (*what to do*) S: Acquiring *skills* (*how to do it*) CM: Developing *confidence and motivation* (*want to do it*) PS: Developing *problem-solving/coping skills* to overcome barrier (*can do it*)	Immediate outcomes of learning can be measured by patient knowledge testing (paper-and-pen testing, or questioning to determine that patient understands information taught). Immediate outcomes for acquiring a skill can be measured by patient's demonstration of that skill. Following are various methods of measuring immediate outcomes for the self-care behavior of *taking medication*.
Name, dose, and frequency of medication (K)	<u>Subjective:</u> Patient names medication and states proper dose and frequency.
Purpose of medication (K)	<u>Subjective:</u> Patient states purpose of his/her medication.
Medication side effects (K)	<u>Subjective:</u> Patient explains relevant side effects to watch for.
Action to take for side effects (K)	<u>Subjective:</u> Patient describes action to minimize side effects, action to take if side effects occur.
Important precautions about medication (K)	<u>Subjective:</u> Patient demonstrates awareness of relevant precautions about medication.
Recognition of efficacy (K)	<u>Subjective:</u> Patient relates medication efficacy to blood glucose status.
Storage and transport of medication (K)	<u>Subjective:</u> Patient describes proper storage and transport of medication.
Injection preparation and technique (K,S)	<u>Subjective:</u> Patient self-report/description of how injection is prepared and taken. <u>Objective:</u> Patient prepares and takes injection using correct technique.
Handling of used injection equipment (K,S)	<u>Subjective:</u> Patient describes proper disposal of used needles. <u>Objective:</u> Patient demonstrates proper disposal of used needles.
Medication dose adjustment per monitoring results, or changes in eating or activity (K,S)	<u>Subjective:</u> Patient self-report of when, how, and why medication is adjusted. <u>Objective:</u> Review of medication adjustments written in patient documentation (logbook).
Prevention, recognition, and treatment of hypoglycemia related to medication (K,S)	<u>Subjective:</u> Patient self-report of how hypoglycemia is handled.
Potential barriers and facilitators to taking medication (PS)	<u>Subjective:</u> Considering his/her individual situation, patient describes anticipated obstacle(s) that may limit the ability to take medications appropriately. Patient describes facilitators that may help him/her take medications appropriately.
Strategy to overcome potential barriers to taking medication (PS)	<u>Subjective:</u> Patient develops a plan to deal with anticipated obstacle(s) to taking medication.

American Association of Diabetes Educators©

Diabetes Education Curriculum

Self-Care Behavior: Taking Medication Outcomes Measures	Self-Care Behavior: Taking Medication Methods of Measurement
Intermediate outcome: Behavior change	Intermediate outcomes measures can be assessed over time: after the educational encounter and once the patient has had adequate time to implement new behavior(s) in a real-life setting. *Behavior change* is an intermediate outcomes measure. It is the ultimate outcome of DSME/T. At follow-up intervals, knowledge and skills (discussed above) should be reassessed, as well as behavior change.
Medication-Taking Regimen (S)	<u>Subjective:</u> Patient self-report of taking medication—frequency of specific dose. <u>Objective:</u> Pill-count; review of pharmacy refill record.
Preparation and injection technique (S)	<u>Subjective:</u> Patient self-report/description of how injection is prepared and taken. <u>Objective:</u> Patient prepares and takes injection using correct technique.
Medication adjustment per monitoring results, or changes in eating or activity (PS)	<u>Subjective:</u> Patient self-report of when, how, and why medication is adjusted. <u>Objective:</u> Review of medication adjustments documented by patient (eg, notes in logbook).
Barriers and strategies for barrier resolution (PS)	<u>Subjective:</u> Patient self-report of barriers faced, facilitators and strategies used, as patient made efforts to implement medication-taking behaviors.
Plan for future behavior change (PS)	<u>Subjective:</u> Patient self-report of medication-taking goals and behavior strategies going forward.

REFERENCES

1. Odegard PS, Capossia K. Medication taking and diabetes: a systematic review of the literature. Diabetes Educ. 2007;33(6):1014-29.

2. Diabetes Control and Complications Trial Group. The effect of intensive treatment of diabetes on the development and progression of long-term complications in insulin-dependent diabetes mellitus. N Engl J Med. 1993;329:977-86.

3. UK Prospective Diabetes Study Group. Intensive blood glucose control with sulphonylurea or insulin compared with conventional treatment and risk for complications in patients with type 2 diabetes (UKPDS 33). Lancet. 1998; 352:837-53.

4. UK Prospective Diabetes Study Group. Effect of intensive blood glucose control with metformin on complications in overweight patients with type 2 diabetes (UKPDS 34). Lancet. 1998;352:854-62.

5. Ohkubo Y, Kishikawa H, Araki E, et al. Intensive insulin therapy prevents the progression of diabetic microvascular complications in Japanese patients with non-insulin-dependent diabetes mellitus: a randomized prospective 6-year study. Diabetes Res Clin Pract. 1995;28:103-17.

6. Stratton IM, Adler AI, Neil HA, et al. Association of glycaemia with macrovascular and microvascular complications of type 2 diabetes (UKPDS 35): prospective observational study. BMJ. 2000;321:405-12.

7. Hoerger TJ, Segel JE, Gregg EW. Is glycemic control improving in US adults? Diabetes Care. 2008;31(1):81-6.

8. Nathan DM, Buse JB, Davidson MB, et al. Management of hyperglycemia in type 2 diabetes: a consensus algorithm for the initiation and adjustment of therapy. Diabetes Care. 2006;29(8):1963-72.

9. Anderson RJ, Freedland KE, Clouse RE, Lustman PJ. The prevalence of comorbid depression in adults with diabetes. Diabetes Care. 2001;24(6):1069-78.

10. Kilbourne AM, Reynold CF, Good CB, et al. How does depression influence diabetes medication adherence in older patients? Am J Geriatr Psychiatry. 2005;13(3):202-10.

11. Lin EHB, Oliver M, Katon W, et al. Relationship of depression and diabetes self-care, medication adherence, and preventive care. Diabetes Care. 2004;27:2154-60.

12. Odegard PS, Gray SL. Barriers to medication adherence in poorly controlled diabetes mellitus. Diabetes Educ. 2008;34(4):692-7.

13. Morisky DE, Green LW, Levine DM. Concurrent and predictive validity of a self-reported measure of medication adherence. Med Care. 1986;24(1):67-74.

14. Rosen MI, Rigsby MO, Salahi JT, et al. Electronic monitoring and counseling to improve medication adherence. Behav Res Ther. 2004;42:409-22.

15. Dowse R, Ehlers MS. Pictograms for conveying medicine instructions: comprehension in various South African language groups. South African Journal of Science. 2004;100:687-93.

16. Dowse R, Ehlers MS. Pictograms in pharmacy. Int J Pharm Pract. 1998;6:109-18.

17. US Pharmacopeia. USP pictograms (cited 2015 Jul 13). On the Internet at: http://www.usp.org/audiences/consumers/pictograms/form.html.

18. Ary DV, Toobert D, Wilson W, et al. Patient perspective on factors contributing to noncompliance to diabetes regimen. Diabetes Care. 1986;9(2):168-72.

19. Klepser TB, Kelly MW. Metformin hydrochloride: an antihyperglycemic agent. Am J Health Syst Pharm. 1997;54:893.

20. Kirpichnikov D, McFarlane SI, Sowers JR. Metformin: an update. Ann Intern Med. 2002;137:25.

21. Rowan JA, Hague WM, Gao W, Battin MR, Moore MP; MiG Trial Investigators. Metformin versus insulin for the treatment of gestational diabetes. N Engl J Med. 2008;358:2003-15.

22. Gui J, Liu Q, Feng L. Metformin vs insulin in the management of gestational diabetes: a meta-analysis. PLoS One. 2013;8:e64585.

23. Sisson EM, Dixon DL. Pharmacologic therapies for glucose management. In: Mensing C, ed. The Art and Science of Diabetes Self-Management Education Desk Reference. 3rd ed. Chicago: American Association of Diabetes Educators; 2014:491-540.

24. Facts and Comparisons 4.0 Online. St. Louis, Mo: Wolters Kluwer Health, Inc; 2009.

25. Mudaliar S, Henry RR. New oral therapies for type 2 diabetes mellitus: the glitazones for insulin sensitizers. Annu Rev Med. 2001;52:239.

26. Nesto RW, Bell D, Bonow RO, et al. Thiazolidinedione use, fluid retention, and congestive heart failure: a consensus statement of the American Heart Association and the American Diabetes Association. Diabetes Care. 2004;27(1):256-63.

27. Zieve FJ, Kalain MF, Schwartz SL, et al. Results of the glucose-lowering effect of WelChol® study (GLOWS): a randomized, double-blind, placebo-controlled pilot study evaluating the effect of colesevelam hydrochloride on glycemic control in subjects with type 2 diabetes. Clin Ther. 2007;29:74-83.

28. Nathan D, Buse JB, Davidson MB, et al. Management of hyperglycemia in type 2 diabetes: a consensus algorithm for the initiation and adjustment of therapy. Update regarding thiazolidinediones: a consensus statement from the American Diabetes Association and the European Association for the Study of Diabetes. Diabetes Care. 2008;31(1):173-5.

29. Psaty BM, Furberg CD. Rosiglitazone and cardiovascular risk. N Engl J Med. 2007;356:2522-4.

30. Drazen JM, Morrissey S, Curfman GD. Rosiglitazone—continued uncertainty about safety. N Engl J Med. 2007;357:63-4.

31. Nathan DM. Rosiglitazone and cardiotoxicity—weighing the evidence. N Engl J Med. 2007;357:64-6.

32. Psaty BM, Furberg CD. The record on rosiglitazone and the risk of myocardial infarction. N Engl J Med. 2007;357:67-9.

144   Diabetes Education Curriculum

33. Lago RM, Singh PP, Nesto RW. Congestive heart failure and cardiovascular death in patients with prediabetes and type 2 diabetes given thiazolidinediones: a meta-analysis of randomized clinical trials. Lancet. 2007;370: 1129-36.

34. Lincoff AM, Wolski K, Nicholls SJ, Nissen SE. Pioglitazone and risk of cardiovascular events in patients with type 2 diabetes mellitus: a meta-analysis of randomized trials. JAMA. 2007;298:1180-8.

35. Singh S, Loke YK, Furberg CD. Thiazolidinediones and heart failure: a teleoanalysis. Diabetes Care. 2007;30: 2248-53.

36. Raz I, Hanefeld M, Xu L, et al. Efficacy and safety of the dipeptidyl peptidase-4 inhibitor sitagliptin as monotherapy in patients with type 2 diabetes mellitus. Diabetologia. 2006;49:2564-71.

37. Bays HE, Cohen DE. Rationale and design of a prospective clinical trial program to evaluate the glucose-lowering effects of colesevelam HCl in patients with type 2 diabetes mellitus. Curr Med Res Opin. 2007;23:1673-84.

38. Staels B, Kuipers F. Bile acid sequestrants and the treatment of type 2 diabetes mellitus. Drugs. 2007;67:1383-92.

39. Gomez G, Upp JR Jr, Luis F, et al. Regulation of the release of cholecystokinin by bile salts in dogs and humans. Gastroenterology. 1988;94:1036-46.

40. Kogire M, Gomez G, Uchida T, et al. Chronic effect of oral cholestyramine, a bile salt sequestrant, and exogenous cholecystokinin on insulin release in rats. Pancreas. 1992;7:15-20.

41. Sibai BM. Treatment of hypertension in pregnancy. N Engl J Med. 1996;335:257-65.

42. How to use Afrezza® inhaled insulin (cited 2015 Jul 13). On the Internet at: https://www.afrezzapro.com/using-afrezza-insulin.

43. American Diabetes Association. Insulin storage (cited 2015 Jul 13). On the Internet at: http://www.diabetes.org/living-with-diabetes/treatment-and-care/medication/insulin/insulin-storage-and-syringe-safety.html.

44. Eli Lilly and Company. Lilly product information (cited 2015 Jul 13). On the Internet at: http://www.lillydiabetes.com/lilly-diabetes-medicines.aspx.

45. Takiya L, Dougherty T. Pharmacist's guide to insulin preparations: a comprehensive review. Pharmacy Times. 2005;71:90.

46. Carroll MF, Schade DS. The dawn phenomenon revisited: implications for diabetes therapy. Endocr Pract. 2005; 11(1):55-64.

47. Pickup JC, Renard E. Long-acting insulin analogs versus insulin pump therapy for the treatment of type 1 and type 2 diabetes. Diabetes Care. 2008;31 Suppl 2:S140-5.

48. American Diabetes Association. Continuous subcutaneous insulin infusion (position statement). Diabetes Care. 2004:27 Suppl 1:S110.

49. Ronsin O, Jannot-Lamotte MF, Vague P, et al. Factors related to CSII compliance. Diabetes Metab. 2005;31(1):90-5.

50. Sanfield JKA, Hegstad M, Hanna RS. Protocol for outpatient screening and initiation of continuous subcutaneous insulin infusion therapy: impact on cost and quality. Diabetes Educ. 2002;28(4):599-607.

51. Wredling R, Lins PE, Adamson U. Factors influencing the clinical outcome of continuous subcutaneous insulin infusion in routine practice. Diabetes Res Clin Pract. 1993;19:59-67.

52. Franz MJ. Diabetes nutrition recommendations: grading the evidence. Diabetes Educ. 2002;28(5):756-66.

53. Hinnen D, Tomky DM. Combating clinical inertia through pattern management and intensifying therapy. In: Mensing C, ed. The Art and Science of Diabetes Self-Management Education Desk Reference. 2nd ed. Chicago: American Association of Diabetes Educators; 2011:531-75.

54. Gonzalez C, Beruto V, Keller G, Santoro S, Di Girolamo G. Investigational treatments for type 2 diabetes mellitus: exenatide and liraglutide. Expert Opin Investig Drugs. 2006;15:887-95.

55. Meier JJ, Nauck MA. Glucagon-like peptide 1 (GLP-1) in biology and pathology. Diabetes Metab Res Rev. 2005; 21:91-117.

56. Flint A, Raben A, Astrup A, Holst JJ. Glucagon-like peptide 1 promotes satiety and suppresses energy intake in humans. J Clin Invest. 1998;101:515-20.

American Association of Diabetes Educators©

57. BYETTA® exenatide injection. Patient information (cited 2015 Jul 13). On the Internet at: http://pi.lilly.com/us/trulicity-uspi.pdf.

58. Barnett AH. Exenatide. Drugs Today. 2005;41:563.

59. Amylin Pharmaceuticals, Inc. BYETTA® exenatide injection. Patient information. Revised 2007 Dec.

60. DeFronzo RA, Ratner RE, Han J, et al. Effects of exenatide (synthetic exendin-4) on glycemic control and weight over 30 weeks in metformin-treated patients with type 2 diabetes. Diabetes Care. 2005;28:1092.

61. SYMLIN® pramlintide injection. Important update about the vial (cited 2015 Jul 13). On the Internet at: http://www.symlin.com.

62. Kruger DF, Gatcomb PM, Owen SK. Clinical implications of amylin and amylin deficiency. Diabetes Educ. 1999;25(3):389-97.

63. Kolterman OG, Gottlieb A, Moyses C, et al. Reduction of postprandial hyperglycemia in subjects with IDDM by intravenous infusion of AC137, a human amylin analogue. Diabetes Care.1995;18:1179-82.

64. Kong M-F, King P, Macdonald IA, et al. Infusion of pramlintide, a human amylin analogue delays gastric emptying in men with IDDM. Diabetologia. 1997;40:82-8.

65. Kong M-F, Stubbs TA, King P, et al. The effect of single doses of pramlintide on gastric emptying of two meals in men with IDDM. Diabetologia. 1998;41:577-83.

66. SYMLIN® pramlintide injection. Approved uses: SymlinPen60 Pen-Injector instructions for use (cited 2015 Jul 13). On the Internet at: http://www.azpicentral.com/symlin/symlinpen_60_piu_medguide_814002-01.pdf#page=1.

67. SYMLIN® pramlintide injection. Approved uses: SymlinPen120 Pen-Injector instructions for use (cited 2015 Jul 13). On the Internet at: http://www.azpicentral.com/symlin/symlinpen_120_piu_medguide_814003-01.pdf#page=1.

68. Hussar DA. New drugs: exenatide, pramlintide acetate, and micafungin sodium. J Am Pharm Assoc. 2005;45:524.

69. American Diabetes Association. Insulin administration (position statement). Diabetes Care. 2004;27 Suppl 1: S106-9.

70. Transportation Safety Administration. Hidden disabilities: travelers with disabilities and medical conditions (cited 2008 13 Oct). On the Internet at: http://www.tsa.gov/travel/special-procedures.

71. American Diabetes Association. Nutrition recommendations and interventions. Diabetes Care. 2008;31 Suppl 1: S61-78.

72. Joslin EP, Kahn CR, Weir GC, et al. Medical nutrition therapy. In: Kahn CR, Weir GC, King GL, et al, eds. Joslin's Diabetes Mellitus. New York: Lippincott Williams & Wilkins; 2004:624.

73. Franz MJ, Bantle JP, Beebe CA, et al. Evidence-based nutrition principles and recommendations for the treatment and prevention of diabetes and related complications. Diabetes Care. 2002;25:148-98.

74. Institute of Medicine Food and Nutrition Board: Dietary Reference Intakes for Vitamin C, Vitamin E, Selenium, and Carotenoids. Washington, DC: National Academy Press; 2000.

75. Hasanain B, Mooradian AD. Antioxidants and their influences in diabetes. Curr Diabetes Reports. 2002;2:448-56.

76. Food and Drug Administration. Center for Food Safety and Applied Nutrition. Qualified health claims: letter of enforcement discretion—chromium picolinate and insulin resistance (cited 2009 Jan 6). On the Internet at: http://www.fda.gov/Food/IngredientsPackagingLabeling/LabelingNutrition/ucm073017.htm.

77. Srivastava AK, Mehdi MZ. Insulino-mimetic and anti-diabetic effects of vanadium compounds. Diabet Med. 2005;22:2-13.

78. Cohen N, Halberstam M, Shlimovich P, et al. Oral vanadyl sulfate improves hepatic and peripheral insulin sensitivity in patients with noninsulin-dependent diabetes mellitus. J Clin Invest. 1995;95:2501-9.

79. Boden G, Chen X, Ruiz J, et al. Effects of vanadyl sulfate on carbohydrate and lipid metabolism in patients with non-insulin dependent diabetes mellitus. Metabolism. 1996;45:1130-5.

80. Goldfine AB, Simonson DC, Folli F, et al. Metabolic effects of sodium meta-vanadate in humans with insulin-dependent and non-insulin-dependent diabetes mellitus: in vivo and in vitro studies. J Clin Endocrinol Metab. 1995;80:3311-20.

146   Diabetes Education Curriculum

81. Packer L, Witt EH, Tritschler HJ. Alpha-lipoic acid as a biological antioxidant. Free Radic Biol Med. 1995;19: 227-50.

82. Foster TS. Efficacy and safety of α-lipoic acid supplementation in the treatment of symptomatic diabetic neuropathy. Diabetes Educ. 2007;33(1):111-7.

83. US Department of Health and Human Services, National Institutes of Health, National Center for Complementary and Alternative Medicine. NCCAM facts-at-a-glance and mission (cited 2009 Mar 2). On the Internet at: http://nccam.nih.gov/about/ataglance/.

84. Barnes PM, Bloom B, Nahin R. CDC National Health Statistics Report #12. Complementary and alternative medicine use among adults and children: United States, 2007. Hyattsville, MD: National Center for Health Statistics; 2008.

85. Shaw D, Leon C, Koley S, et al. Traditional remedies and food supplements: a 5-year toxicological study (1991-1995). Drug Safety. 1997;17:342-56.

86. Boullata JI, Nace AM. Safety issues with herbal medicine. Pharmacotherapy. 2000;20:257-69.

87. Miller LG. Herbal medicinal: selected clinical considerations focusing on known or potential drug-herb interactions. Arch Intern Med. 1998;158:220-2.

88. Fugh-Berman A. Herb-drug interactions. Lancet. 2000;355:134-8.

89. Eisenberg DM, Davis RB, Ettner SL, et al. Trends in alternative medicine use in the United States, 1990-1997: results of a follow-up national survey. JAMA. 1998;280:1569-75.

90. Lee A, Chui PT, Aun CST, et al. Possible interaction between sevoflurance and Aloe vera. Ann Pharmacother. 2004;38:1651-4.

91. Basch E, Gabardi S, Ulbricht C. Bitter melon (Momordica charantia): a review of safety and efficacy. Am J Health Syst Pharm. 2003;60:356-9.

92. Ludvik B, Neuffer B, Pacini G. Efficacy of Ipomoea batatas (Caiapo) on diabetes control in type 2 diabetes subjects treated with diet. Diabetes Care. 2004;27:436-40.

93. Khan A, Safdar M, Ali Khan MM, et al. Cinnamon improves glucose and lipids of people with type 2 diabetes. Diabetes Care. 2003;26:3215-8.

94. Vuksan V, Sievenpiper JL, Koo VY, et al. American ginseng (Panax quinquefolius L) reduces postprandial glycemia in nondiabetic subjects and subjects with type 2 diabetes mellitus. Arch Intern Med. 2000;160:1009-13.

95. Sotaniemi EA, Haapakoski E, Rautio A. Ginseng therapy in non-insulin dependent diabetic patients. Diabetes Care. 1995;18:1373-5.

96. Vuksan V, Stavro MP, Sievenpiper JL, et al. Similar postprandial glycemic reductions with escalation of dose and administration time of American ginseng in type 2 diabetes. Diabetes Care. 2000;23:1221-6.

97. Pepping J. Alternative therapies—milk thistle: silybum marianum. Am J Health Syst Pharm. 1999;56:1195-7.

98. Knowles MS, Holton EF, Swanson RA, eds. The Adult Learner: The Definitive Classic in Adult Education and Human Resource Development. Houston, Tex: Gulf Professional Publishing; 1998.

American Association of Diabetes Educators©

Module 4 *Taking Medication* 147

TAKING MEDICATION: RESOURCES

Resources for Assistance With Free and Low-Cost Medications. 147

Taking Medication Activity Handout (English). 148

Taking Medication Activity Handout (Spanish) 150

Insulin Injection Know-How Handouts 152

Resources for Assistance With Free and Low-Cost Medications

RxAssist

RxAssist is an online resource of all patient assistance programs in the United States. Search for specific medications by typing in the name of the drug or the drug company that makes it. Call 401-729-3284; www.rxassist.org.

> Drug Discount Card FAQs: http://www.rxassist.org/faqs/drug-discount-cards
> Frequently Asked Questions About Patient Assistance Programs: http://www.rxassist.org/faqs
> Patient Assistance Program Directory: http://www.rxassist.org/pap-info
> Statewide Drug Assistance Programs: http://www.rxassist.org/patients/res-state-programs

Partnership for Prescription Assistance (PPA)

The PPA's mission is to increase awareness of patient assistance programs and boost enrollment of those who are eligible. The site is a single point of access to more than 475 public and private programs, including nearly 200 offered by biopharmaceutical companies. Web site: https://www.pparx.org/.

NeedyMeds

The mission of NeedyMeds is to make information about assistance programs available to low-income patients and their advocates at no cost. Databases such as Patient Assistance Programs, Disease-Based Assistance, Free and Low-Cost Clinics, government programs, and other types of assistance programs are the crux of the free information offered online. Web site: http://www.needymeds.org.

> Brand Name Drugs List: http://www.needymeds.org/drug_list.taf
> Diagnosis-Based Assistance: http://www.needymeds.org/copay_branch.taf
> Drug Coupons, Rebates & More Information: http://www.needymeds.org/inclusions/coupon.htm
> Free/Low-Cost/Sliding-Scale Clinics: http://www.needymeds.org/free_clinics.taf
> NeedyMeds: First-Time Users: http://www.needymeds.org/inclusions/newuser.htm

American Association of Diabetes Educators©

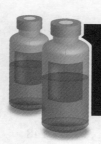

AADE7™ SELF-CARE BEHAVIORS
TAKING MEDICATION

There are several types of medications that are often recommended for people with diabetes. Insulin, pills that lower your blood sugar, aspirin, blood pressure medication, cholesterol-lowering medication, or a number of others may work together to help you lower your blood sugar levels, reduce your risk of complications and help you feel better.

Your medications come with specific instructions for use—and they can affect your body differently depending on when and how you take them. It may take a while to figure out which medicines work best with your body. So it's important for you to pay attention to how you feel and how your body reacts to each new medicine or treatment. It's up to <u>you</u> to tell your pharmacist, doctor, nurse practitioner, or diabetes educator if you've noticed any side effects.

It's important to know the names, doses and instructions for the medications you're taking, as well as the reasons they are recommended for you.

REMEMBER TO:

» **Ask your doctor, nurse practitioner or pharmacist** why this medication was recommended for you.

» **Ask your diabetes educator** to help you fit your medication routine into your daily schedule. Be sure to bring all medications or labels with you when you go to health appointments.

» **Ask a family member** to go with you to an appointment and take notes about any medication instructions. Or, ask someone to remind you to take your medications if you have difficulty remembering to take them.

DID YOU KNOW?

Some over-the-counter products, supplements, or natural remedies can interfere with the effectiveness of your prescribed medicines. Tell your diabetes educator about ANY supplements you are taking so that he/she can make the best recommendations for your care.

TRUE OR FALSE?

When you inject insulin, you need to rotate your injection sites.

TRUE. If you inject insulin in the same spot every time, your tissue can become damaged and won't absorb insulin as well. Be sure to rotate your injection sites between the fattier parts of your upper arm, outer thighs, buttocks, or abdomen.

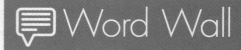

Word Wall

INSULIN:
A hormone that helps the body use glucose (sugar) for energy

SIDE EFFECT:
An effect that a drug has on your body that it is not intended (i.e. diarrhea, nausea, headache)

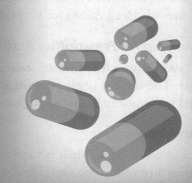

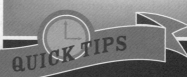

QUICK TIPS

If you often forget to take your medication, try to remind yourself by linking it to a specific activity—like watching the news every night or brushing your teeth—or by setting an alarm on your watch or cell phone.

Take a pen and some paper with you to your healthcare visit and take notes when your provider tells you about your medicine.

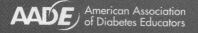

Supported by an educational grant from Eli Lilly and Company.

ACTIVITIES

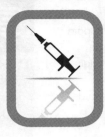
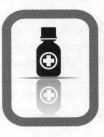
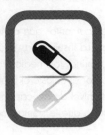

How do you feel about having to take insulin or other medicines?

_____

What is the hardest part about taking your medications?

_____

Name one of your medications.

How much are you supposed to take?

When are you supposed to take it and how often?

Why do you have to take this medication?

What are some of the possible side effects?

What are you supposed to do if you experience side effects?

Anything else you need to know?

What do you do if you forget to take this medication?

*Repeat this exercise for every medication. Be sure to ask your pharmacist or diabetes educator if you do not know the answers.

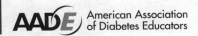

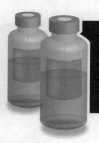

CONDUCTAS PARA EL CUIDADO PERSONA DE AADE7™

TOMAR MEDICAMENTOS

Hay diversos tipos de medicamentos que generalmente se recomiendan para las personas con diabetes. La insulina, las píldoras para bajar tu nivel de azúcar en la sangre, la aspirina, los medicamentos para la presión arterial, los medicamentos para bajar el colesterol u otros medicamentos pueden actuar juntos para bajar tu nivel de azúcar en la sangre, reducir el riesgo de complicaciones y ayudarte a que te sientas mejor.

Tus medicamentos vienen con indicaciones específicas de uso y pueden afectar a tu cuerpo de manera diferente según cuándo y cómo los tomes. Necesitarás cierto tiempo para darte cuenta qué medicamentos funcionan mejor con tu cuerpo. Por eso es importante que prestes atención a cómo te sientes y cómo reacciona tu cuerpo a cada medicamento o tratamiento nuevo. Deberás comunicarle a tu farmacéutico, médico, profesional de enfermería o educador en diabetes si notas efectos secundarios.

Es importante que conozcas los nombres, las dosis y las indicaciones de los medicamentos que estás tomando, y también los motivos por los que están recomendados para ti.

RECUERDA:

- » Pregúntale a tu médico, profesional de enfermería o farmacéutico por qué este medicamento fue recomendado para ti.
- » Pídele a tu educador en diabetes que te ayude a incluir tu rutina de medicamentos en tu programa diario. Asegúrate de llevar todos los medicamentos o las etiquetas cuando vas a las citas médicas.
- » Pídele a un familiar que te acompañe a una cita y toma nota de las indicaciones de los medicamentos. O pídele a alguien que te recuerde tomar tus medicamentos si tienes dificultad para acordarte de tomarlos.

¿LO SABÍAS?

Algunos productos, suplementos o remedios naturales de venta libre pueden interferir en la eficacia de tus medicamentos recetados. Cuéntale a tu educador en diabetes sobre CUALQUIER suplemento que estés tomando para que él pueda darte las mejores recomendaciones para tu atención.

¿VERDADERO O FALSO?

Cuando te inyectas insulina, debes cambiar los lugares de inyección.

VERDADERO. Si te inyectas insulina siempre en el mismo lugar, tu tejido se puede dañar y no absorberá la insulina. Asegúrate de alternar el lugar donde te inyectas entre las partes con más grasa en la parte superior de tu brazo, la parte externa del muslo, las nalgas, o el abdomen.

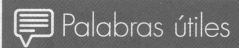

Palabras útiles

INSULINA:
Una hormona que ayuda al cuerpo a utilizar la glucosa (azúcar) para generar energía

EFECTO SECUNDARIO:
Un efecto que tiene un fármaco en tu cuerpo que no está previsto (por ej., diarrea, náuseas, dolor de cabeza).

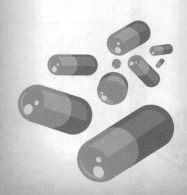

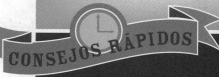

Si a menudo te olvidas de tomar tu medicamento, trata de recordarlo relacionándolo con una actividad específica — como mirar las noticias todas las noches o cepillarte los dientes — o poniendo una alarma en tu reloj o en tu teléfono celular.

Lleva un papel y un bolígrafo a tu visita de atención médica y toma nota cuando tu proveedor de atención médica te dé información sobre tu medicamento.

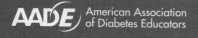

Supported by an educational grant from Lilly USA, LLC.

ACTIVIDADES

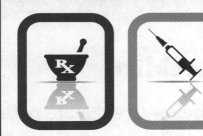
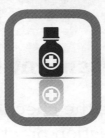
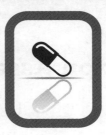

¿Cómo te sientes acerca de tener que tomar insulina u otros medicamentos?

_____

¿Cuál es la parte más difícil de tomar tus medicamentos?

_____

Nombra uno de tus medicamentos.

¿Cuánto debes tomar?

¿Cuándo y con qué frecuencia debes tomarlo?

¿Por qué tienes que tomar este medicamento?

¿Cuáles son algunos de los efectos secundarios posibles?

¿Qué debes hacer si experimentas efectos secundarios?

¿Hay algo más que debes saber?

¿Qué haces si te olvidas de tomar este medicamento?

*Repite este ejercicio para todos tus medicamentos. Asegúrate de preguntarle a tu farmacéutico o a tu educador en diabetes si no sabes las respuestas.

AADE American Association of Diabetes Educators

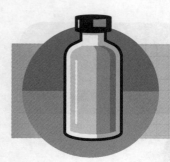

INSULIN INJECTION KNOW-HOW

Injection Assessment Checklist

Use the checklist below to evaluate patients' injection practices and determine areas of educational need.

Demonstrates Competency	Education Indicated	
☐	☐	**SITE MANAGEMENT** Injection site(s): _____ Evidence of: ☐ Lipohypertrophy ☐ Lipotrophy ☐ Bruising ☐ Infection Describe injection rotation pattern: _____ Skin Preparation Technique: _____
☐	☐	**INJECTION PROCEDURE** ☐ Sterile technique ☐ Rolling to uniformity (if necessary) ☐ Pre-injection priming (pen only) ☐ Air into vial (syringe only) ☐ Correct order for mixing in same syringe (if necessary) ☐ Dosing accuracy ☐ Needle insertion ☐ Complete injection ☐ Needle withdrawal (with waiting time)

  American Association of Diabetes Educators   Supported by BD Diabetes Care

insulin injection know-how
insulin assessment checklist

Demonstrates Competency	Education Indicated	
☐	☐	**DISPOSAL PROCEDURE** Local regulations: _____ Aware of local regulations? ☐ Yes ☐ No Has sharps container or needle clip? ☐ Yes ☐ No Uses sharps container or needle clip? ☐ Yes ☐ No
☐	☐	**NEEDLE REUSE** Re-using pen or syringe needles? ☐ Yes ☐ No Wiping needle? ☐ Yes ☐ No Recapping? ☐ Yes ☐ No Aware of potential for air in pen? ☐ Yes ☐ No Using same needle for >1 insulin type? ☐ Yes ☐ No ☐ N/A
☐	☐	**INJECTION DEVICE SELECTION** ☐ Appropriate needle size ☐ Sufficient volume ☐ Appropriate dosing increments ☐ Suited to physical limitations
☐	☐	**INJECTION ADHERENCE** How often do you miss taking an injection? ☐ Daily ☐ Weekly ☐ Monthly ☐ Almost Never

  American Association of Diabetes Educators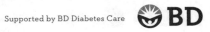

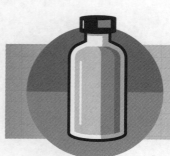

INSULIN INJECTION KNOW-HOW

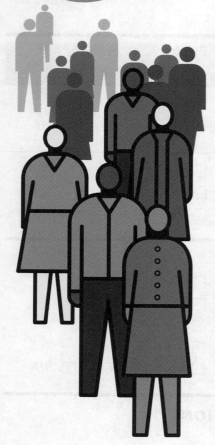

Understanding Insulin

Welcome to the ranks of nearly 26 million Americans diagnosed with diabetes. By now you've probably been given enough information about diabetes to make your head spin. But two important facts should stand out:

 DIABETES CAN BE CONTROLLED, AND IT IS VERY IMPORTANT TO DO SO.

No doubt, you and your healthcare team will develop a plan for managing your diabetes. The plan may include some changes to the way you eat, the way you move, and the medications you take. Even if insulin injections are not currently part of the plan, it is important that you familiarize yourself with the concept of taking insulin. Here's why.

DIABETES IS EVER-CHANGING

Insulin is a hormone produced by the pancreas. Insulin's job is to shuttle glucose (sugar) out of the bloodstream and into the body's cells (the tiny components of all parts of our bodies). This helps to nourish the body's cells and keep the blood sugar level from climbing too high.

All people with type 1 diabetes require insulin—not just to control blood sugar levels, but simply to stay alive. The human body cannot survive without insulin, and people with type 1 diabetes produce little or no insulin of their own. Upon diagnosis, some people with type 1 diabetes still make a small amount of insulin. This is called a "honeymoon" phase. However, no honeymoon lasts forever. After a period of weeks or months, insulin injections almost always become necessary.

  American Association of Diabetes Educators

Supported by BD Diabetes Care

insulin injection know-how
understanding insulin

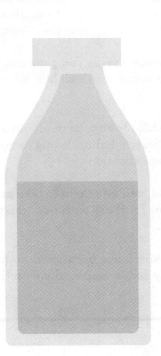

More than 90% of people with diabetes have type 2 diabetes. Type 2 is very different from type 1 in that the pancreas continues to produce insulin. The problem is that the body's cells don't utilize the insulin very well. This is called insulin resistance, and may be the root cause of type 2 diabetes. Insulin resistance develops as a result of faulty genes (our heredity) and an unhealthy lifestyle. Excess body fat is perhaps the greatest contributor to insulin resistance. The aging process plays a role as well.

When insulin resistance is present, the pancreas needs to produce more insulin than usual to keep blood sugar levels within a normal range, kind of like an air conditioner that has to work extra hard to keep the house cool on a hot summer day. Over time the pancreas, like an overworked air conditioner, begins to break down. It starts losing the ability to produce insulin. Although very few people with type 2 diabetes require insulin when they are first diagnosed, nearly one in three will eventually require insulin to control their diabetes.

A FEW FACTS ABOUT TAKING INSULIN

Fear of the unknown is common in our society. Remember the first time you tried a strange, new type of food? Chances are that once you gave it a try, you found it wasn't so bad. It might have even become a personal favorite. How about the first time you were introduced to a computer? What seemed intimidating at first has probably become an important part of your daily life.

We all have preconceived (and often incorrect) notions of what it means to take an insulin injection. Here are a few common assumptions, and the honest facts:

 American Association of Diabetes Educators

Supported by BD Diabetes Care

insulin injection know-how
understanding insulin

ASSUMPTION	FACT
Going on insulin means I've failed at taking care of my diabetes.	As described above, it is perfectly natural for many people with diabetes to eventually need insulin–especially those who have had diabetes for quite some time.
Taking insulin puts me one step closer to the grave.	Just the opposite! What puts people with diabetes at risk of serious health problems and death is uncontrolled blood sugar. By improving blood sugar control, insulin reduces these risks.
Insulin injections hurt like the dickens.	Insulin is injected into the fat below the skin, where there are no nerve endings. Today's insulin syringes and pen needles are so small and thin that most people feel no discomfort at all when giving their injections.
Insulin will make me gain weight.	Eating more calories than you burn is what makes you gain weight. if you get more exercise and eat less, you can lose weight even when taking insulin.
Once I start taking insulin, I'll be on it forever.	Many people with type 2 diabetes are able to reduce or eliminate their need for insulin by adopting healthy lifestyle habits, losing weight, and using other newly-developed diabetes medications.
I'll never be able to give myself a shot.	Just about anyone, from age four to 104, can be taught to take an injection. There are special adaptive devices for those with poor dexterity, limited vision, or fear of sharp objects.
Insulin can make my blood sugar go too low.	While anyone who takes insulin can experience occasional bouts of low blood sugar, the chances are extremely small – especially with the new long-acting insulin products.

  American Association of Diabetes Educators   Supported by BD Diabetes Care

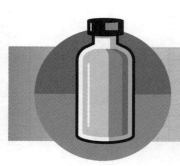

INSULIN INJECTION KNOW-HOW

Learning How to Inject Insulin

Congratulations for making the move to insulin therapy. It won't be long before you start enjoying better blood sugar control, more energy, and a host of other benefits.

The prospect of taking insulin injections may have you feeling a bit anxious. That's OK! Just about everyone feels that way. Just know that your anxiety will vanish soon enough. Here are some valuable facts and tips to help make your transition to insulin smooth and easy.

WAYS TO GIVE INSULIN

Because insulin is broken down by digestive enzymes, it cannot be taken in pill form. Instead, it is delivered with a syringe into the layer of fat below the skin, also called the "subcutaneous" tissue. The layer of fat on the stomach, hips, thighs, buttocks and backs of the arms are common sites for injecting insulin. From there, the insulin absorbs into the bloodstream where it circulates to the cells throughout the body.

The really good news about delivering insulin into the layer of fat below the skin is that there are no nerve endings in this area, so injections are usually painless. There are a number of options for administering insulin:

SYRINGES

Disposable plastic insulin syringes are still widely used, but the popularity of pens and pumps (see next page) is growing. Syringes vary in terms of how much insulin they hold as well as the length and thickness of the needle. Syringes can be used to deliver insulin directly into the layer of fat below the skin, or they can inject insulin into a temporary "port" that sits on the skin. The port, which is changed every 2-3 days, features a small flexible plastic tube that sits below the skin. A needle is used to place the tube under the skin, so only one needle stick is required every 2-3 days when a port is used.

  American Association of Diabetes Educators

Supported by BD Diabetes Care

157

insulin injection know-how
learning how to inject insulin

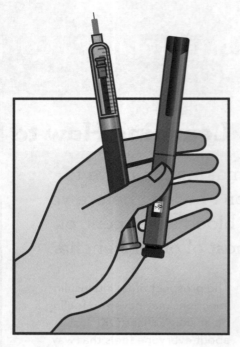

PENS

Insulin pens got their name because they are about the size and shape of a writing pen. They contain insulin (instead of ink) and have a dial for setting the dose. A disposable pen needle is attached to the end of the pen prior to injecting. As was the case with syringes, pen needles are available in a variety of lengths and thicknesses. Because they cut down on medical waste and are considered by most to be more convenient, accurate and easy to use than syringes, insulin pens are growing in popularity among people of all ages.

PUMPS

Insulin pumps are electronic devices that are worn continuously and deliver insulin into the fat layer below the skin by way of a flexible plastic tube (similar to the "port" described above). Insulin pumps are popular among those who require multiple daily injections of insulin. Safe and successful use of a pump requires considerable education and training, and their cost can be relatively high. Insulin pumps are not typically used by those who are new to insulin, but can be an effective option once you have a bit more experience.

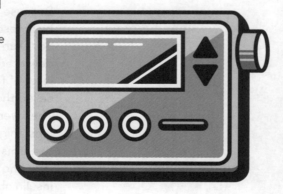

  American Association of Diabetes Educators   Supported by BD Diabetes Care

insulin injection know-how
learning how to inject insulin

CHOOSING AN INJECTION DEVICE

The decision to use syringes or pens is a personal one. If you have an opportunity to sample both at your healthcare provider's office, certainly do so. It is best to speak with your healthcare provider and check with your health insurance to find out what is covered under your plan.

Most pens hold 300 units of insulin and allow delivery of up to 60 to 80 units at a time. "Prefilled" disposable pens deliver in single-unit increments. "Durable" pens utilize replaceable/ insulin cartridges, and may deliver insulin in ½ unit increments. Pens can be used to deliver a variety of long-acting and rapid-acting insulin types, as well as premixed insulin formulations.

Disposable syringes hold up to 100 units per injection. If you decide to use syringes, select a type that holds enough to cover your largest dose with a little room to spare. The markings on a syringe allow dosing in 2-unit, 1-unit, or ½-unit increments. Once you have a size that meets your needs, select a type that allows you to dose as precisely as possible.

The needles on syringes vary as well. Syringe and pen needles as short as 4mm and as long as 12.7mm are available. Thickness is measured in gauge. The higher the gauge, the thinner the needle. Gauges as high as 32 and as low as 28-gauge can be obtained. In general, it is best to use the shortest, thinnest (highest gauge) needles available. Skin thickness doesn't vary much from person to person. Even if you are overweight or obese, it is unlikely that you will need a needle longer than 6mm. Needles that are too long may produce painful intramuscular injections, with insulin absorbing faster than it should.

  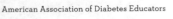 American Association of Diabetes Educators

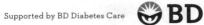 Supported by BD Diabetes Care

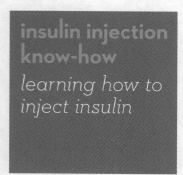

insulin injection know-how
learning how to inject insulin

INJECTION TECHNIQUE

Technique is everything when it comes to making insulin injections easy.

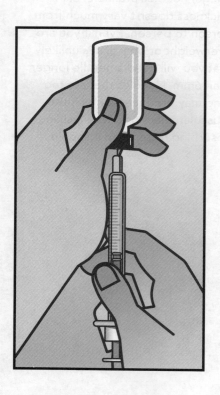

TO DRAW ONE TYPE OF INSULIN INTO A SYRINGE:

* **Gather your insulin supplies:** Get your insulin vial and a fresh syringe. Check the insulin vial to make sure it is the right kind of insulin and that there are no clumps or particles in it. Also make sure the insulin is not being used past its expiration date.

* **Gently stir intermediate or premixed insulin:** Turn the bottle on its side and roll it between the palms of your hands. Clear (fast-acting, long-acting) insulin generally does not need to be mixed.

* **Prepare the insulin bottle:** If the insulin bottle is new, remove the cap. It is not necessary to wipe the top of the bottle with alcohol as long as it is clean.

* **Pull air into the syringe:** Remove the cap from the needle. Pull back the plunger on the syringe to draw in an amount of air that is equal to your insulin dose. The TIP of the black plunger should correspond to the number on the syringe.

* **Inject air into the vial:** Hold the syringe like a pencil and insert the needle into the rubber stopper on the top of the vial. Push the plunger down until all of the air is in the bottle. This helps to keep the right amount of pressure in the bottle and makes it easier to draw up the insulin.

* **Draw up the insulin into the syringe:** With the needle still in the vial, turn the bottle and syringe upside down (vial above syringe). Pull the plunger to fill the syringe to the desired amount.

* **Check the syringe for air bubbles:** If you see any large bubbles, push the plunger until the air is purged out of the syringe. Pull the plunger back down to the desired dose.

* **Remove the needle from the bottle:** Be careful to not let the needle touch anything until you are ready to inject!

  American Association of Diabetes Educators

Supported by BD Diabetes Care

insulin injection know-how
learning how to inject insulin

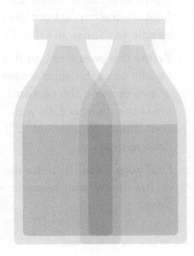

WHEN COMBINING TWO TYPES OF INSULIN (INTERMEDIATE AND RAPID) IN THE SAME SYRINGE:

- **Gather your insulin supplies:** Get your insulin vial and a fresh syringe. Check the insulin vial to make sure it is the right kind of insulin and that there are no clumps or particles in it, and that the expiration date has not passed.

- **Gently stir intermediate or premixed insulin:** Turn the vial on its side and roll it between the palms of your hands. Clear (fast-acting, long-acting) insulin generally does not need to be mixed.

- **Prepare the insulin vials:** If the insulin vial is new, remove the cap. It is not necessary to wipe the top of the bottle with alcohol as long as it is clean.

- **Inject air into the intermediate insulin vial:** Remove the cap from the needle. With the vial of insulin below the syringe, inject an amount of air equal to the dose of intermediate insulin that you will be taking. Do not draw out the insulin into the syringe yet. Remove the needle from the vial.

- **Inject air into the rapid-acting insulin vial:** Only inject an amount equal to the rapid-acting insulin dose. Leave the needle in the vial.

- **Draw up the rapid-acting insulin:** With the needle still in the vial, turn the vial upside down (vial above the syringe) and pull the plunger to fill the syringe with the desired dose.

- **Check the syringe for air bubbles:** If you see any large bubbles, push the plunger until the air is purged out of the syringe. Pull the plunger back down to the desired dose.

- **Remove the needle from the vial:** Recheck your dose.

- **Draw up the intermediate-acting insulin:** Insert the needle into the vial of cloudy insulin. Turn the vial upside down (vial above syringe) and pull the plunger to draw the dose of intermediate-acting

  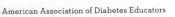

insulin injection know-how
learning how to inject insulin

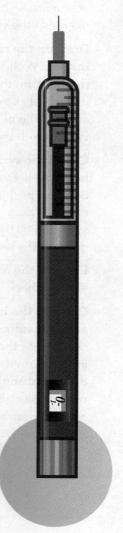

insulin. Because the short-acting insulin is already in the syringe, pull the plunger to the total number of units you need. Do not inject any of the insulin back into the vial, since the syringe now contains a mixture of intermediate and rapid-acting insulin.

* **Remove the needle from the vial:** Be careful to not let the needle touch anything until you are ready to inject!

PREPARING A PEN FOR INJECTION:

* **Check the pen:** Ensure that it contains the proper type of insulin and contains enough to cover your full dose. Also check to make sure that the expiration date has not passed.

* **Gently stir intermediate or premixed insulin:** Turn the pen on its side and roll it between the palms of your hands. Clear (fast-acting, long-acting) insulin generally does not need to be mixed.

* **Attach a fresh pen needle:** Screw or click the needle securely in place according to the manufacturer's instructions. Remove the cap(s) from the pen needle to expose the needle.

* **Prime the pen:** Pointing the needle up in the air, dial one or two units on the pen and press the plunger fully with your thumb. Repeat until a drop appears.

* **Dial your dose:** Turn the dial on the pen to your prescribed dose.

 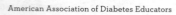 American Association of Diabetes Educators   Supported by BD Diabetes Care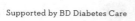

insulin injection know-how
learning how to inject insulin

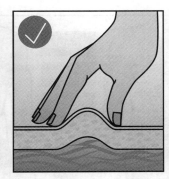 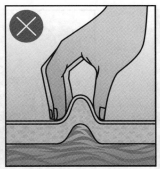 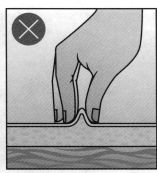

Correct (left) and incorrect (right) ways of performing the skin fold.

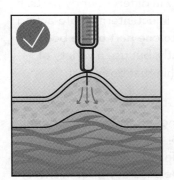

The correct angle of injection when lifting a skin fold is 90°

DELIVERING AN INJECTION:

* **Select a site:** Choose a spot on your skin that you can see and reach. It is important to not "overuse" any particular area of skin. See the information below on "rotating" injection sites.

* **Make sure skin is clean:** It is generally not necessary to wipe the skin with alcohol before injecting. Those at a high risk of infection should discuss site-preparation procedures with their healthcare team.

* **Pinch the skin:** Pinch a one-to-two-inch portion of skin and fat between your thumb and first finger.

* **Push the needle into the skin:** With your other hand, hold the syringe or pen like a pencil at a 90-degree angle to the skin and insert the needle with one quick motion. Make sure the needle is all the way in.

* **Inject the insulin:** Let go of the skin pinch before you inject the insulin. Push the plunger with your thumb at a moderate, steady pace until the insulin is fully injected. If using a syringe, keep the needle in the skin for 5 seconds. If using a pen, keep the needle in the skin for 10 seconds.

* **Pull out the needle:** Remove at the same 90-degree angle at which you inserted the needle. Press your injection site with your finger for 5-10 seconds to keep insulin from leaking out.

* **Remove the needle:** If using a pen, remove the needle from the pen by replacing the large cover and unscrewing. Leaving the needle on the pen can result in leakage or air bubbles.

* **Dispose of your used needle:** It is important to protect yourself, your loved ones, sanitation workers and pets from accidental needle sticks. Do not recap syringes before throwing them away. Place used syringes and pen needles in a thick plastic container (sharps container, detergent bottle, etc.). When nearly full, close the container tightly with a screw-on cap and tape closed. Dispose according to standards set forth by your local department of sanitation.

 American Association of Diabetes Educators   Supported by BD Diabetes Care

insulin injection know-how
learning how to inject insulin

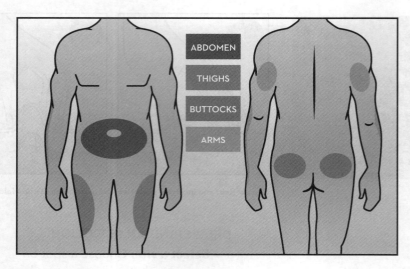

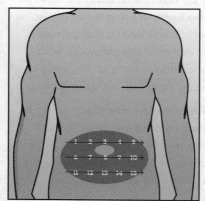

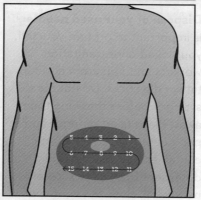

Recommended way to rotate injection sites.

ROTATING INJECTION SITES:

Insulin is injected into the fat layer below the skin on the abdomen (staying two fingers or a few inches away from the belly button), outer thighs, hips, buttocks, or backs of the arms. Although insulin injections are usually painless, injecting the same spot repeatedly can cause inflammation or fat tissue breakdown. Lipodystrophy, as this is called, can cause lumps/swelling and thickened skin, and it may keep insulin from absorbing properly. Nearly half of all people who take insulin develop lipodystrophy, particularly when injection sites are not rotated properly.

Most forms of rapid and long-acting insulin absorb consistently from just about any body part, so feel free to use a variety of body parts for your injections, and use a variety of spots within each body part.

Intermediate-acting (cloudy) insulin and premixed insulin absorbs differently in different body parts. It is best to inject intermediate-acting insulin into one part of the body consistently, but use a variety of spots within that body part.

NEEDLE RE-USE

Use of a new, fresh syringe or pen needle for each injection is the best way to minimize discomfort and ensure the accuracy/effectiveness of the insulin dose. Using someone else's needle puts you at danger of contracting Hepatitis and HIV.

American Association of Diabetes Educators

Supported by BD Diabetes Care

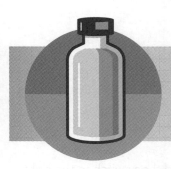

INSULIN INJECTION KNOW-HOW

Pro Tips (and Tricks) for Easier and Better Insulin Injections

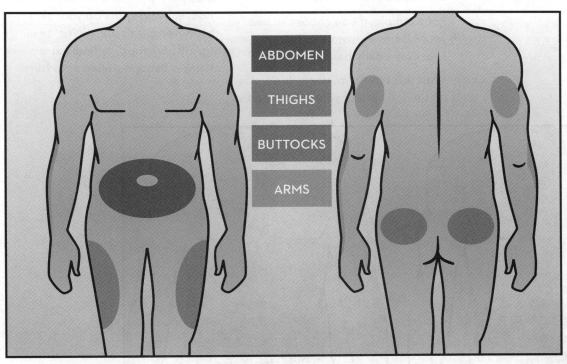

Recommended injection sites

WHERE IS THE BEST PLACE TO GIVE INJECTIONS?

Insulin and other injected diabetes medications are meant to be delivered into the fat layer just under the skin. Popular injection sites include the abdomen (staying two fingers or a few inches away from the belly button), outer thighs, hips, upper buttocks, lower back, and backs of the arms. Modern insulin products are well absorbed and act about the same regardless of where they are injected. However, for best results it is important to stick with a consistent body part for your injections in order to avoid variations in insulin action. Ultimately, the choice is up to you. Select a part of your body that you can see, reach, and access easily. But be sure to use a number of different

  American Association of Diabetes Educators

Supported by BD Diabetes Care

insulin injection know-how
pro tips and tricks for easier and better insulin injections

spots within that body part. This is called "rotating" injection sites. Injecting into the same spot too often can cause skin problems and can impair insulin absorption.

For example, if you choose to use your abdomen, rotate injection spots on a daily basis like these:

With this type of pattern, you'll stay on the left side of your abdomen for 12 days and then switch to the right side for 12 days. That way, each spot has 24 days to "heal" before you use it again! Regardless of which body part and rotation pattern you choose, avoid spots on your skin that have scar tissue, moles, swelling/inflammation, or unusual changes in appearance or texture.

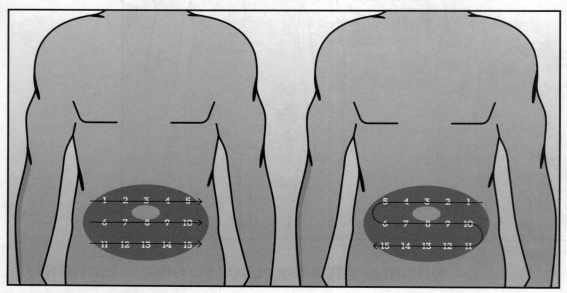

Recommended way to rotate injection sites.

  American Association of Diabetes Educators

Supported by BD Diabetes Care

insulin injection know-how
pro tips and tricks for easier and better insulin injections

IS THERE A TRICK FOR REMEMBERING TO TAKE MY INJECTIONS?

Missed injections (or taking injections much too late) can cause serious blood sugar control problems. Research has shown that missing just one insulin injection per week can raise your A1c by more than 0.5%!

Here are some techniques for helping you to remember to take your injections:

* Attitude is important, so take your diabetes seriously!
* Write down your injection doses after taking them
* Use reminder alarms on a watch or cellular phone
* Take your injection at the same time that you perform another daily ritual, such as taking oral medication or brushing your teeth
* Keep your injection materials in a strategic location so that you notice them at the right times
* If you take insulin at mealtimes, take it before eating (with your doctor's approval).

DO I HAVE TO KEEP MY INSULIN REFRIGERATED ALL THE TIME?

Yes and no. Insulin is a large protein molecule that breaks down gradually when exposed to warm temperatures. It is best to keep your extra insulin and other injected diabetes medications refrigerated. However, once you begin to use a vial or pen, it is usually fine to keep it at room temperature for up to a month. Do not store your insulin near extreme heat (above 86°) or extreme cold (below 36°). (3) Never store insulin in the freezer, direct sunlight, or in the glove compartment of a car.

All insulin vials and pens should be replaced monthly, if not more often, to ensure that they are working at full potency. Be sure to check the expiration date before opening the box, and do not use insulin past its expiration date without your physician's approval. Examine the insulin closely to make sure it looks normal. Clear insulin should not have crystals or discoloration, and cloudy insulin should not have clumps or pieces stuck to the sides of the vial/pen.

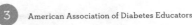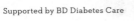

insulin injection know-how
pro tips and tricks for easier and better insulin injections

IS IT NECESSARY TO MIX INSULIN BEFORE INJECTING IT?

In general, clear insulin does not need to be mixed before injecting. This includes Regular insulin, rapid-acting insulin analogs (aspart, lispro and glulisine) and long-acting basal insulin (glargine and detemir). However, any vial or pen that contains NPH — including premixed formulations such as 75/25 and 70/30 — must be mixed until they are uniformly cloudy before injecting. The best way to ensure an even mixture is to roll the pen or vial between your palms ten times, then inspect to make sure there are no "clumps" settling at the bottom. Injecting insulin that is not properly mixed can result is serious high or low blood sugar.

HOW CAN I KEEP THE INJECTIONS FROM HURTING?

In most cases, insulin injections hurt very little, if at all. However, there are a few things you can do to make the injections as painless as possible:

* Use fresh needles for each injection. Even after just one or two uses, syringe and pen needles can become dull. Sharp needles cause the least amount of trauma to the skin.
* Inject your insulin at room temperature. Cold insulin has a tendency to sting. When using a pen or vial for the first time, take it out of the fridge a half hour early so that it has time to warm up to room temperature.
* Relax the muscles in the area where you are injecting. Tense muscles make the nerves in the area more sensitive.
* Pinch the area where you will inject so that the skin surface is hard. This ensures a quick, clean injection. A quick needle insertion causes the least amount of pain.
* If you clean your skin with an alcohol pad, wait until it has dried completely before you inject.
* Doses of 30 units or more may cause pressure to build up under the skin. Ask your physician if you can split large doses.
* Avoid injecting into sensitive muscle by using a short needle (6mm or less).
* Choose the thinnest needle possible. Remember, the higher the gauge, the thinner the needle.

  American Association of Diabetes Educators

Supported by BD Diabetes Care

insulin injection know-how

pro tips and tricks for easier and better insulin injections

* If pain persists despite using these techniques, try rubbing ice on your skin for a few minutes before injecting, or ask your doctor about using an injection port instead of injecting directly into your skin.

WHAT SHOULD I DO IF INSULIN LEAKS OUT AFTER THE INJECTION?

Occasionally, insulin may leak out of the skin after you remove the needle, even if you have left the needle in the skin for 5-10 seconds. Research has shown that the amount of insulin lost in these situations is usually minimal and will probably not affect blood sugar control. Unless large drops appear that run down your skin, you should not have to worry about replacing what is lost.

However, to ensure accurate and consistent dosing, it is best to do what you can to prevent leakage. Here are a few tricks:

1. When injecting, release the "pinch" on your skin before pressing down on the plunger.
2. Keep the needle in your skin a few seconds longer than usual.
3. If leakage occurs often, insert the needle and inject at a 45-degree angle rather than going straight into the skin.
4. After removing the needle, put mild pressure on the injection site (with a clean finger) for 5-8 seconds.

IS IT OK TO THROW MY USED NEEDLES IN THE TRASH?

There are two things to consider when it comes to disposing sharp objects such as syringes, pen needles and lancets:

Local ordinances

Every municipality has its own rules about the handling of medical waste. Check with your local department of sanitation for details. Each state also has established guidelines regarding sharps disposal. The Centers for Disease Control (CDC) has more information about safe needle disposal in your area: www.cdc.gov/needledisposal.

The safety of those around you

Being a responsible person with diabetes means taking steps to ensure the safety of family, friends, domestic employees, sanitation workers and yes, even pets. Accidental needle sticks can produce serious pain and infections. One way to protect those around you is to place your used syringes, pen needles and lancets in a non-clear heavy-duty plastic jug with a secure screw-on cap. Don't bother recap-

  American Association of Diabetes Educators

Supported by BD Diabetes Care

insulin injection know-how
pro tips and tricks for easier and better insulin injections

ping the needles... just throw them into the jug, and keep the jug in an out-of-the-way place. When the jug is full, seal the cap with strong tape and dispose according to local regulations (usually it is OK to just place in your normal trash). When traveling, bring a smaller container with you for your used items, and bring it home with you for safe disposal.

Another way to protect those around you is to purchase and use a device that clips, catches, and contains the needles. Do not break the needles off with your fingers, as you can easily stick yourself. And do not use scissors to clip off needles — the flying needle could hurt someone or become lost.

ARE LONGER NEEDLES BETTER THAN SHORTER NEEDLES?

Good news! In almost all cases, shorter needles are better than longer ones. For insulin to work, it only needs to get into the fat layer below the skin. While the amount of fat varies from person to person, skin thickness tends to be about the same — around 2mm. So needles that are at least 4mm long do the job quite well, producing normal absorption/action and no increase in leakage back onto the skin surface. Glucose control does not suffer when switching from long to short needles, even in those who are obese. Needles that are too long can cause accidental injection into muscle, which alters the normal action of the medication and can be quite painful.

For these reasons, most healthcare organizations now recommend the use of shorter needles. Rarely is there a medical reason to use needles longer than 6mm. For those with a great deal of fat below the skin, use of short needles also eliminates the need to pinch the skin when administering the injection.

 American Association of Diabetes Educators

Supported by BD Diabetes Care

MODULE 5

Monitoring

Table of Contents

MONITORING: AN EDUCATOR'S OVERVIEW 172

    AADE Systematic Review of the Literature. 172

    Background Information and Instructions for the Educator 172

        Terminology Matters 172

        Discussing the "Numbers" 173

        Required Skill Sets for Successful Monitoring 173

    Learning Objectives 173

        Knowledge. 173

        Skills 174

        Barriers and Facilitators 174

    Behavioral Objective 174

MONITORING: INSTRUCTIONAL PLAN 174

    There's More to Monitoring Than Checking Blood Glucose 174

    Identifying Participant Thoughts and Feelings About Monitoring 175

        Benefits of Monitoring. 175

        Why Monitor Blood Glucose? 176

    Target Blood Glucose Levels. 176

        Glucose Targets for Pregnant Women With Diabetes. 177

        Glucose Targets for Children 177

    Selecting a Glucose Meter. 179

        Continuous Glucose Monitoring System 180

    General Guidelines for Monitoring. 180

        Control Testing: Checking the System for Quality. 180

        Storage of Monitoring Supplies 181

        Traveling With Monitoring Supplies 181

        Hand-washing 181

172   Diabetes Education Curriculum

Tips for Getting an Adequate Blood Sample 181

Alternate Site Testing..182

Disposal of Used Lancets 183

Recording and Sharing Your Results...183

When and How Often to Monitor Blood Glucose 185

How Often Are You Willing and Able to Monitor? 188

Interpreting and Responding to Blood Glucose Results 189

Identifying Barriers to Monitoring 192

Identifying Facilitators for Monitoring 193

Common Facilitators 194

Long-Term Monitoring to Prevent Complications: A Brief Overview.....................194

Measuring Long-Term Glucose Control..194

eAG: Estimated Average Glucose 195

Fructosamine 196

1,5-Anhydroglucitrol (1,5-AG) 196

Monitoring Cardiovascular Health..196

Monitoring Kidney Health 197

Monitoring Eye Health 197

Monitoring Foot (Nerve) Health 197

Setting a SMART Goal for Monitoring 197

Follow-up/Outcomes Measurement 197

REFERENCES 199

MONITORING: RESOURCES...200

MONITORING: AN EDUCATOR'S OVERVIEW

AADE Systematic Review of the Literature

A systematic review of the literature was conducted by the American Association of Diabetes Educators (AADE) to first assess the impact of self-monitoring of blood glucose (SMBG) on A1C levels for patients with type 2 diabetes. A second reason for the review was to explore mediators and moderators, those factors that influence a patient's decision to voluntarily self-monitor his or her blood glucose and then respond to the reading. The review concluded that "SMBG may be effective in controlling blood glucose for patients with type 2 diabetes. There is a need for studies that implement all the components of the process for self-regulation of SMBG to assess whether patient use of SMBG will improve HbA1c levels."[1]

Background Information and Instructions for the Educator

Terminology Matters

The words *test* and *testing* insinuate a pass/fail outcome. When discussing the results of monitoring, educators should avoid descriptors such as *good* or *bad*, which imply a mistake was made. Patients may subconsciously transfer these value judgments to their worth as a manager of their diabetes. This can add to their emotional burden.

American Association of Diabetes Educators©

For patients who have repeatedly seen unacceptable results, use of such terminology may cause discouragement and lower their confidence in their diabetes self-management abilities. The terms *monitor* or *check* or *measure* rather than *test* are better accepted by patients. Guide patients to use neutral words like *above or below target* or *above or below range*. *Target* or *range* suggests a level to strive for and suggests that action is needed to move toward that desired level.[2(p240)]

Discussing the "Numbers"

Diabetes educators should be attentive to *how* patients refer to their monitoring results. Listening for "monitor talk" can yield valuable information for the educator, information that is beyond the clinical significance of glucose results. Monitor talk is a phenomenon wherein the patient experiences a negative emotional response when glucose results are outside the range that is acceptable to him or her. Asking what the numbers mean to the patient will help the educator learn more about the patient's life with diabetes. Listening for, and responding to, the emotional context is affirming to the person. It builds trust in the patient-provider relationship. Interest in how the patient feels in relation to monitoring results helps validate his or her experience with a condition that is unrelenting and frequently frustrating. This deeper understanding can, in turn, help the educator better guide interventions.

Required Skill Sets for Successful Monitoring

Two skill sets are required to successfully perform SMBG with the goal of improving diabetes outcomes. Patients must be comfortable and confident in their ability to operate the blood glucose meter (*operational* skills) and to use the SMBG data (*interpretation* skills) to make behavior change (a problem-solving skill). The educator may be involved in teaching both or just one of the skills, but both skills should be assessed at the time of diabetes education, and the educator should be aware of possible barriers to successful SMBG.[2(pp200-16)]

Learning Objectives

Knowledge

The participant will:

- state how to obtain a blood glucose meter and supplies
- explain how to operate a glucose meter
- state how to care for monitoring supplies
- explain the purpose of quality control testing for the meter and describe how and when to do it
- describe proper disposal of used lancets, listing household items that may be used
- list target blood glucose values
- describe appropriate monitoring times for his or her individual situation
- describe how to log blood glucose results and share with healthcare provider

For Type 1 Diabetes or During Pregnancy

The participant will:

- explain how to perform ketone testing
- describe appropriate ketone testing times
- explain relevance of ketone monitoring results and describe appropriate action to take when ketone results are out of range

American Association of Diabetes Educators©

174   Diabetes Education Curriculum

Skills

The participant will:

- demonstrate proper glucose monitoring technique
- demonstrate proper care of monitoring supplies
- demonstrate accurate quality control testing
- demonstrate proper disposal of used lancets
- document glucose results appropriately (eg, record in logbook, flag results in meter, or use a mobile application)
- track, log, and share other important medical data
- explain relevance of glucose monitoring results and describe appropriate action to take when glucose results are out of range

Barriers and Facilitators

The participant will:

- identify potential barriers/facilitators which may impact his or her ability to implement an appropriate monitoring plan
- develop strategies for reducing barriers and increasing facilitators in order to successfully implement an appropriate monitoring plan

Behavioral Objective

The participant will set realistic, measurable individual goals for monitoring.

MONITORING: INSTRUCTIONAL PLAN

There's More to Monitoring Than Checking Glucose

When you talk about monitoring and diabetes, most people automatically think about checking the blood glucose level. It's true that checking your glucose is an important part of diabetes self-care. But monitoring your overall health includes keeping tabs on lots of other things too. That's because diabetes can have an effect on many parts of your body.

To lower your risk of diabetes complications, there are actions you can take every day. And there are tests and exams that you need to have done on a periodic basis:

- Measuring long-term glucose control—A1C, eAG, fructosamine, and 1,5 Anhydroglucitol
- Cardiovascular health—blood pressure and lipid testing
- Liver health—liver enzyme testing
- Kidney health—urine and blood testing
- Eye health—dilated eye exams
- Foot health—foot exams and sensory testing
- Weight

You should work with your provider to make sure that your long-term health is being monitored in a timely manner.

American Association of Diabetes Educators©

Module 5 *Monitoring*   175

Refer to Module 8: Reducing Risks for more detailed information on prevention and treatment strategies for long-term complications.

Identifying Participant Thoughts and Feelings About Monitoring

> *In what ways can you monitor diabetes?*
> *How important is monitoring your blood glucose level? Why?*
> *What do you want to learn today about monitoring?*
> *What is your greatest concern/frustration about monitoring?*
> *What is the hardest part about monitoring?*
> *For you, what is the best part about monitoring?*
> *What do you need to help you be successful in monitoring your blood glucose?*
> *How do you think monitoring your blood glucose level will affect your pregnancy?*

Benefits of Monitoring

Consider using analogies to everyday life that can help describe the benefits of monitoring. One analogy, "Driving a Car," is provided below.

Driving a Car

If you drive a car, you already have experience using monitors. When driving, you look at the instrument panel to tell you what the next step should be. To know how fast you are going, you look at the numbers on the speedometer. If you see that you are going above the speed limit (your target), you step on the brake. If you need to speed up, you press on the accelerator. To know your fuel level, you look at the gas gauge. If it is low, you stop at the gas station and refuel. If you see the engine light come on, you know that something needs attention. You then take a look under the hood and correct it. If it's beyond your ability, you can get help from a mechanic. If you drove your car without a speedometer, gas gauge, or engine light, sooner or later you'd get a ticket for speeding, or you'd run out of gas. You may even run out of oil, burn up your oil pan, and ruin the engine.

Trying to manage diabetes without monitoring is like driving without these instruments. You may be able to get along OK for a while. But sooner or later, the lack of information, and not taking corrective action, would probably cause serious health problems. Your blood glucose monitor is your instrument panel. Knowing what the monitoring results mean will help guide your next step.

If you experience certain symptoms, you can monitor to see if your blood glucose level is the cause. If your blood glucose is above your target, you can take steps to lower it or at least limit the rise. If your blood glucose is below your target, you can take steps to bring it up. If it's beyond your ability, you can get help from your healthcare provider. If you know what the numbers mean, you can make wiser choices in managing your diabetes. And just like driving a car, using monitoring results to manage diabetes is a skill that takes time to master. You will learn by trial and error.

American Association of Diabetes Educators©

Why Monitor Blood Glucose?

Why am I asked to check my blood glucose at different times of the day? Why can't I check every morning? That is what my brother does each day.

Monitoring your blood glucose can help in a lot of ways:

- Monitoring glucose in the blood is much more accurate than testing urine for glucose. In the past, urine testing was the only way to measure glucose at home. The amount of glucose in the urine only gives an estimate of the amount of glucose that was in the blood hours earlier. Also, urine testing cannot measure hypoglycemia (low blood glucose).
- Monitoring can help you reach your target goals for blood glucose. Keeping blood glucose near normal most of the time helps lower the chance of complications. Research shows that monitoring blood glucose related to meals helps improve long-term diabetes control (lowering A1C).[3,4]
- For those who are pregnant or planning to become pregnant, monitoring helps prevent poor outcomes with the pregnancy.
- Monitoring can help you prevent or detect low blood glucose (hypoglycemia). Extremely low blood glucose may require a visit to the hospital.
- Monitoring can help you prevent or detect extremely high blood glucose (hyperglycemia), such as when you are ill. Checking blood glucose during times of illness is especially important if you have type 1 diabetes. Extremely high glucose may require a visit to the hospital.
- Monitoring can help you learn how food affects your blood glucose. What type of food? What amount of food?
- Monitoring can help you learn how activity affects your blood glucose. What type of activity? What amount of activity?
- Monitoring can help you know the right amount of insulin to take (with your provider's guidance).
- Monitoring can help you and your healthcare provider know whether any changes are needed in your medication(s).

Target Blood Glucose Levels

What blood glucose level is advised for a person with diabetes?

Has your doctor recommended any specific goals for your blood glucose?

What glucose level is advised for a pregnant woman with diabetes?

When a person does not have diabetes, the blood glucose stays in a narrow range:

- Before meals: 70 to 100 mg/dL (3.9 to 5.6 mmol/L)
- 2 hours after meals: <140 mg/dL (<7.8 mmol/L)

Research shows that if people with diabetes keep their blood glucose close to normal, it helps prevent complications. If a person already has diabetes complications, keeping the glucose close to normal helps keep him or her from getting worse.[5-10] Your diabetes self-care plan is meant to help get your glucose within a near-normal range. This range is called your *target*.

American Association of Diabetes Educators©

Different professional organizations—eg, the American Diabetes Association (ADA) and the American Association of Clinical Endocrinologists (AACE)—recommend glucose targets for those with diabetes. Even though they may differ slightly, they are still close enough to normal to give you major health benefits. Or, if you have certain conditions, your provider may make adjustments to the target to keep you safe. For example, if you are unable to recognize when blood glucose is dropping too low, your provider may recommend a slightly higher target.

Glucose Targets for Nonpregnant Adults With Diabetes	
American Diabetes Association*	**American Association of Clinical Endocrinologists[†]**
Before meals: 80–130 mg/dL (4.4–7.2 mmol/L)	Before meals: <110 mg/dL (<5.6 mmol/L)
1 to 2 hours after meals: <180 mg/dL (<10 mmol/L)	2 hours after meals: <140 mg/dL (<7.8 mmol/L)
A1C: <7% in general for individuals, as close to 6.5% as possible without hypoglycemia; <8.0% for multiple comorbidities	A1C: <6.5%

*American Diabetes Association, "Standards of medical care in diabetes—2015," *Diabetes Care* 38, Suppl 1 (2015): S1-94.
[†]American Association of Clinical Endocrinologists Diabetes Mellitus Clinical Practice Guidelines Task Force, "Medical guidelines for clinical practice for the management of diabetes mellitus," *Endocr Pract* 13, Suppl 1 (2007): 1-68.

Glucose Targets for Pregnant Women With Diabetes

Controlling blood glucose during pregnancy is extremely important to prevent complications with the growing baby. Table 5.1 has the recommended blood glucose targets from the ADA. Other professional organizations recommend different glucose targets for pregnant women with diabetes. Even though they differ, they are still close enough to normal to help prevent complications with the pregnancy. Your healthcare provider may recommend one target or the other.

The American College of Obstetricians and Gynecologists (ACOG) recommends the targets shown in Table 5.2. The ADA recommends slightly higher targets if the risk for hypoglycemia is high. The ADA recommends setting targets based on clinical experience and individualizing care.[11(p578)]

Glucose Targets for Children

The recommended blood glucose targets in children are higher than those for adults. (See Table 5.3.) A higher target lowers the chance of hypoglycemia, which can be very dangerous in a child. Babies and small children are unable to recognize hypoglycemia and make it known to others. Children who have hypoglycemia unawareness—a condition where the symptoms of low blood glucose are delayed or absent—will need even higher targets in order to remain safe. All goals should be individualized; lower or higher goals may be reasonable based on benefit-risk assessment. Consider checking postprandial blood glucoses if there is a discrepancy between preprandial blood glucose and expected A1C levels.

The ADA releases the updated Standards of Medical Care in Diabetes *each January.* Refer to this resource to update your curriculum each year.

TABLE 5.1 Recommended Target Blood Glucose During Pregnancy*

	Women With Preexisting Type 1 or Type 2 Diabetes[‡]	Women With Gestational Diabetes[§]
Premeal	60–99 mg/dL (3.3–5.4 mmol/L)	<95 mg/dL (<5.3 mmol/L)
1-hour postmeal (peak postprandial)	100–129 mg/dL (5.5–7.1 mmol/L)	<140 mg/dL (<7.8 mmol/L)
2-hour postmeal (peak postprandial)	100–129 mg/dL (5.5–7.2 mmol/L)	<120 mg/dL (<6.7 mmol/L)
Bedtime/overnight	60–99 mg/dL (3.3–5.4 mmol/L)	
A1C[†]	<6%	

*Plasma values.

[†]Due to the increase in red blood cells during pregnancy, A1C levels fall during pregnancy. A1C should be used as a secondary measure after self-blood glucose monitoring. A1C levels may need to be monitored more frequently in pregnancy (eg, monthly).

[‡]American Diabetes Association, "Standards of medical care in diabetes—2015," *Diabetes Care* 38, Suppl 1 (2015): S1-94; American Association of Clinical Endocrinologists Diabetes Mellitus Clinical Practice Guidelines Task Force, "Medical guidelines for clinical practice for the management of diabetes mellitus," *Endocr Pract* 13, Suppl 1 (2007): 1-68; JL Kitzmiller, JM Block, FM Brown, et al, "Managing preexisting diabetes for pregnancy: summary of evidence and consensus recommendations for care," *Diabetes Care* 31 (2008): 1060-79.

[§]JL Kitzmiller, JM Block, FM Brown, et al, "Managing preexisting diabetes for pregnancy: summary of evidence and consensus recommendations for care," *Diabetes Care* 31 (2008): 1060-79; BE Metzger, TA Buchanan, DR Coustan, et al, "Summary and recommendations of the Fifth International Workshop—Conference on Gestational Diabetes Mellitus," *Diabetes Care* 30, Suppl 2 (2007): S251-60.

TABLE 5.2 ADA and ACOG Glucose Targets Compared

	American Diabetes Association (ADA)*	American College of Obstetrics and Gynecologists (ACOG)[†]
Fasting	<150 mg/dL (8.3 mmol/L)	<90 mg/dL (5.0 mmol/L)
Preprandial	60–99 mg/dL (3.3–5.5 mmol/L)	<105 mg/dL (5.8 mmol/L)
1-hour postprandial	<155 mg/dL (8.6 mmol/L)	<130–140 mg/dL (7.2–7.8 mmol/L)
2-hour postprandial	<130 mg/dL (7.2 mmol/L)	<120 mg/dL (<6.7 mmol/L)

*American Diabetes Association, "Standards of medical care in diabetes—2015," *Diabetes Care* 38, Suppl 1 (2015): S1-94.

[†]MB Landon, SG Gabbe, "Gestational diabetes mellitus," *Obstet Gynecol* 118 (2011): 1386.

TABLE 5.3 Recommended Target Blood Glucose for Children of All Age Groups

Premeal	90–130 mg/dL (5.0–7.2 mmol/L)
Bedtime/overnight	90–150 mg/dL (5.0–8.3 mmol/L)
A1C	<7.5%*

*A lower A1C goal (<7.0%) is reasonable if achievable without excessive hypoglycemia.

Source: American Diabetes Association, "Standards of medical care in diabetes—2015," *Diabetes Care* 38, Suppl 1 (2015): S1-94.

Selecting a Glucose Meter

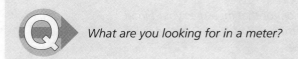
What are you looking for in a meter?

Every glucose meter is different. The best meter for you is the one that meets *your* needs, the one that you can operate correctly. All glucose meters on the market have met federal guidelines for accuracy. The US Food and Drug Administration (FDA) regulates glucose meters and their test strips. Let's look at several factors that may help you decide on the right meter for you:

- **Meter selection offered by your insurance plan:** Sometimes an insurance plan will cover only certain meters, or it may cover any meter, but some at a higher co-pay than others.
- **Cost of meter and strips:** If your supplies are covered by insurance, you will need to find out how much you will have to pay—a set co-pay or a percentage of the total cost?
- **Size and shape of meter:** Do you want a meter small enough to put in a purse or backpack? Do you want something that's easy to hold in your hands?
- **Steps to do a glucose check:** Can you easily operate the meter? Can you handle the test strips? Is loading of the lancing device easy enough to do?
- **How long it takes for results:** Some meters offer results in as little as a few seconds; some may take several seconds. Does time matter to you?
- **Size of the readout:** Can you easily read the prompts and the results on the screen?
- **Blood sample size required:** Meters differ in the size of the blood drop required. The lancing device can be adjusted to get just enough blood for the test.
- **Maintaining the equipment (cleaning, calibrating, coding):** Meters differ in the need to code for each batch of test strips. Those that require the blood to be inserted inside the meter will require cleaning.
- **Marking of test results:** Can you mark results to show that it was a pre- or postmeal reading?
- **Memory and averaging of test results:** Nearly all of today's meters have memory; that is, they can recall past test results. How much memory do you want? Some meters can show you an average of all readings, or an average of readings done at a certain time (for example, an average of postmeal readings).
- **Computer download feature:** Do you want to connect your meter to a computer and download your results? Most meters have download capability. You can obtain software and a download cable from the meter company. With the software, you can show results in many different formats—pie charts, line graphs, a format similar to a logbook, etc. These printouts are useful in helping you and your healthcare provider understand your blood glucose patterns.
- **Interface with mobile application:** Some meters have the capability of interfacing with a mobile application, which may allow for additional tracking of data, analysis and display of data, and sharing of data.
- **Special features:** There are meters that have audio capability. These are the "talking meters" that are useful for those with vision problems or who want the instructions spoken aloud during the procedure. Some meters have a backlight, so monitoring can be done in the dark. Some meters can interact with an insulin pump to coordinate monitoring and insulin.

Continuous Glucose Monitoring System (CGMS)[11(ppS33-4)]

I heard that there is a monitor that measures your blood sugar constantly. Is this true, and how can I get one? I'm tired of poking my fingers.

Continuous glucose monitoring is another method of monitoring glucose *trends*. A tiny probe in the skin measures the glucose content in the fluid of your skin. This system can measure glucose every few minutes for up to 72 hours. The effect of food, exercise, and insulin on blood glucose can be better understood than with standard monitoring. The CGMS alarms when glucose levels go lower or higher than programmed limits.

The CGMS sensor is placed during a healthcare provider office visit for trending and diagnostic purposes. The patient keeps the sensor on for up to 3 days. Finger-stick monitoring must be done each day with a standard glucose monitor, following the recommendations of the sensor manufacturer for testing frequency, in order to calibrate the sensor. Any diabetes treatment decisions that need to be made should be based on a finger-stick glucose reading. After 3 days, the patient returns to the provider's office. The sensor is removed, and the provider analyzes the glucose patterns. This helps the patient and the healthcare provider decide on the best plan of care.

Continuous glucose monitoring is also available for home use. Many CGMS sensors are paired with insulin pumps to help in making lifestyle decisions based on more complete glucose information. The sensor may be used for varying amounts of time and can show more blood glucose trends than is possible with standard monitoring. The cost of a CGMS can be a factor in patient use.

General Guidelines for Monitoring

How do you know your meter is working correctly?
How can you check to see if your strips are OK?
What's control range?

Different meters will vary in their operating instructions. But the following basic guidelines for monitoring generally apply: control solution testing, storage of testing supplies, disposing used lancets, hand-washing, getting an adequate drop of blood, alternate testing sites, and recording results.

Control Testing: Checking the System for Quality

You can run a quality check on your meter and strips to see if they are working properly. These quality checks are called *control testing*. Some meters will automatically run a quality check each time you turn the meter on. Follow the meter manufacturer's instruction for control solution testing.

Some new meters come with control solution; others require the control solution to be purchased separately. Every monitoring system uses its own brand of control solution. It's important to do a control test whenever you open a new container of test strips. Another time you should consider control testing is when your blood glucose results are unusual and do not match how you feel. Follow the meter manufacturer's specific guidelines for how often you should do control testing.

An unopened vial of control solution can be used until the expiration date. Once opened, it is only good for a few months. Check the product insert for each specific brand, as brands may vary. To keep track of when you need to discard the control solution, mark the date on the side of the vial.

Storage of Monitoring Supplies

Testing supplies need to be kept in a certain temperature and humidity range to keep working correctly. The user's manual will give specifics for each brand of meter. In general, though, the following are guidelines for safe storage of testing supplies:

- Strips that are unopened are good until the printed expiration date. If you receive a shipment of test strips from a mail order company, check the expiration date on all boxes of strips. Be sure to first use the strips that expire the soonest. Once the strip container is opened, the strips must be used within a certain time frame. Check the product insert for each specific brand, as brands may vary.
- Keep strips in a dry place.
- Avoid storing strips or meter in areas of high humidity, like the bathroom.
- Keep the strip container tightly capped to protect the strips from light, heat, and humidity. If strips are individually wrapped, *do not* unwrap until ready to use a strip.
- Never leave the meter or strips where they can be exposed to extreme temperatures, eg, in a parked car or in the cargo hold of a bus, train, or airplane.

Traveling With Monitoring Supplies[12]

When you travel, take extra care to keep your meter and monitoring supplies safe from harm. The cargo compartments of buses, airplanes, and trains, as well as the trunk of a car, may be too hot or too cold for your meter and supplies. Carry your meter and all monitoring supplies on board with you when traveling by these modes of transportation.

Notify the Transportation Safety Administration (TSA) officer that you have diabetes and that you have monitoring supplies with you. Be aware of the current TSA regulations that apply to most modes of public transportation.

Hand-washing

Washing your hands before monitoring is important for 2 reasons. First, it removes any residue from your skin that could cause inaccurate results. Second, hand-washing helps prevent infection. You may use an alcohol pad, but it is not necessary. Alcohol can be very drying to the skin. Waterless hand rinses tend to be high in alcohol content.

Whether you use soap and water, alcohol, or waterless hand rinse, be sure to thoroughly dry the skin before monitoring. If you try to get a blood sample while the skin is still moist, the blood tends to run into the grooves of the skin. When this happens, it is hard to get a usable drop to place on the test strip.

Tips for Getting an Adequate Blood Sample

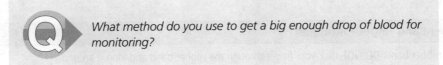

What method do you use to get a big enough drop of blood for monitoring?

The most common cause of inaccurate monitoring results is an inadequate blood sample. Some meters will not start unless there is enough blood. Other meters give an error message when the blood sample is too small to start the procedure. Even if your meter has these safeguards, it's still important to get an adequate drop of blood, just to be sure. Follow these steps to get an adequate drop of blood from your fingertip:

- Use warm water to wash the hands. Vigorously rub hands together to increase blood circulation to the fingertips.
- Shake the hand to force blood to the fingertips.

- Help blood run to the fingertips by holding your hand at your side for about 30 seconds.
- Set the lancing device to puncture just deep enough to get the size of blood drop you need.
- Lance on the sides of the finger rather than the fingertip. This causes less discomfort because there are fewer nerve endings on the sides. Also, the blood vessels on the sides of the finger are closer to the surface of the skin. On the fingertip, there is a fat pad that may prevent the lancet from reaching the vessel.
- If your lancet does not puncture deeply enough, use a larger gauge; if your lancet punctures too deeply, use a smaller gauge. **Note:** the larger the gauge number, the smaller the thickness of the lancet.

After the finger is lanced, gently milk blood toward the fingertip. Apply pressure to the base of the finger where it meets the palm, and move toward the tip. This is more effective than squeezing just the tip of the finger.

If the steps outlined above are not effective, consider placing a rubber band around your dangling finger just above the first joint to make a tourniquet, trapping blood in the fingertip.

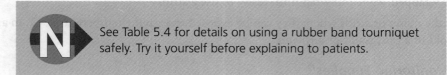

See Table 5.4 for details on using a rubber band tourniquet safely. Try it yourself before explaining to patients.

Alternate Site Testing

You may have seen or heard advertising about meters that don't require you to stick your finger. This refers to *alternate site testing*. It's true that you can monitor your blood glucose without lancing the *finger*. *But* you have to lance *someplace*.

In alternate site testing, the meter and strips have been designed to allow blood from places such as the palm, forearm, upper arm, or thigh. These areas of the body have far fewer nerve endings than the fingers. If you plan to use alternate sites, you must understand the limits of this kind of monitoring.

Blood flows more quickly through the finger vessels than in the smaller vessels in the skin in these other (alternate) areas. Because of this lag in blood flow to alternate sites, there can be a big difference when you compare glucose results from alternate sites with those from the finger. Differences of up to 100 mg/dL (5.6 mmol/L) have been reported. When your blood glucose level is rapidly changing, the difference is greater. An exception is the base of the thumb, which does not experience this significant lag in blood flow. If you use alternate sites, this area is recommended.[13]

Finger-stick monitoring is the best in pregnancy because of the rapid changes in blood glucose concentration that occur in pregnancy.

TABLE 5.4 Rubber Band Finger Tourniquet
• Get a fairly large rubber band. DO NOT stick your finger through the rubber band and loop it around.
• First, pinch the "hole" of the rubber band shut so you have two parallel lengths of rubber.
• Then, wrap the double strip of rubber once around the middle section of your finger, just above the first joint.
• Pull the rubber band just snugly enough to slow the circulation through your finger. DO NOT pull so tightly as to cut off circulation to your finger completely.
• Hold the overlapping area of rubber band between the finger and your thumb. This leaves your other hand free to lance your finger.
• Lance your finger when it becomes engorged with blood.
• Lift your thumb to release the tourniquet, but be sure not to disturb the drop of blood.

Source: Diabetes Self-Management, "Rubber band tourniquet" (cited 2015 July 12), on the Internet at: http://static.diabetesselfmanagement.com/pdfs/pdf_2250.pdf.

When It's OK to Use an Alternate Site

Alternate site testing may be done when glucose levels are fairly steady, such as before a meal and the 2 hours after a meal. Always note on your blood glucose logbook if the check was done using an alternate site.

When It's *Not OK* to Use an Alternate Site

Blood glucose levels are expected to change quickly in certain situations. In the following instances, alternate site testing is *not recommended*.

When Blood Glucose Is Rising Quickly	When Blood Glucose Is Falling Quickly
• within the 2 hours after a meal • when you are sick	• when insulin reaches its "peak" activity (rapid-, short-, and intermediate-acting insulin) • after exercise • during a hypoglycemic (low blood glucose) episode

To be on the safe side, it is also *not recommended* to use alternate sites for pre-driving glucose checks. People who have *hypoglycemia unawareness* (a condition where one cannot properly feel the symptoms of hypoglycemia) should not use alternate sites for monitoring.

Few patients use alternate site testing. Address if a specific concern is verbalized in your group.

Disposal of Used Lancets

Used lancets are a health hazard. They should be stored in a container that is shatterproof and has a lid that holds firm if the container is dropped.

What type of containers could you find at home that would be suitable to store used lancets?

Heavy plastic containers like detergent or bleach jugs are ideal for storing used lancets. When the lancets are ready for disposal, the top of the container should be tightly closed and the words *medical sharps* written on the container. Another option is to use a store-bought sharps disposal unit. Follow your local sanitation department rules for disposal of either type of container. Some areas allow marked sharps containers to be placed in the regular trash. **Sharps containers should never be placed in the recycle bin.**

Recording and Sharing Your Results

What do you think you can learn from logging your glucose results?

Ask any participants who have learned from their results to share their experience with others in the group.

American Association of Diabetes Educators©

184   Diabetes Education Curriculum

Monitoring and logging results is not just busywork to please your provider. By reviewing your results over time, you can learn to spot a pattern or trend. This will help you see whether changes in eating, activity, or medication (with your provider's guidance) need to be made in your diabetes self-care. Results can be recorded manually by writing them in a glucose logbook (diary). If you can't log a result right away, use your meter's memory to look it up later. It is important to discuss your blood glucose targets and share your blood glucose results with your healthcare provider.

Using Meter Memory

Most meters have a memory function that stores past readings. How these results are displayed varies meter by meter.

 ◆ *Scrolling one result at a time*—You can view results, one by one, from the most recent to the oldest saved reading. When you see results by scrolling, it is very hard to detect a pattern or trend, even if the date and time are included with each result.

 ◆ *Average*—Most meters will average results. Averages may show for the past 7, 14, or 30 days. Some meters also average results that have been marked for a certain time, like premeal or postmeal.

 ◆ *Downloaded memory*—You might want to use software to download meter results. It can be obtained from your meter company. After downloading, you can print them out in the same format as a written logbook. You can display your results in several other ways. For example, you may want to know the percentage of time your fasting blood glucose results are within target. Download programs can display a pie chart to show you the percentage within target, below target, or above target. Or, they can show results from a certain time frame as a line graph.

 ◆ *Mobile app interface with blood glucose meter*—Some meters have the capability of interfacing with a mobile application which may allow for additional tracking of data, analysis and display of data, and sharing of data. They can provide you with the additional capability trending data.

Using a Manual/Electronic Logbook

It is important to record your results, whether you choose to use a paper form or an electronic logbook. There are a number of mobile apps and wearables on the market that can be used to track results. It is important to organize the blood glucose data so that you and your healthcare provider can understand the results. The following guidelines can help.

Day and Date

You should include the date for each entry. Also include the day of the week. This will help you begin to see whether certain results tend to occur on certain days. For many people, their daily schedule changes on the weekends. Blood glucose readings may reflect this change in activity. It is recommended that you enter day and date on the left-hand side of the page. Any glucose readings on that day will be recorded left to right.

Time/Relationship to Meal

Logging the time of a glucose reading is essential. It's especially useful to indicate whether the reading was done just prior to a meal or afterward. Most logbooks label columns with *Breakfast*, *Lunch*, and *Dinner*. Some also include a *Bedtime* or *Other* column. Having the results separated into columns by mealtime is especially helpful if you want to average your results at the end of the week.

Comments/Notes

A comments/notes section allows you to record what may have affected your glucose levels on a certain day. This way you don't have to rely on your memory for details. Comments are meant to help you put "two and two together," so to speak, to learn what affects your glucose levels and when. Then you can make changes, and later

American Association of Diabetes Educators©

> **Advanced Detail**
>
> **American Diabetes Association Guidelines for Monitoring**[11(ppS33-40)]
>
> Self-monitoring of blood glucose has been demonstrated to be an integral component of effective therapy for insulin-treated patients.
>
> Integrating SMBG into diabetes management can be a useful tool for both patients and providers by:
>
> - Providing a tool for assessing whether glycemic targets are being met
> - Guiding adjustments of food and physical activity
> - Preventing hypoglycemia
> - Adjusting medications (particularly mealtime insulin doses)
>
> The recommended frequency and timing of SMBG should be based on the patient's specific needs and goals, which should be reevaluated at each routine visit. Evidence supports a correlation between greater SMBG frequency and lower A1C.
>
> - Patients on an intensive insulin therapy regimen may benefit from SMBG prior to meals and snacks, occasionally postprandially, at bedtime, prior to physical activity, whenever they suspect low blood glucose and after treating low blood glucose, and prior to critical tasks such as driving.
> - While the evidence is insufficient regarding when to prescribe SMBG for patients using basal insulin or oral agents, it should be considered that SMBG itself does not lower blood glucose levels. To be effective, it is essential that the SMBG data be integrated into the diabetes care plan.
>
> It is important to evaluate each patient's monitoring technique when first starting to monitor and at frequent intervals thereafter to ensure consistently accurate results are obtained.
>
> Ongoing review and interpretation of the data by both the patient and the provider are required. Patients should be taught how to use SMBG data to adjust food intake, physical activity, or medications to achieve glycemic goals.
>
> Similar recommendations regarding SMBG are available in the AACE Clinical Practice Guidelines (American Association of Clinical Endocrinologists Medical Guidelines for clinical practice for developing a diabetes mellitus comprehensive care plan. Endocr Pract. 2011;17(Suppl 2):S27).

you can see whether those changes helped bring your glucose levels toward your target. If your adjustments in eating or activity do not correct the problem, your provider may need to change your medication dosage or timing.

 What blood glucose trends are you able to see using your own blood glucose results?

Do you have enough data points to see trends?

When and How Often to Monitor Blood Glucose

 See American Diabetes Association Guidelines for Monitoring. See also the examples of "staggered," paired, and 3-, 5-, and 7-point profile blood glucose checking regimens in Table 5.5.

186 Diabetes Education Curriculum

TABLE 5.5 Examples of SMBG Regimens

3-point SMBG profile to check fasting and effect of largest meal

	Pre-breakfast	Post-breakfast	Pre-lunch	Post-lunch	Pre-supper	Post-supper	Bedtime
Monday	X				X	X	
Tuesday	X				X	X	
Wednesday	X				X	X	
Thursday	X				X	X	
Friday	X				X	X	
Saturday	X				X	X	
Sunday	X				X	X	

5-point SMBG profile

	Pre-breakfast	Post-breakfast	Pre-lunch	Post-lunch	Pre-supper	Post-supper	Bedtime
Monday	X	X		X	X	X	
Tuesday	X	X		X	X	X	
Wednesday							
Thursday							
Friday							
Saturday							
Sunday	X	X		X	X	X	

7-point SMBG profile

	Pre-breakfast	Post-breakfast	Pre-lunch	Post-lunch	Pre-supper	Post-supper	Bedtime
Monday							
Tuesday							
Wednesday							
Thursday	X	X	X	X	X	X	X
Friday	X	X	X	X	X	X	X
Saturday	X	X	X	X	X	X	X
Sunday							

American Association of Diabetes Educators©

TABLE 5.5   Examples of SMBG Regimens (*continued*)

"Staggered" SMBG profile

	Pre-breakfast	Post-breakfast	Pre-lunch	Post-lunch	Pre-supper	Post-supper	Bedtime
Monday	X	X					
Tuesday			X	X			
Wednesday					X	X	
Thursday	X	X					
Friday			X	X			
Saturday					X	X	
Sunday	X	X					

Meal-based SMBG profile (less intensive)

	Pre-breakfast	Post-breakfast	Pre-lunch	Post-lunch	Pre-supper	Post-supper	Bedtime
Monday	X	X					
Tuesday							
Wednesday			X	X			
Thursday							
Friday							
Saturday					X	X	
Sunday							

SMBG profile to assess or detect fasting hyperglycemia

	Pre-breakfast	Post-breakfast	Pre-lunch	Post-lunch	Pre-supper	Post-supper	Bedtime
Monday							X
Tuesday	X						
Wednesday							X
Thursday	X						
Friday							X
Saturday	X						
Sunday							

Note: Ensure that the patient's food and activity tracking are consistent in order to appropriately interpret the glucose data.

Source: MM Austin, N D'Hondt, "Monitoring," in C Mensing, ed, *The Art and Science of Diabetes Self-Management Education: A Desk Reference for Healthcare Professionals*, 3rd ed (Chicago: American Association of Diabetes Educators, 2014), 211-2.

American Association of Diabetes Educators©

There are no standard guidelines for how often a person should monitor his or her blood glucose. Different professional organizations publish their own recommendations. How often and when *you* should monitor should be a decision made between you and your diabetes team. Your provider may recommend a monitoring schedule. If not, here are some questions that will help you decide *when* and *how often* you should monitor.

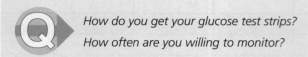

How do you get your glucose test strips?
How often are you willing to monitor?

How Often Are You Willing and Able to Monitor?

Your health plan may limit the number of strips it will cover. Typically, persons who do not use insulin are provided with 100 testing strips every 3 months; those who use insulin are provided with 3 testing strips per day. More than 3 testing strips per day may require additional documentation from the healthcare provider showing that more testing is needed.

If you can monitor only once per day, vary the times you do it. On some days, check before the first meal of the day (fasting). On other days, check 2 hours after a meal. Rotate the postmeal readings between breakfast, lunch, and dinner.

If you plan to monitor twice a day, do it just before a meal *and* 2 hours after the same meal. From day to day, rotate these checks between breakfast, lunch, and dinner. On the days that you are monitoring pre- and post-breakfast, you will capture the fasting blood glucose level.

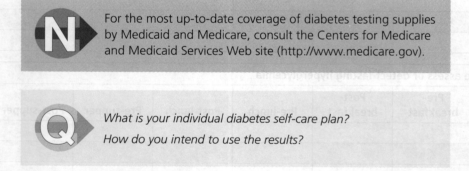

For the most up-to-date coverage of diabetes testing supplies by Medicaid and Medicare, consult the Centers for Medicare and Medicaid Services Web site (http://www.medicare.gov).

What is your individual diabetes self-care plan?
How do you intend to use the results?

If you want to learn the effect of food portions on your glucose levels, you can check 2 hours after the start of a meal. Pregnant women should generally monitor 1 or 2 hours after the start of a meal. Frequent elevated readings may reflect too much carbohydrate intake at meals; a change in the carbohydrate intake at meals may help normalize your glucose levels. Experiment and see for yourself. If postmeal blood glucoses continue to be elevated despite a reduction in carbohydrate intake, a change in medication dosage or additional medication may need to be considered. Share your results with your healthcare provider.

If you want to find out if your oral or injected diabetes medication is effective, you can check your glucose when the medication is supposed to have its biggest impact (see Table 5.6).

- If your diabetes medication is meant to help control the postmeal blood glucose rise, then it makes sense to check the glucose level 2 hours after eating. If these readings frequently remain out of range, it could mean the medication needs adjustment. Consult your provider for any medication adjustments.
- If your diabetes medication is meant to help control the fasting blood glucose (by limiting glucose from the liver), then it makes sense to check the glucose level upon waking. If these readings frequently remain out of range, it could mean the medication needs adjustment. Consult your provider for any medication adjustments.

TABLE 5.6 Medication Effects on Blood Glucose

Medication	Fasting	Postprandial
Biguanides (metformin)	X	X (mild)
Insulin secretagogues:		
• Sulfonylureas (glyburide, glimepiride, glipizide)	X	X
• Meglitinides (nateglinide, repaglinide)		X
Alpha-glucosidase inhibitors (acarbose, miglitol)		X
Thiazolidinediones (pioglitazone)	X	X
Sodium-glucose co-transporter 2 (SGLT2) inhibitors (canagliflozin, dapaglifozin)	X	X
Incretin mimetics:		
• GLP-1 receptor agonists (exenatide, liraglutide)	X (mild)	X
• Amylin analogs (pramlintide)		X
• DPP-IV inhibitors (sitagliptin, vildagliptin, linagliptin, saxagliptin, alogliptin)		X
Insulin:		
• Premeal insulins (lispro, aspart, glulisine, Regular)	X	X
• Basal insulins (glargine, detemir, NPH, Ultralente)	X	X
• Premixed insulins (NPH/Regular, 70/30; NPH/lispro, 75/25 or 50/50; NPH/aspart, 70/30		X

Source: MM Austin, N D'Hondt, "Monitoring," in C Mensing, ed, *The Art and Science of Diabetes Self-Management Education: A Desk Reference for Healthcare Professionals*, 3rd ed (Chicago: American Association of Diabetes Educators, 2014), 213.

For a comprehensive listing of current diabetes medications and their primary physiological action, refer to Module 4: Taking Medication. Additionally, refer to ADA Standards of Care *each year* to keep your curriculum updated.

Interpreting and Responding to Blood Glucose Results

Sometimes it is easy to understand what your glucose results mean and what you should do in response. For example, when you have symptoms of hypoglycemia (low blood glucose), a single blood glucose reading can confirm your suspicions. In this situation, you should know that your next action should be to take a 15-g carbohydrate snack.

In most cases, making decisions about your diabetes self-care will require that you take multiple glucose readings over time. This will help you identify a *trend* or *pattern*. When you see similar results repeatedly after a certain action (food, activity, medication), you can begin to make a connection.

Always insist that your provider review the past few weeks or so of your blood glucose results. If you use a logbook and circle or highlight readings that are out of range, your provider will be able to more easily notice any patterns or trends. This helps the provider quickly zero in on areas that may need adjustment. Your written comments will show the provider that you are invested in your diabetes self-care.

An alternative to a paper logbook is the use of mobile prescription therapy (MPT), where you electronically log your blood glucose results, notes, and other health information into a smartphone or other device and are able to share results for use by the healthcare provider at any time.[14,15] The ADA recognizes MPT as a new category of therapy. MPT products are not simple health apps for your phone or tablet. They can provide real-time guidance that typical apps are not allowed to do. MPT products are regulated by the FDA.

For technology tools to be successful in engaging individuals with diabetes, changing behavior, and improving outcomes, it is necessary that they be based on evidence-based content and methods. It is also critical that these technologies and tools link the individual with diabetes with his or her provider for the ongoing support, coaching, and treatment modifications that are essential to ongoing long-term diabetes control.[15]

Too often patients keep their blood glucose results from their provider for fear of being scolded. The review of the logbook or electronically transmitted blood glucose results should not be viewed as an opportunity to cast blame. **It should be a time to discover how your self-care or your medical care can be adjusted.**

What Would You Do? Problem-Solving Activity

Below are 5 real-life scenarios that patients might face. Ask the questions in the box and encourage patients to brainstorm for solutions. Or, if patients are willing to share their own blood glucose results, utilize their data for the scenarios. Reasonable responses for how to deal with the situation follow, with the understanding that there may well be other possible solutions.

Reality Scenario #1

Your pre-breakfast glucose readings are usually within range. But most days, your readings taken 2 hours after breakfast are above range.

What do you think could be causing the elevated glucose readings after breakfast?

What could you do to keep track of possible causes for the elevated results?

Reasonable response: Too much carbohydrate at breakfast might be causing the elevated readings. Jot down or input information on carbohydrate intake on days when glucose is above range.

Once you figure out possible causes, what could you do to prevent future elevated readings after breakfast?

What could you do to keep track of possible causes for the elevated results?

Reasonable response: Make a change in type or amount of carbohydrate choices at breakfast.

Reality Scenario #2

Your pre-dinner readings are usually above target. You know that dinner will raise it more, even if you follow your meal plan.

What do you think might have caused your glucose to already be elevated before dinner?

Reasonable responses: Too much carbohydrate at lunch (or afternoon snack, if taken). Diabetes medication not at optimum dose.

What could you do to limit the rise in glucose after dinner?
How will you know if your plan works or not?

Reasonable responses: Increase activity (eg, take a walk) after dinner. Check blood glucose before bedtime. Record activity in the comments section of the logbook. If this becomes a trend, contact healthcare provider with results for possible medication adjustment.

What could you do to prevent future elevated readings before dinner?

Reasonable responses: Make a change in amount of carbohydrate at lunch (or afternoon snack, if taken). Show provider logbook trends. If carbohydrate intake at lunch (or afternoon snack, if taken) is not the cause of elevated readings before dinner, ask if diabetes medication needs adjustment.

Reality Scenario #3

On 3 days of 1 week, you had an episode of low blood glucose (hypoglycemia) sometime between lunch and dinner. You treated each episode properly and recovered within 15 to 30 minutes. You record or input the glucose level and the time of each event in the comments section of your monitoring logbook or mobile device.

What do you think may have caused the episodes of low blood glucose?

Reasonable response: More than 6 hours between meals (eg, ate early lunch and/or late dinner).

Once you figure out possible causes, what could you do to prevent future episodes of low blood glucose?

Reasonable response: Shift some carbohydrates from breakfast or dinner to midafternoon for a snack.

Reality Scenario #4

You plan to check your blood glucose after meals, but you keep forgetting.

What can you do to help you remember to check your glucose after meals?

American Association of Diabetes Educators©

192 Diabetes Education Curriculum

Reasonable responses: Set an alarm on your watch or mobile device. Post a reminder note where you will see it later. Ask someone to remind you.

Reality Scenario #5

Your MPT program has alerted you that you had elevated fasting blood glucoses over the past week, but you haven't shared your results with your healthcare provider.

Why is it important to share your results with your healthcare provider?

Reasonable response: Have a clear understanding of what your blood glucose targets are and share your results with your healthcare provider when your results are consistently above your target range.

Identifying Barriers to Monitoring[2(p203)]

Even though you know that monitoring is useful, there may be barriers that prevent you from making healthy choices about monitoring. For every barrier there may be many possible solutions.

What might work to overcome this barrier? Let's brainstorm together and learn from one another's experiences.

Poor health literacy and numeracy skills can negatively impact successful monitoring. Consider screening for literacy and numeracy skills.[16]

Reality Scenario	Problem Solving Possible Solutions/What Would *You* Do?
Financial	
I can't afford to monitor. The strips are too expensive and I don't have any (or enough) insurance coverage.	Some glucose test strip companies offer coupons (some can be applied to your insurance co-pay). Call the toll-free number on the back of your meter to see if coupons for strips are available for your meter. Check your insurance benefits to see if you are using the brand of glucose meter that requires the lowest co-pay for your plan or if you are required to use a mail order service. Consider any other sources of support besides insurance that may be able to assist.
Physical limitations	
I have arthritis/neuropathy in my hands. It's hard to open the container that the test strips come in. And they're so tiny, I usually drop the strip once I get one out.	Work with your diabetes educator to find a meter that can be operated easily with hand problems such as arthritis or neuropathy. Look for a meter with hands-free test strips (disk) or whose test strip containers are easily opened.
I have trouble monitoring because of my vision.	Work with your diabetes educator to find a meter that you can use. Consider a meter with a large digital readout or a nonvisual glucose meter. See Module 8: Reducing Risks for more on resources for visual impairment.

American Association of Diabetes Educators©

Reality Scenario	Problem Solving Possible Solutions/What Would *You* Do?
Time constraints	
I'm so busy, I just don't have time to be checking my blood sugar.	Review the times for monitoring. What information do you need to gather? Can you do it? If not, let's work together to make a plan that you can live with.
	Consider your priorities. Think of how you can use your time differently. Delegate less important tasks to others if possible.
I only get a lunch break at work. If I take extra time to go do testing, my boss gets after me.	Explain your medical needs to your boss, and ask that a "reasonable accommodation" be made to allow you to stay healthy with your condition.
Inconvenience	
I get so busy doing other things, I don't think of it till it's too late. Or, when I do think of it, I don't want to stop what I'm doing.	Build in some reminders: alarm on your watch or mobile device. Post reminder notes where you'll see them. Remind yourself that your needs are important, that you are worth the effort to monitor.
At the jobsite, there's nowhere to wash my hands. And besides, I work outside and it's too hot to keep the testing supplies out there.	Consider waterless hand rinse, such as hand sanitizer. Use an insulated storage container for your testing supplies. Monitor when you are home.
Emotional	
Those sticks hurt! I just can't stand to poke myself.	Lance the side of the finger, where there are fewer nerve endings. Learn how to "milk" blood down to your fingertips. Adjust the depth control on your lancing device. Use a lancet with a thinner gauge.
If I have to do a check at work/school/practice, everybody looks at me.	Find a private place to monitor. Learn to monitor discreetly.
My numbers are bad all the time anyway, so what's the point? It just brings me down. I don't want to be reminded of having diabetes.	Put the numbers in perspective. Monitoring results do not reflect your worth as a person. Above-target numbers don't represent failure. They are an opportunity to learn something about your self-care plan. Focus on the positives, on what you are doing that is working. Try to come up with a plan to change the things that are working against achieving your target glucose. Tackle one thing at a time: work on monitoring at a certain time of the day (for example, morning). Once monitoring at that time becomes more routine, add monitoring at other times of the day. If your self-care efforts do not result in improved blood glucose results, consider discussing your efforts with your healthcare provider for possible dosage, or medication change.
My husband hounds me whenever I test. He always wants to know what the result is, and then he makes me feel bad if it's high, like I'm to blame.	Acknowledge your husband's interest in your diabetes. Thank him for his concern. Ask him to help you come up with a plan to prevent above-target results. Ask for his support in carrying out the plan.

Identifying Facilitators for Monitoring

What are some things that help you monitor your blood glucose on a regular basis?

As important as it is to identify barriers to monitoring, it's just as important to consider the positives in our situation—facilitators. Looking deeper, you may find that there are more positives than you thought.

Common Facilitators

- Social support—family members, coworkers, etc
- Community resources—coupons for purchasing glucose testing strips, resources for nonvisual glucose meters
- Reminders and cues—reminder notes, reminder alarms, visual reminders, notes of encouragement (positive affirmations)
- Rewards—incentives to maintain motivation

Long-Term Monitoring to Prevent Complications: A Brief Overview

See Module 8: Reducing Risks for more detailed instructional content on monitoring to prevent complications.

Other than checking your glucose, in what other ways can you monitor the status of your diabetes and your overall heath?

Measuring Long-Term Glucose Control

When you check your blood glucose with a meter, you learn what your glucose level is *at that very moment in time*. It's like you have taken a snapshot. If you check your level several times a day, you learn about *several moments in time* (you have taken several snapshots). Since you can't yet check your level constantly, there are bound to be gaps in what you know. There are certain blood tests that give you a better idea about your overall glucose control during a specific time frame.

A1C

Some of the following content about A1C is duplicated in Module 8: Reducing Risks.

What does the A1C test tell you?
How often should your A1C be measured?
Do you know your target for A1C?

The A1C blood test reflects glucose control over the past 2 to 3 months. A1C results are expressed as a number followed by a percent sign.

Red blood cells circulate throughout your bloodstream for 2 to 3 months, then they die. Your body is always making fresh red blood cells. During their lifespan, some of the glucose in your blood gets stuck to the red blood cells. If the glucose levels are normal, a normal amount of glucose will be found on the red blood cells. If the glucose levels are often higher than normal, a higher amount of glucose will be found on the red blood cells. By measuring the amount of glucose on the red blood cells, overall glucose control for the past 2 to 3 months can be determined.

Different professional groups have slightly different opinions about A1C targets; for example, see Glucose Targets for Nonpregnant Adults with Diabetes (page 177). The different groups do agree that the attempt to achieve these targets should not put a person at risk for having too many episodes of hypoglycemia (low blood sugar).

Numerous studies show that keeping the A1C near normal most of the time drastically lowers your risk of long-term diabetes complications.[5-7] In fact, people who keep nearly normal glucose levels for an extended period tend to have more protection against complications years later, even if their glucose levels begin to creep up during those later years. This lasting (*legacy*) effect of early control emphasizes how important it is to get to goal early in the course of diabetes.[8,9]

> **Standard of Medical Care in Diabetes**
>
> - If your baseline A1C is within target and glucose control is stable, you should have an A1C test done at least twice a year.
>
> - If your A1C is above target or if your diabetes therapy has changed, you should have an A1C test done at least quarterly (4 times a year).
>
> *Source:* American Diabetes Association, "Standards of medical care in diabetes—2015," *Diabetes Care* 38 Suppl 1 (2015): S1-94.

My A1C is higher than target, but my glucose is always normal when I check it at home. How can this be?

Sometimes there is a mismatch between the A1C result and glucose results from home monitoring. If your A1C result does not match your home monitoring, you may not be monitoring at the right time.

A person who monitors before meals with normal results most of the time may believe that his or her diabetes is in control. But since that person does not monitor after any meals, he or she never captures the moment in time when the glucose level is above target. The A1C test will reflect these accumulated upward swings in glucose that premeal monitoring fails to show.

You can't just rely on home monitoring alone *or* on A1C alone. You need both. They are 2 sides of the same coin. The combined information from home monitoring and A1C gives you the *big picture*, rather than just a single snapshot.

The accuracy of the A1C test is affected by the level of red blood cells. People who have too few or too many red blood cells may not have an accurate A1C reading.

eAG: Estimated Average Glucose

Your provider may report your A1C results as *estimated average glucose*, or eAG.[11(pS35)] The eAG shows you what your A1C results mean in terms of an *average* glucose during the past 2 to 3 months. Your doctor may say that "your A1C of 7% shows that your estimated average glucose is 154 mg/dL (8.6 mmol/L)." (See Table 5.7.)

TABLE 5.7 American Diabetes Association Estimated Average Glucose (eAG) Calculator

A1C (%)	eAG mg/dL	eAG mmol/L
6	126	7
6.5	140	7.8
7	154	8.6
7.5	169	9.4
8	183	10.2
8.5	197	10.9
9	212	11.8
9.5	226	12.6
10	240	13.4
10.5	255	14.1
11	269	14.9
11.5	283	15.7
12	298	16.5
12.5	312	17.3
13	326	18.1
13.5	341	18.9
14	355	19.7
14.5	369	20.5
15	384	21.3

Source: American Diabetes Association, "A1C and eAG" (cited 2015 July 12), on the Internet at: http://www.diabetes.org/living-with-diabetes/treatment-and-care/blood-glucose-control/a1c/?loc=lwd-slabnav and http://professional.diabetes.org/GlucoseCalculator.aspx.

Fructosamine

Fructosamine is a test that reflects the overall glucose level over the past 2 to 3 weeks. This test is useful when it is not practical to wait 2 to 3 months for an A1C test, such as during pregnancy.

1,5-Anhydroglucitrol (1,5-AG)

Approved by the FDA in 2003, the 1,5-AG test measures a specific sugar, 1,5 anhydroglucitrol, in the blood. 1,5-AG detects if blood glucoses spike after meals over a period of 2 weeks. It is known as the Glycomark test.

See Module 8: Reducing Risks for more detail about the following aspects of health monitoring.

Monitoring Cardiovascular Health

Your individual cardiovascular risk factors should be discussed with your healthcare provider annually.

- Blood pressure should be measured at every visit to your provider. TARGET: <140/90 mm Hg; <130/80 mm Hg for younger patients if achievable without undue treatment burden.

American Association of Diabetes Educators©

◆ Lipids should be measured at least once a year. TARGETS for most adults with diabetes:

—LDL <100 mg/dL (<2.6 mmol/L)

—HDL for men >40 mg/dL (>1.0 mmol/L)

—HDL for women >50 mg/dL (>1.3 mmol/L)

—Triglycerides <150 mg/dL (<1.7 mmol/L)

Monitoring Kidney Health

Your urine should be tested at least annually to measure the amount of protein.

Monitoring Eye Health

You should have a yearly diabetic eye examination.

Monitoring Foot (Nerve) Health

◆ At each routine visit to your provider, he or she should inspect your feet.

◆ Once a year, your provider should do a comprehensive foot examination. In this examination, the sensitivity of the nerves in the feet is assessed as well as your circulation.

Setting a SMART Goal for Monitoring

S—Specific: not vague

M—Measurable: you can measure it (how much, how often, etc)

A—Attainable: challenging but not out of reach

R—Realistic: given person's situation, can it be done?

T—Timeline: short term, for next week or two

The participant sets an individual goal for monitoring. The educator and the participant schedule a date in which to evaluate progress with behavior change.

Follow-up/Outcomes Measurement

Per the Standards for Outcomes Measurement of Diabetes Self-Management Education, the **first follow-up should be conducted within 2 to 4 weeks** after the initial teaching session on monitoring. At this follow-up, success in implementing monitoring behavior can be assessed. **Subsequent follow-up is recommended at 3- to 6-month intervals thereafter**. Use the following table as a guide for identifying outcomes measures and how to measure them. Measurement of these outcomes may be objective or subjective.[17]

The exception to this schedule would be during pregnancy. The first follow-up should be conducted within 1 week and subsequent visits at 2 to 4 weeks.

Self-Care Behavior: Monitoring Outcomes Measures	Self-Care Behavior: Monitoring Methods of Measurement
Immediate outcome: Learning Immediate outcomes of learning can be assessed right away after the educational encounter. Immediate outcomes include: K: Acquiring *knowledge* (*what to do*) S: Acquiring *skills* (*how to do it*) CM: Developing *confidence and motivation* (*want to do it*) PS: Develop *problem-solving/coping skills* to overcome barrier (*can do it*)	Immediate outcomes of learning can be measured by patient knowledge testing (paper-and-pen testing, or questioning to determine that patient understands information taught). Immediate outcomes for acquiring a skill can be measured by patient's demonstration of that skill. Following are various methods of measuring immediate outcomes for the self-care behavior of *monitoring*.

American Association of Diabetes Educators©

Self-Care Behavior: Monitoring Outcomes Measures	Self-Care Behavior: Monitoring Methods of Measurement
Self-monitoring of blood glucose (K,S)	<u>Subjective:</u> Patient explains how to operate glucose meter. <u>Objective:</u> Patient demonstrates proper glucose monitoring technique.
Care of monitoring supplies (K,S)	<u>Subjective:</u> Patient states how to care for monitoring supplies. <u>Objective:</u> Patient demonstrates proper care of monitoring supplies.
Quality control testing (K,S)	<u>Subjective:</u> Patient explains the purpose of quality control testing for his/her meter and describes how and when to do it. <u>Objective:</u> Patient demonstrates accurate quality control testing.
Disposal of used lancets (K,S)	<u>Subjective:</u> Patient describes proper disposal of used lancets and lists household items that may be used for disposal of used lancets. <u>Objective:</u> Patient demonstrates proper disposal of used lancets.
Target blood glucose values (K)	<u>Subjective:</u> Patient lists target blood glucose values.
Blood glucose monitoring schedule (K,PS)	<u>Subjective:</u> Patient describes appropriate monitoring times for his/her individual situation.
Recording monitoring results (S)	<u>Objective:</u> Patient records results in logbook. Patient marks (flags) results in meter. Patient demonstrates retrieving results from meter memory.
Interpretation and use of glucose results (K,PS)	<u>Subjective:</u> Patient explains relevance of glucose monitoring results, and describes appropriate action to take when results are out of range.
Ketone testing [for type 1, pregnancy] (K,S)	<u>Subjective:</u> Patient explains how to perform ketone testing. Patient explains purpose of quality control testing. <u>Objective:</u> Patient demonstrates correct ketone testing technique.
Testing schedule for ketones [for type 1, pregnancy] (K,PS)	<u>Subjective:</u> Patient describes appropriate ketone testing times.
Interpretation and use of ketone results [for type 1, pregnancy] (K,PS)	<u>Subjective:</u> Patient explains relevance of ketone monitoring results, and describes appropriate action to take when results are out of range.
Potential barriers (physical, financial, cognitive, time, inconvenience, emotional) and facilitators to monitoring (PS)	<u>Subjective:</u> Considering his/her individual situation, patient describes anticipated obstacle(s) that may limit the ability to monitor appropriately. Patient describes facilitators which may help him/her to monitor appropriately.
Strategy to overcome potential barriers to monitoring (PS)	<u>Subjective:</u> Patient develops a plan to deal with anticipated obstacle(s) to monitoring.
Intermediate outcome: Behavior change	Intermediate outcomes measures can be assessed over time: after the educational encounter and once the patient has had adequate time to implement new behavior(s) in a real-life setting. *Behavior change* is an intermediate outcomes measure. It is the ultimate outcome of DSME/T. At follow-up intervals, knowledge and skills (discussed above) should be reassessed, as well as behavior change.
Frequency of monitoring (K,PS)	<u>Subjective:</u> Patient self-report of the frequency of monitoring. <u>Objective:</u> Review of logbook, computer printout of downloaded blood glucose data, and/or manual retrieval of meter (or insulin pump) memory data. Review for frequency and consistency of monitoring.

American Association of Diabetes Educators©

Self-Care Behavior: Monitoring Outcomes Measures	Self-Care Behavior: Monitoring Methods of Measurement
Schedule of monitoring and usage of data (PS)	Subjective: Patient self-report of when monitoring was done and how data are used to make self-care adjustments (carbohydrate intake, insulin dose, activity, etc). Objective: Review of "comments" section in logbook or meter memory for patient interpretation of out-of-range results.
Planned and unplanned monitoring (PS)	Subjective: Patient self-report of planned schedule and actual monitoring. Objective: Review of logbook, computer printout of downloaded blood glucose data, and/or manual retrieval of meter (or insulin pump) memory data. Review of "comments" section in logbook or meter memory for patient interpretation of out-of-range results.
Level of data documentation (PS)	Objective: Are there written results (manual logbook or downloaded computer printout of data from meter or insulin pump), or does patient solely rely on scrolling through meter memory?
Barrier identification and resolution (PS)	Subjective: Patient self-report of barriers faced and of facilitators and strategies used, as patient made efforts to implement monitoring behaviors.
Plan for future behavior change (PS)	Subjective: Patient self-report of monitoring goals and behavior strategies going forward.

REFERENCES

1. McAndrew L, Schneider SH, Burns E, et al. Does patient blood glucose monitoring improve diabetes control? A systematic review of the literature. Diabetes Educ. 2007;33(6):1005-13.

2. Austin MM, D'Hondt N. Chapter 7—Monitoring. In: Mensing C., ed. The Art and Science of Diabetes Self-Management Education Desk Reference. 3rd ed. American Association of Diabetes Educators: Chicago; 2014: 197-245.

3. Schwedes U, Siebolds M, Mertes G. Meal-related structured self-monitoring of blood glucose: effect on diabetes control in noninsulin-treated type 2 diabetic patients. Diabetes Care. 2002;25:1928-32.

4. Polonsky WH, Fisher L, Schikman CH, et al. Structured self-monitoring of blood glucose significantly reduces A1C levels in poorly controlled, non-insulin-treated type 2 diabetes. Diabetes Care. 2011;34:262-7.

5. Diabetes Control and Complications Trial Group. The effect of intensive treatment of diabetes on the development and progression of long-term complications in insulin-dependent diabetes mellitus. N Engl J Med. 1993;329: 977-86.

6. UK Prospective Diabetes Study Group. Intensive blood glucose control with sulphonylurea or insulin compared with conventional treatment and risk for complications in patients with type 2 diabetes (UKPDS 33). Lancet. 1998;352:837-53.

7. Ohkubo Y, Kishikawa H, Araki E, et al. Intensive insulin therapy prevents the progression of diabetic microvascular complications in Japanese patients with non-insulin-dependent diabetes mellitus: a randomized prospective 6-year study. Diabetes Res Clin Pract. 1995;28:103-17.

8. The DCCT Trial/Epidemiology of Diabetes and Complications (EDIC) Research Group. Retinopathy and nephropathy in patients with type 1 diabetes 4 years after a trial of intensive therapy. N Engl J Med. 2000;342:381-9.

9. Holman RR, Paul SK, Bethel MA, et al. 10-year follow-up of intensive glucose control in type 2 diabetes. N Engl J Med. 2008;359:1577-89.

American Association of Diabetes Educators©

200   Diabetes Education Curriculum

10. Skyler JS, Bergenstal R, Bonow RO, et al. Intensive glycemic control and the prevention of cardiovascular events: implications of the ACCORD, ADVANCE, and VA Diabetes Trials: a position statement of the American Diabetes Association and a scientific statement of the American College of Cardiology Foundation and the American Heart Association. Diabetes Care. 2009;32:187-92.

11. American Diabetes Association. Standards of medical care in diabetes—2015. Diabetes Care. 2015;38 Suppl 1: S1-94.

12. Transportation Security Administration. Travelers with disabilities and medical conditions (cited 2015 Jul 12). On the Internet at: http://www.tsa.gov/traveler-information/travelers-disabilities-and-medical-conditions.

13. Bina DM, Anderson RL, Johnson ML, et al. Clinical impact of prandial state, exercise, and site preparation. AADE position statement on the equivalence of alternative-site blood glucose testing. Diabetes Care. 2003;26:981-5.

14. Peeples M, Iyer A. Mobile prescription therapy: a case study. In: Krohn R, Metcalf D, eds. Health Innovation: Best Practices From the Mobile Frontier. Chicago: Healthcare Information Management System Society (HIMSS); 2014:131-42.

15. Greenwood D. Better type 2 diabetes self-management using paired testing and remote monitoring. AJN. 2015; 115(2):58-65.

16. Bailey SC, Brega AG, Crutchfield TM, et al. Update on health literacy and diabetes. Diabetes Educ. 2014;40:581-604.

17. Mulcahy K, Maryniuk M, Peeples M, et al. Diabetes self-management education core outcomes measures: technical review. Diabetes Educ. 2003;29(5):768-803.

MONITORING: RESOURCES

Monitoring Activity Handout (English) 201

Monitoring Activity Handout (Spanish) 203

Monitoring Checklist for Healthcare Professionals 205

Checklist for SMBG Education. 205

Common Factors Affecting Accuracy of Blood Glucose Results. 205

Identifying Barriers to SMBG 206

Securing an Adequate Blood Sample 207

Factors That May Raise or Lower Blood Glucose. 207

Positive Glucose Questioning 207

Blood Glucose Monitoring Problem Solving for the Person With Diabetes 208

Blood Glucose Monitoring Problem Solving for the Diabetes Educator 209

American Association of Diabetes Educators©

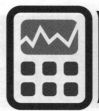

AADE7™ SELF-CARE BEHAVIORS
MONITORING

Checking your blood sugar levels regularly gives you vital information about your diabetes control. Monitoring helps you know when your blood sugar levels are on target. It helps you make food and activity adjustments so that your body can perform at its best. It takes some time and experience to figure out how your daily activities and actions affect your blood sugar.

Your diabetes educator can help you learn:

» How to use a blood sugar (glucose) meter.
» When to check your blood sugar and what the numbers mean.
» What to do when your numbers are out of your target range.
» How to record your blood sugar results.

Checking your blood sugar is an important part of diabetes self-care, but monitoring your overall health includes a lot of other things too, especially when you have diabetes. You and your healthcare team will also need to monitor your:

» Long-term blood sugar control—A1C, eAG
» Cardiovascular health—blood pressure, weight, cholesterol levels
» Kidney health—urine and blood testing
» Eye health—dilated eye exams
» Foot health—foot exams and sensory testing

DID YOU KNOW?

The American Diabetes Association recommends an A1C target below 7% (an eAG of 154 mg/dl); the American Association of Clinical Endocrinologists recommends less than 6.5% (an eAG of 140 mg/dl).

TRUE OR FALSE?

If you want to see how your body responds to your meal, wait 1-2 hours after eating to check your blood sugar levels.

TRUE. Your blood sugar rises in response to what you've eaten. It takes about 2 hours for the numbers to reflect the full rise.

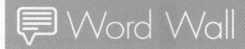

Word Wall

METER:
A small device that is used to check blood sugar levels

LANCET:
A small needle used to get a blood sample

A1C:
A test that measures your average blood sugar levels during the past 2-3 months

ESTIMATED AVERAGE GLUCOSE (eAG):
The number of the A1C test changed into mg/dl like the blood sugar levels shown on your glucose meter

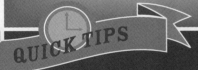

QUICK TIPS

Wash your hands with soap and water and dry them thoroughly before checking your blood sugar. Substances on your skin (like dirt, food, or lotion) can cause inaccurate results.

When traveling, keep your supplies with you. Advise security personnel that you are carrying diabetes supplies.

If you have trouble affording the test strips, call the toll-free number on the back of your meter to see if coupons are available, or ask your diabetes educator about other resources.

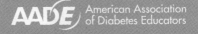

Supported by an educational grant from Eli Lilly and Company.

ACTIVITIES

Remember, the way you feel does not always reflect what your blood sugar is doing. The only way you know is to check your numbers!

» Check your blood sugar levels as directed to share with your doctor or diabetes educator.
» Follow a schedule, keep a record of your daily levels, and use the numbers to make decisions about your diabetes care.
» Check your blood sugar levels if you think you're getting sick.

When you check your blood sugar levels:

» Keep a record and bring it to every health appointment.
» Try to identify patterns when your blood sugar goes up or down.

If your numbers aren't at goal, don't get down. This is useful information that can help your healthcare provider match your treatment to your needs.

If you develop a regular schedule and follow it closely, you'll learn how your blood sugar levels affect how you feel. You'll start to recognize unhealthy blood sugar trends before they get out of control.

What is your typical day like, in terms of eating, activity, and diabetes medication? *(Record it in the space below)*

Time	Activity	Eating	Medication
6:00 a.m.			
7:00 a.m.			
8:00 a.m.			
9:00 a.m.			
10:00 a.m.			
11:00 a.m.			
12:00 p.m.			
1:00 p.m.			
2:00 p.m.			
3:00 p.m.			
4:00 p.m.			
5:00 p.m.			
6:00 p.m.			
7:00 p.m.			
8:00 p.m.			
9:00 p.m.			
10:00 p.m.			

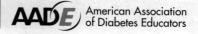

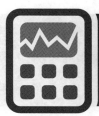

CONDUCTAS PARA EL CUIDADO PERSONA DE AADE7™
CONTROL

La medición regular de tus niveles de azúcar en la sangre te brinda información vital sobre el control de tu diabetes. Te ayuda a saber cuándo tus niveles de azúcar en la sangre están dentro de los valores previstos. Te ayuda a hacer ajustes en las comidas y en las actividades para que tu cuerpo pueda funcionar de la mejor manera. Necesitarás tiempo y experiencia para darte cuenta cómo tus actividades y acciones diarias afectan tu nivel de azúcar en la sangre.

Tu educador en diabetes puede ayudarte a aprender:

» Cómo usar un medidor de azúcar en la sangre (glucosa).
» Cuándo debes controlar tu nivel de azúcar en la sangre y qué significan los valores.
» Qué hacer cuando tus valores están fuera del rango previsto.
» Cómo registrar los resultados de tu nivel de azúcar en la sangre.

El control de tus niveles de azúcar en la sangre es una parte importante de la atención personal de la diabetes, pero el control de tu salud general incluye muchas otras cosas también, especialmente cuando tienes diabetes. Tú y tu equipo de atención médica también deberán controlar lo siguiente:

» Control del nivel de azúcar en la sangre a largo plazo: prueba A1C y eAG.
» Tu salud cardiovascular: la presión arterial, el peso y los niveles de colesterol.
» Tu salud renal: análisis de orina y de sangre.
» Tu salud ocular: exámenes oculares con dilatación.
» La salud de tus pies: exámenes de los pies y prueba sensorial.

¿LO SABÍAS?

La American Diabetes Association recomienda un valor de A1C por debajo del 7% (un eAG de 154 mg/dl), y la American Association of Clinical Endocrinologists recomienda menos del 6,5% (un eAG de 140 mg/dl).

¿VERDADERO O FALSO?

Si quieres ver cómo tu cuerpo responde a tu comida, espera 1 a 2 horas después de comer y luego controla tus niveles de azúcar en la sangre.

VERDADERO. Tu nivel de azúcar en la sangre sube en respuesta a lo que comiste. Deben pasar unas 2 horas para que las cifras reflejen el aumento completo.

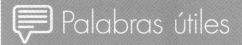

Palabras útiles

GLUCÓMETRO:
Un dispositivo pequeño que se utiliza para controlar los niveles de azúcar en la sangre.

LANCETA:
Una aguja pequeña que se utiliza para obtener una muestra de sangre.

A1C:
Una prueba que mide tus niveles promedio de azúcar en la sangre durante los últimos 2 a 3 meses.

GLUCOSA PROMEDIO ESTIMADA (Estimated Average Glucose, eAG):
El valor de la prueba A1C cambiado a mg/dl, como los niveles de azúcar en la sangre que se muestran en tu glucómetro.

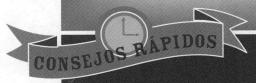

Antes de controlar tu nivel de azúcar en la sangre, lávate las manos con agua y jabón y sécalas bien. Las sustancias presentes en tu piel (como suciedad, alimentos o loción) pueden producir resultados imprecisos.

Cuando viajes, lleva tus suministros contigo. Comunica al personal de seguridad que llevas suministros para la diabetes.

Si no tienes dinero suficiente para pagar las tiras reactivas, llama al número gratuito que figura en la parte posterior de tu glucómetro para ver si hay cupones disponibles, o pregunta a tu educador en diabetes sobre otros recursos.

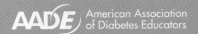

Supported by an educational grant from Lilly USA, LLC.

ACTIVIDADES

Recuerda que la manera en que te sientes no siempre refleja tu nivel de azúcar en la sangre. La única manera de saberlo es controlando tus valores!

» Controla tus niveles de azúcar en la sangre según se te indicó para compartirlos con tu médico o tu educador en diabetes.

» Sigue un programa, lleva un registro de tus niveles diarios y usa las cifras para tomar decisiones sobre la atención de tu diabetes.

» Controla tus niveles de azúcar en la sangre si crees que te estás enfermando.

Cuando controles tus niveles de azúcar en la sangre:

» Conserva un registro y llévalo a todas las citas médicas.

» Trata de identificar patrones cuando tu nivel de azúcar en la sangre sube o baja.

Si tus cifras no están dentro de los valores establecidos, no te desalientes. Ésta es información útil que puede ayudar a tu proveedor de atención médica a adaptar tu tratamiento a tus necesidades.

Si desarrollas un programa regular y lo sigues en detalle, aprenderás cómo tus niveles de azúcar en la sangre afectan la manera en que te sientes. Comenzarás a reconocer las tendencias no saludables del nivel de azúcar en la sangre antes de que estén fuera de control.

¿Cómo es un día típico para ti en cuanto a comidas, actividad física y medicamentos para la diabetes?
(Anótalo en el espacio siguiente)

	Actividad	Comidas	Medicamentos
6:00 a.m.			
7:00 a.m.			
8:00 a.m.			
9:00 a.m.			
10:00 a.m.			
11:00 a.m.			
12:00 p.m.			
1:00 p.m.			
2:00 p.m.			
3:00 p.m.			
4:00 p.m.			
5:00 p.m.			
6:00 p.m.			
7:00 p.m.			
8:00 p.m.			
9:00 p.m.			
10:00 p.m.			

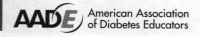

Monitoring Checklist for Healthcare Professionals

Clinical	• A1C • Lipids • Blood pressure
Microvascular	• Neuropathy • Nephropathy • Retinopathy
Macrovascular	• Smoking • Antiplatelet
DSMES	• Nutrition • Activity • Support • SMBG • Medication adherence

Acute complications	• Hypoglycemia • DKA • Hyperosmolar hyperglycemic state
Psychosocial	• Depression • Preconception planning • Transitional care

Checklist for SMBG Education

Using the Meter—Operational Skills	Using the Data—Interpretation Skills
• Select a meter • Ensure meter accuracy • Obtain adequate blood sample • Document the SMBG data • Address individual needs	• Know blood glucose targets or goals • Understand frequency and timing of tests • Use pattern management

Common Factors Affecting Accuracy of Blood Glucose Results

Problem	Result	Recommendation
Sensor strip not fully inserted into meter	False low	Always be sure strip is fully inserted into meter
Sample site (eg, the fingertip) is contaminated with a glucose source (eg, juice)	False high	Always clean test site before sampling
Not enough blood applied to strip	False low	Repeat test with a new sample
Batteries low on power	Error codes	Change batteries and repeat sample collection
Test strips/control solution stored at temperature extremes	False high/low	Store kit according to directions
Person is dehydrated	False high	Stat venous sample on main lab analyzer
Person is in shock	False low	Stat venous sample on main lab analyzer
Squeezing fingertip too hard because blood is not flowing	False low	Repeat test with a new sample from a new stick
Sites other than fingertips	High/low	Results from alternative sites may not match finger-stick results
Test strip/control solution vial cracked	False high/low	Always inspect package for cracks, leaks, etc
Anemia/decreased hematocrit	False high	Venous sample on main lab analyzer
Polycythemia/increased hematocrit	False low	Venous sample on main lab analyzer

Source: US Food and Drug Administration, "Common problems with the use of glucose meters at the point of care" (updated 2013 Mar 21; cited 2014 Apr 1), on the Internet at http://www.fda.gov/MedicalDevices/Safety/AlertsandNotices/TipsandArticlesonDeviceSafety/ucm109449.htm.

Identifying Barriers to SMBG

Type of Potential Barrier	Description	Possible Solution (depends on the real cause of the barrier)*
Physical	Lack of manual dexterity or visual deficits	• Select meter and strips that are easy to handle and maneuver • Select meter with large numbers and backlighting or specialty meter for visually impaired
Financial	Inadequate or lack of insurance coverage for testing supplies	• Focus testing times to maximize use of strips • Ensure testing technique does not waste strips • Explore programs offered by meter companies and social service agencies to provide supplies • Find a pharmacy or medical equipment supplier that is enrolled in Medicare (as applicable) and accepts assignment
Cognitive	Cognitive deficits that make it impossible to carry out the testing procedure without assistance	• Engage significant others or assistants in education and provide written directions at the level of the user and assistants • Adjust testing time and frequency to fit schedule of the assistants • Suggest reminder aids
Time constraints	Real or perceived lack of time to perform blood glucose checks	• Review operational skills to increase confidence in technique • Reinforce that the SMBG results are not a "test" but rather feedback to be used along with other information • Engage others to help perform the blood glucose check
Health literacy/ numeracy[†]	Difficulty understanding steps, recording SMBG data, and interpreting results	• Ask patient how to do SMBG and record the description using the patient's own words and/or pictures • Practice completing a logbook that the patient designs with you • Assess patient's numeracy skills[‡]
Inconvenience	Choosing not to stop current activity to check blood glucose, limited access to hand-washing facilities, working in climate extremes that make access to blood glucose meter challenging	• Problem-solve what would help the individual to do the blood glucose check • Provide suggestions to keep the meter and strips within recommended temperature guidelines
Emotional	Fear of performing SMBG checks due to anticipated pain, fear of being noticed as being different, denial of diabetes, lack of support from family or caregivers	• Listen to patient fears and concerns and acknowledge that others have felt the same way • Suggest the patient access support by joining a diabetes support group or by receiving counseling to address concerns

*Be sure to determine the root cause of the barrier to ensure the solution addresses the appropriate need. Additionally, ask the individual how he or she feels about doing the blood glucose check and whether he or she is confident in performing the test and using the results. Determine whether the individual has the basic operational and interpretive skills necessary for successful SMBG.

[†]CY Osborn, K Cavanaugh, KA Wallston, RO White, RL Rothman, "Diabetes numeracy: an overlooked factor in understanding racial disparities in glycemic control," *Diabetes Care* 32, no. 9 (2009): 1614-9.

[‡]K Cavanaugh, MM Huizinga, KA Wallston, et al, "Association of numeracy and diabetes control," *Ann Intern Med* 148 (2008): 737-46.

Securing an Adequate Blood Sample

Using the Meter—Operational Skills

Each person should be taught to follow specific directions for securing an adequate blood sample.[14] For example, when using the fingertips as a puncture site, the person should be aware of the following procedures to help increase sample size:

- Vigorously wash hands with warm water to increase circulation to fingertips.
- Hang the hand at your side for 30 seconds so blood pools in that hand.
- Shake the hand to be pricked as though you were shaking down a thermometer.
- Use either a larger gauge lancet or a lancing device or end-cap that will allow a deeper puncture.
- Puncture the sides of the fingertips rather than the pads in the center of the fingers, as this produces less pain.
- After your finger is punctured, gently milk the blood from the bottom to the tip of the finger until the blood sample is the correct size. Milking the finger with a press/release, press/release repetition assists blood flow, whereas just squeezing the fingertip may obstruct blood flow.

Factors that May Raise or Lower Blood Glucose

Factors that May Raise Blood Glucose	Factors that May Lower Blood Glucose
• Insulin/oral agent—not enough • Other medications • Physical activity • Stress (dehydration, etc) • Carbohydrate—more than usual	• Insulin/oral agent—too much • Other medications • Physical activity • Stress • Carbohydrate—less than usual

Positive Glucose Questioning

Instead of	Consider
What is the most difficult part of blood glucose monitoring?	What is the easiest part of blood glucose monitoring for you? What would make blood glucose monitoring easier for you? How would you know when you were successful with blood glucose monitoring?
Why did you forget to test in the morning?	What helps you remember to test?
Your numbers are running high in the morning; what do you think you are doing wrong?	Look how great your numbers are on these days (or times). Let's talk about what you do then.
Why aren't you checking your blood glucoses?	How important is blood glucose monitoring to you?
Why are your post-dinner blood glucoses always high?	Tell me about your dinner meal. Tell me about what happens the hour or two before dinner.
Why are you checking only fasting blood glucose?	Tell me what your fasting blood glucoses are telling you.
Why aren't you checking your blood glucose at least twice per day?	What part of your day would you most like to know something about your blood glucose results? How often do you think you would want to look at (check) your blood glucose results in a week?
Do you think checking your blood sugar 3 times a day is realistic?	On a scale of 1–10, how confident are you that you can check your blood glucose 3 times a day every day of the week? (If not confident, ask the patient if she or he would like to change the goal to one in which she or he felt confident.)

Blood Glucose Monitoring Problem Solving Tool For the Person With Diabetes

Why is my blood sugar out of the target range? These things can make your blood sugar go up or down. Do you see anything that might explain your blood sugar? Are blood sugars out of range for several days at the same time?

Eating	Physical Activity	Monitoring Blood Sugar	Taking Medication	Coping Skills	Problem Solving	Complications or Risks
Blood Sugar Too High—Questions to Ask						
Ate more food?	Got less exercise?	Missed checking?	Took after eating?	Stressed out?	Been sick?	Stomach problems?
Ate out or special occasion?	Changed schedule?	Got off schedule?	Missed meds/insulin?	Family problems?	Got a sore?	Chest pain?
Snacking or nibbling on food?	BG was >300 mg before starting exercise?	Not enough blood?	Problems drawing up insulin?	Financial problems?	Over treated low blood sugar?	Hard to draw up insulin with poor vision?
Drank alcohol?		Hands were not clean?	Took too little?	Depressed?		Pregnant?
Type of food?			Need more oral medication?	Work problems?		
			Insulin too hot/cold?			
Blood Sugar Too Low—Questions to Ask						
Ate less food?	Changed schedule?	Missed checking?	Problems drawing up insulin?	Stressed out?	Over treated high blood sugar?	Stomach problems?
Drank alcohol?	Got more exercise?	Got off schedule?	Took too much?	Took extra insulin to cover high BG from stress?		Kidneys are failing?
Missed snack?	Exercise was more intense?	Not enough blood?	Need less medication?			Hard to draw up insulin with poor vision?
Delayed or missed meal?	BG low before exercise?	Meter/strips too hot or cold?	Took wrong insulin at wrong time?			

Source: Developed by Donna Tomky, MSN, RN, CNP, CDE, FAADE and Sue Perry, PhD, CDE for the New Mexico Department of Health, Diabetes Prevention & Control Program. Version 2006. Reprinted with permission.

Blood Glucose Monitoring Assessment Tool For the Diabetes Educator

More reasons to consider why the patient's blood glucoses are out of target ranges. Review several days of BG levels and look for patterns.

Eating	Physical Activity	Monitoring Blood Sugar	Taking Medication	Coping Skills	Problem Solving	Complications or Risks
Blood Glucose Too High—Questions to Ask						
Gastroparesis? Inaccurate carb counting? Snacking? Large or high- fat meal with slow digestion?	Insufficient insulin with counter-regulatory hormones release? Intense workout with elevated BG?	Integrity of strips? Meter/technique? Data accuracy? Insufficient data? Somogyi or dawn phenomenon?	Lipohypertrophy? Timing of meds/insulin? Absorption of meds or insulin? Insulin/pill integrity?	Stress hormones? Memory loss/ forgetfulness? Untreated psych disorder?	Recent infection? Silent infection? Oral or injection of steroids? Pubertal or growth hormones? Hyperthyroidism?	2nd or 3rd trimester of pregnancy? Recent myocardial infarction? Visual acuity? Dexterity problems? Gastroparesis?
Blood Glucose Too Low—Questions to Ask						
Inconsistent carb intake? Inaccurate carb counting? Alcohol consumption? High-fat meal with rapid insulin absorption, and slow digestion?	Injection site near active extremity? Timing of med or insulin in relationship to activity? Weight loss?	Data accuracy? Integrity of strips? Meter/technique? Insufficient data?	Timing of insulin? Wrong med? Inconsistent taking of meds/insulin? No access to medication?	Depression? Anxious? Memory loss/ forgetfulness? Untreated psych disorder?	Hypoglycemia unawareness? Missed other meds, ie steroids? Hypothyroidism?	1st trimester of pregnancy? Gastroparesis? Visual acuity? Dexterity problems? Renal insufficiency?

Source: Developed by Donna Tomky, MSN, RN, CNP, CDE, FAADE and Sue Perry, PhD, CDE for the New Mexico Department of Health, Diabetes Prevention & Control Program. Version 2006. Reprinted with permission.

MODULE 6

Problem Solving

Table of Contents

PROBLEM SOLVING: AN EDUCATOR'S OVERVIEW	212
AADE Systematic Review of the Literature	212
Background Information and Instructions for the Educator	212
Problem-Solving Skills	212
Hypoglycemia, Hyperglycemia, and Sick-Day Management	214
Learning Objectives	214
Knowledge	214
Skills	215
Barriers and Facilitators	215
Behavioral Objectives	215
Problem Solving	215
Hypoglycemia/Hyperglycemia/Sick-Day Management	215
PROBLEM SOLVING: INSTRUCTIONAL PLAN	215
Problem-Solving Skills	215
Steps in Problem Solving	216
Setting SMART Goals	218
Goal-Setting Activity	219
Tips for the Educator: Using Motivational Interviewing Techniques to Enhance Confidence and Conviction	220
Hypoglycemia Management	222
Identifying Participant Thoughts and Priorities About Hypoglycemia	222
Hypoglycemia Defined: Know Your Target	222
Signs of Hypoglycemia: Know Your Symptoms	222
Nocturnal Hypoglycemia	223
Treatment of Hypoglycemia: Know Your Plan	223
Prevention of Hypoglycemia: Know Your Risk	225
Identifying Barriers to Hypoglycemia Management	227
Identifying Facilitators for Managing Hypoglycemia	228

211

212   Diabetes Education Curriculum

Hyperglycemia Management 228

    Identifying Participant Thoughts and Priorities About Hyperglycemia. 228

    Hyperglycemia Defined: Know Your Target 229

    Causes of Hyperglycemia 229

    Signs of Hyperglycemia: Know Your Symptoms. 229

    Prevention and Treatment of Hyperglycemia: Know Your Plan 230

    Identifying Barriers to Hyperglycemia Management. 230

    Identifying Facilitators for Managing Hyperglycemia 232

Sick-Day Management 233

    Sick-Day Guidelines 233

Setting a SMART Goal for Problem Solving for Hypoglycemia, Hyperglycemia, and Sick Days. 235

Follow-up/Outcomes Measurement 236

REFERENCES 238

PROBLEM SOLVING: RESOURCES 239

PROBLEM SOLVING: AN EDUCATOR'S OVERVIEW

AADE Systematic Review of the Literature

A systematic review of the literature was conducted by AADE "to assess the published literature on problem solving and its associations with diabetes self-management and control, as the state of evidence exists. Problem solving is a multidimensional construct encompassing verbal reasoning/rational problem solving, quantitative problem solving, and coping."[1]

Background Information and Instructions for the Educator

In this module, problem solving is approached differently in each of 2 parts: "Problem-Solving Skills" and "Hypoglycemia, Hyperglycemia, and Sick-Day Management."

Problem-Solving Skills

Problem solving is a skill that can be learned and applied to *all* diabetes self-care behaviors. There are logical step-by-step approaches for solving problems: identifying the problem; coming up with options for action; choosing, planning, and enacting one option; and evaluating its effectiveness.[2(p247)] Even so, problem solving involves several other dimensions. Focused problem-solving skills training is one of the components of a formal diabetes education program. Alternatively, situational problem solving for the various self-care behaviors may be incorporated into educational interventions. The first section of this module covers problem-solving skills training. Situational problem-solving activities are integrated throughout all of the other modules in this curriculum.

    There is a dearth of studies focusing on problem solving in diabetes self-management. Despite this fact, the evidence is clear that a problem-based approach to diabetes education leads to improved behavioral and clinical outcomes.[3]

Assessment in Problem Solving

In the educator-patient relationship, there should be initial and ongoing assessment of how the patient is solving problems that he or she encounters as part of living with a chronic disease. By asking the patient pertinent questions such as "In the past month, if you woke up and found your fasting glucose was high, how did you respond to that?" the educator can help the patient uncover problems and existing barriers. Role playing, talking about

American Association of Diabetes Educators©

real-life situations that the patient has been in, or discussing a "case study" can be used to assess the patient's current ability to problem solve. This information forms the basis of a problem-solving intervention.

Direct Instruction Versus Facilitating Problem Solving

Considering the patient to be the "expert" of his or her life, the educator should encourage the patient to be creative in determining the best course of action for a given problem. The patient's personal goals, lifestyle, and preference should be respected as he or she learns from experience what works and what doesn't. Only when trial and error or failure would be dangerous (eg, hypoglycemia treatment) should the educator choose the best strategy for the patient to pursue. In such cases, direct instruction trumps patient-centered problem solving.

Identifying and Assessing Problems and Barriers[2(p249)]

While the patient's problem list may be extensive, problems should be prioritized *by the patient* and then dealt with one at a time. An educator can always say, "I'm concerned that if we work on the problem you chose, you would still be at risk for a low blood sugar event. Do you mind if we set aside some time so we can also talk about treating low blood glucose?" Educators should avoid the tendency to address all of the problems at once. Depending on the patient's abilities and capacity, the educator may serve as collaborator, facilitator, or confidant during the problem-solving process.

Educators should match the problem-solving approach to the patient's needs and learning preferences.

- ❖ For patients who already possess effective problem-solving skills, intervention may be aimed at reinforcing those skills to promote maintenance.
- ❖ For those with ineffective problem-solving skills due to a lack of diabetes knowledge, intervention must first address filling those knowledge gaps.
- ❖ When dealing with patients who have ineffective problem-solving skills because of negative past experiences, educators should frame each failure as an opportunity to learn something valuable. When subsequent attempts to problem solve have a positive outcome, educator and patient should revisit, step-by-step, what occurred to produce the desired outcome. When attempts fail, the educator should help the patient analyze what went wrong and focus on making a different choice in future problem-solving situations.
- ❖ For patients with ineffective problem-solving skills stemming from emotional or attitudinal factors, educators can intervene in several ways:
  - —Discuss how emotions can help or hinder the problem-solving process.
  - —Determine whether a referral for professional counseling is warranted.
  - —Recommend techniques to curb negative thoughts or replace them with different cognitions.
  - —Help patients build on each small success ("Nothing succeeds like success").
- ❖ For patients who have outside factors that hinder problem solving, provide referrals to relevant external resources. See the Diabetes Resources Appendix for a list of agencies that can provide resources. Table 6.1 provides a list of individuals that can help with resolving patient problems.

TABLE 6.1 Who Is on Your Healthcare Team?	
Person with diabetes and his or her family	Ophthalmologist
Primary care provider (eg, physician, nurse practitioner, advanced nurse practitioner)	Podiatrist
	Dentist
Board Certified-Advanced Diabetes Management (BC-ADM)	Social worker
Certified Diabetes Educator® (CDE®)	Psychologist
Nurse educator	Psychiatrist
Registered dietitian	Marriage/family therapist
Registered pharmacist	Exercise physiologist

Source: Adapted with permission from G Kanzer-Lewis, *10 Steps to Better Living With Diabetes* (Alexandria, Va: American Diabetes Association, 2007), 17.

American Association of Diabetes Educators©

Factors That Influence Problem Solving

Factors such as age, cognitive development, education level, ethnicity, and patient willingness can influence the ability to problem solve. The educator should consider the following guidelines relating to these influencing factors:

- For patients with cognitive impairment, the educator should involve support person(s) to the extent necessary to ensure safe problem solving.

- Educators should appropriately align the problem-solving approach with the stage of cognitive development (eg, early childhood, late childhood, adolescence, older adult), keeping in mind the patient's ability to think abstractly and to independently follow through with enactment of a plan.

- Educators should avoid the tendency to assume that education level equates to problem-solving skill. Although higher education generally results in higher scores in problem solving, this is not always the case. In a study by Hill-Briggs et al, individuals with lower literacy but whose life experiences prepared them to effectively problem solve showed problem-solving scores that were similar to those of the college students and professionals who made up the control group.[4]

- The educator should employ cultural competency when working with unacculturated minorities to help them learn the problem-solving skill itself or to utilize the skill to try to resolve a current problem affecting their diabetes self-care.

- For patients who actively choose not to independently problem solve, the educator should provide prepared guidelines that can be accessed in an emergency situation. The educator should involve support person(s) in the education process.

Hypoglycemia, Hyperglycemia, and Sick-Day Management

People with diabetes must constantly apply their problem-solving skills to effectively manage their condition. Changes in blood glucose levels often require quick decisions about eating, activity, and medications. The second section of this module includes educational content relating to the management of hypoglycemia, hyperglycemia, and sick days. A variety of questions are included to stimulate active discussion around problem solving related to hypoglycemia, hyperglycemia, and sick days.

Learning Objectives

Knowledge

Problem Solving

The participant will:

- list the steps to take in problem solving
- describe the steps in setting a SMART goal for behavior change: **S**pecific, **M**easurable, **A**ttainable, **R**elevant,[5,6(pp51-2)] **T**imely

Note: There is a newer version of the acronym SMART used in both health care and corporate management. In this alternative version, used in this module, *Realistic* is replaced by *Relevant* and *Timeline* is replaced by *Timely*. *Realistic* is seen as too similar to *Attainable*, while *Relevant* is seen as more patient-focused; ie, is the goal relevant to the patient? *Timeline* is seen as a literal series of events, while *Timely* is seen as better reflecting the idea of something being done at a favorable or opportune time for the patient.

Hypoglycemia/Hyperglycemia/Sick-Day Management

The participant will:

- differentiate the symptoms of hypoglycemia and hyperglycemia
- describe the appropriate prevention and treatment of hypoglycemia and hyperglycemia

American Association of Diabetes Educators©

- list appropriate self-care actions to take during sick days
- explain when to contact the healthcare provider regarding unresolved hypoglycemia or hyperglycemia

Skills

The participant will:

- demonstrate using his or her problem-solving skills for correctly managing hypoglycemic and hyperglycemic situations
- along with significant other(s), demonstrate correct use of a glucagon emergency kit (as appropriate)

Barriers and Facilitators

Problem Solving

The participant will:

- develop strategies for reducing barriers and increasing facilitators in order to successfully problem solve in diabetes self-care situations

Hypoglycemia/Hyperglycemia/Sick-Day Management

The participant will

- identify potential barriers and facilitators that may impact his or her ability to respond to episodes of hypoglycemia, hyperglycemia, and sick days

Behavioral Objectives

Problem Solving

The participant will:

- apply situational problem-solving skills to diabetes self-care
- demonstrate skill in each step of problem solving: identifying a problem; coming up with options for action; choosing, planning, and enacting one option; and evaluating its effectiveness
- set behavior change goals following SMART guidelines

Hypoglycemia/Hyperglycemia/Sick-Day Management

The participant will:

- appropriately respond to unanticipated situations that occur in his or her diabetes self-management (eg, hypoglycemia, hyperglycemia, and sick days)

PROBLEM SOLVING: INSTRUCTIONAL PLAN

Problem-Solving Skills

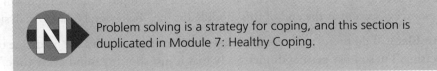

Problem solving is a strategy for coping, and this section is duplicated in Module 7: Healthy Coping.

Steps in Problem Solving

Directions for Role-Playing Activity:

- Guide participants through an example of problem solving (See the "Resources" section at the end of this module) before having them commence solving a problem of their own.
- If in a one-on-one session, the educator reads the part of both the guide and the diabetes educator, and the participant reads the part of the person with the problem.
- If in a group setting, ask if there are 2 participants who would be willing to role-play: one reading the part of the guide, and the other reading the part of the person with the problem. The educator will read the part of the diabetes educator. If there is no participant to play the part of the guide, the educator will read this part also.
- Distribute the script to each willing participant.

Managing your diabetes involves actively dealing with the problems that come up every day. There may be lots of areas in your diabetes care that need attention—physical activity, eating, taking medication, monitoring your blood glucose level, etc. If you try to address them all at once, it can be overwhelming.

Hearing the script as it is read aloud—or better yet, reading something aloud to others—appeals to those with verbal/auditory intelligence. Those with social/interpersonal intelligence learn well in role-playing activities.

Start with the one area in your diabetes care that you feel is a *challenge* right now. Think of a challenge that you feel ready and able to take on at this time. Once you have found some success solving problems in a small area, take on a bigger challenge. The old saying "Nothing succeeds like success" is true. Choose something achievable to try first, and then build on that accomplishment. Problem solving is a method for putting together a behavior change plan. The steps in problem solving can be remembered by the acronym SOAR, which was coined by David B. Rosengren and stands for[7(pp282-6)]:

Set goals
Sort **O**ptions
Arrive at a plan
Reaffirm commitment

SOAR can guide you as you go through the steps in problem solving. Let's go through an example of problem solving together.

Step 1: SET THE GOAL in general terms

Setting the goal is the flip side of identifying the problem. Describe the problem you are facing. Be very specific. The more specific you can be, the more likely you are to find a solution that works. Here's an example of identifying and then clarifying the problem:

Problem: "I can't remember to take my meds."

This is a start, but it's too vague. It's important to drill down to the "sticking point," the one area that has tripped you up over and over again. Creating a behavior chain is a technique to help drill down to the barrier or obstacle. See the "Resources" section at the end of this module for the "Behavioral Chain Analysis."

More specific problem: "I do pretty well remembering the morning meds. It's the medicine before *dinner* that I keep forgetting. I'm so busy getting dinner ready that it just slips my mind every time."

Set the goal in general terms: "I will remember to take my meds before dinner."

Step 2: Sort the OPTIONS

Start off by thinking of possible solutions. Brainstorm things that you can do to remember to take the pre-dinner meds.

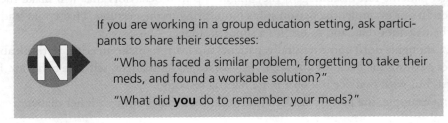

If you are working in a group education setting, ask participants to share their successes:

"Who has faced a similar problem, forgetting to take their meds, and found a workable solution?"

"What did **you** do to remember your meds?"

Other possible solutions:

1. Place the bottle of meds where you always eat dinner, next to the salt and pepper shakers.
2. Set the alarm on your cell phone for 5 PM.
3. Buy a medication reminder alarm from the pharmacy and set it for 5 PM.
4. Place a note in the kitchen to remind you to take the meds.
5. Make getting dinner ready less stressful by planning ahead and doing some of the work earlier in the day or earlier in the week. For example, some people cook several meals at one time on a Sunday afternoon. Others do the cutting and chopping in advance and leave the cooking for right before dinner.

If working with an individual, ask about similar situations when he or she forgot to do something and what solutions he or she came up with that worked. Perhaps that solution will work this time. Build on any prior successes.

Before going on to Step 3, choose which solution will be tried first.

Step 3: ARRIVE AT A PLAN in specific terms

Arriving at a plan is done by collaborating on thinking of all the steps involved to enact the plan and then thinking of the potential barriers to successfully carrying out the plan.

"What will you do first?"
"What specific steps need to be done?"

Step 4: REAFFIRM commitment

Some patients find that writing out the steps can be very helpful. It can clarify what they will do, act as a memory aid, and even reinforce commitment to change. You can give feedback if their plan seems underdeveloped. At times, you may want to offer a worksheet or form for the patient to use in creating a written document.

It is important to discuss with the patient his or her feelings, thoughts, and attitudes that come with the problem.

Ask the patient to recall thoughts or attitudes that he or she experienced when this problem happened before, and what happened next. Examples that your patients may provide:

"I'll realize *after dinner* that I forgot my diabetes medicine. Now it's too late to take it. I feel so stupid! Why can't I get it right?"

"This diabetes is too hard to deal with! No way am I going to check my blood sugar tonight; I know it'll be high because I forgot the medicine *again*. So why even bother? I get so discouraged, I just want to forget it all."

Work with patients to help them practice more positive thoughts. This is a skill that can be learned and that patients can get better at with practice. Focus on *any* progress the patient has made, even if it's a little thing. Focus on something he or she can feel good about.

American Association of Diabetes Educators©

Help patients realize that negative expectations may discourage them from trying to cope with diabetes-related problems in the future. Negative thoughts about their ability to manage diabetes can easily lead to negative actions in the future. When patients feel discouraged, they might slip into behaviors that will make their blood glucose level go even higher. In our example, the person stops monitoring in the evening. That could lead to less monitoring the next day, the day after that, and so on. It's a slippery slope.

Even if positive thoughts don't come naturally, patients can learn to make an effort to think about the positives and give themselves a pat on the back for *any small step* toward better diabetes self-care behavior. It may feel corny and artificial at first, but with practice it'll be a more natural response.

In the following example, the person thinks about what she's doing *right* with her diabetes:

"Well, at least I'm watching my food portions. I do pretty well with that. I haven't gained any weight since I started paying attention to my diet. I guess I'm not a complete failure after all."

Setting SMART Goals

When you go on a road trip, you need a map. Once you decide on a destination, you use your map to set a course and then follow it to get there.

Managing your diabetes is much the same idea. You decide what outcome you want and then you set about making the changes that will help you get there. There is often confusion between a goal and a result. People will say, "My goal is to be healthy," but that is actually the result of behaviors that promote health. Make sure your goals are not the result or outcome you want. Setting SMART goals means being specific about what behavior you will do to achieve the desired result, such as a lower weight or a lower A1C.

When you set a goal, make sure it's something that *you* want to do. It should be something that *you* see a need for. The goal you set should be something that you feel you are *capable* of doing. Think about how meeting that goal is going to help you in the long run.

Using a mnemonic like SMART to help remember an idea can be a useful teaching tool, especially for those with verbal/auditory intelligence.

Follow these SMART steps to set your goal[8(p605)]:

S— Specific: The goal is not vague. What exactly are you going to do?
M— Measurable: You should be able to measure (how much, how often, etc) whether you have achieved your goal.
A— Attainable: Your goal should be challenging but not out of reach.
R— Relevant: You can see a clear link between your goal and your health or how you feel. You want to make the change.
T— Timely: Set a time frame in which the goal can be achieved. It's best to make it short term, in the next week or two, but if your goal will take longer time to achieve, plan mini-goals to complete for the next session.

Example of a SMART goal: "Starting Monday, I will substitute fresh fruit for junk food for my afternoon snack at least 3 days a week because I want to stop overeating later in the day." (Educator writes goal on board.)

Ask participants to analyze the goal and answer the following questions:

- **How is this goal specific?** It is specific in terms of the type of foods, the time of day, when it starts, and how many days per week.
- **How is it measurable?** It is measurable in terms of the start date and how many days per week but not about which fresh fruits.
- **How do you know if it's attainable?** (This part is always person-specific.) Three days per week is more realistic than 5 days.
- **How do you know if it is relevant?** It includes the reason for setting this goal.
- **Is there a timeline?** Yes. It starts Monday. It'll happen 3 days per week.

Goal-Setting Activity[9(p51)]

Guide participants through the goal-setting example before having them set a goal of their own. If in a one-on-one session, the educator asks the questions, and the participant reads the part of the patient. If in a group setting, ask if there are 2 participants who would be willing to role-play: one asking the questions, and the other playing the part of the patient. Distribute the script to each player. See the "Resources" section at the end of this module for the "Goal-Setting Activity Script."

Those with intrapersonal intelligence learn best when allowed to reflect on their own experiences. This activity urges patients to think of their own situation when applying the steps in goal setting.

It is always possible that you did your best to set a SMART goal but didn't achieve your goal. Think of it as an experiment. You tried it to see how it would work out. If your plan didn't work, don't give up! Try again, revise the goal time frame or specifics, or find another option. Remind yourself that trying is worth the effort. Try to view any failures as opportunities to learn what *doesn't* work.

Thomas Edison tried numerous different metals before he found the one that would make the lightbulb glow. He had a great attitude about failure. He said, "I have not failed. I've just found 10,000 ways that won't work."

Before you set a goal, carefully think it through. The following list of questions can help you figure out an appropriate goal for you to set at this time. Let's work through an example so you can see goal-setting in action.

_____ [make up a name] is a 43-year-old woman who works as a bank teller. She has type 2 diabetes and is overweight.

- What area of diabetes self-care do you feel you need to improve on the most? There may be lots of areas, but try to prioritize.

    "Afternoon snacking is a problem for me. I get real hungry around 3:30 or 4:00 in the afternoon, so I usually buy chips or a candy bar from the employee lounge."

    (Drill down!) Why do you suppose you are so hungry at 4 o'clock?

    "I eat my lunch early, so I know I need a snack in the late afternoon, but if it was a healthy snack that would be better. I'm trying to lose weight."

- On a scale of 0 to 10, how convinced are you that it's important to snack on something healthy?

    "I'd have to give it an 8. I know it's important to do something about this, because once I feel I've already blown my diet, I tend to overeat for the rest of the evening and it's discouraging not to lose weight."

American Association of Diabetes Educators©

220 Diabetes Education Curriculum

♦ What would you have to do differently (or give up) to make this change?

"I'd need to find something different to snack on. There's a vending machine in the lounge, but there's nothing but junk food in there. Also, nearly every day, people bring doughnuts or something sweet to the lounge. I could take my snack at my desk or outside in the covered area next to the building. That way, I wouldn't be tempted by the stuff in the employee lounge."

♦ How will this change help you?

"If I eat a healthier snack in the afternoon, I'll feel better about myself. When I've done the 'right thing' earlier in the day, it helps me want to keep it up into the evening. If I do that, I'll be in a better frame of mind to stick to my meal plan at dinner. Having a piece of fresh fruit instead of high-fat junk food will help me manage my blood sugar level. In the long run, it might help me lose weight or at least not gain any more weight."

♦ Are you willing and able to make the changes? On a scale of 0 to 10, how confident are you that you can make this change?

"As far as the confidence to do this, I think I'm a 7 or 8. I am willing to try it. I think my coworker would do it with me, too. She's always talking about eating better, and she needs to lose weight also."

♦ What change can you start with right away?

"I could buy a bag of apples and oranges over the weekend and take them to work with me on Monday."

So your goal is to keep apples and oranges at work and eat 1 piece of fresh fruit for your afternoon snack on Monday through Friday, so you'll do the "right thing" all day long and prevent yourself from overeating in the evening. Now that you've seen an example of setting a goal for change, set one for yourself!

Tips for the Educator: Using Motivational Interviewing Techniques to Enhance Confidence and Conviction[10(pp62-4),11(pp216-7)]

When patients are setting goals for change, the educator can assess conviction and confidence by asking:

"On a scale of 0 to 10, how *convinced* are you that it is important to make this _____ (specify the behavior to be changed)?"

"On a scale of 0 to 10, how *confident* are you that you can make this _____ (mention the same behavior to be changed)?"

Enhance Conviction

Respond to ambivalence by:

♦ Using reflective listening skills to summarize what the patient has said. This shows you are interested and allows for clarification of patient's intent.

♦ Showing empathy and validating the patient's emotions and thoughts. Respectful acknowledgment of the patient's efforts helps create a safe environment.

♦ Listening for and supporting "change talk." Change talk includes statements made by the patient that express a desire to change. As the patient's commitment to change grows, change talk progresses through 3 phases:

—Early change-talk statements—*"I want to . . ."* and *"I need to . . ."*

—Middle change-talk statements reveal an awareness of need to change—*"I have reason to . . .,"* *"It's possible . . .,"* and *"I know I can . . ."*

—Late change-talk statements show intent—*"I will . . ."*

American Association of Diabetes Educators©

Clarify reasons for choosing a low conviction score by asking:

◆ *"What led you to rate your conviction a [__] and not zero?"*

◆ *"What would have to happen to move your conviction from a [__] to [__] + 1 or 2?"*

◆ *"What could I do to help you understand the importance of making this change?"*

Explore ambivalence by asking:

◆ *"What's the down side of making a change?"*

◆ *"What are the good things about making a change?"*

◆ *"What's the down side of staying the same (not changing)?"*

◆ *"What are the good things about staying the same (not changing)?"*

◆ *"What would you have to give up to make this a higher priority?"*

Expose discrepancies by:

◆ Pointing out differences between the patient's conviction to change and what he or she says is important to him or her.

> *"You said that staying well for your kids' sake is important, yet you rate making this change as a low priority. Tell me more."*

Enhance Confidence

Clarify the patient's reasons for choosing a low confidence score by asking:

◆ *"What led you to rate your confidence a [__] and not zero?"*

◆ *"What would have to happen to move your confidence from a [__] to [__] + 1 or 2?"*

◆ *"What could I do to help you increase your confidence?"*

Help the patient build on past success by asking:

◆ *"Can you think of a time when you were able to make a change?"*

◆ *"What helped you be successful in making the change?"*

Help the patient break the change down into small, realistic steps.
Identify potential barriers by asking:

◆ *"What do you think might get in the way of making this change?"*

◆ *"What else?"* Keep asking until the patient can't think of any other barriers.

Assist the patient with problem solving by asking:

◆ *"What might help you overcome that barrier?"*

◆ *"Did anything help in the past?"*

◆ *"Other people have tried . . ."*

◆ *"Here's what the literature recommends as useful to overcome that barrier."*

Anticipate and plan for slips/lapses by asking:

◆ *"What has happened before that caused you to slip up?"*

◆ *"Is there any specific thing that you think might trigger a slipup this time?"*

◆ *"What can you do differently this time if you see a slipup coming?"*

Reassure the patient by:

- Normalizing feelings of guilt when a lapse occurs
- Reframing lapses as a chance to learn about triggers
- Teaching him or her to think about the positive things he or she is doing, not just about the lapse

Hypoglycemia Management

Identifying Participant Thoughts and Priorities About Hypoglycemia

Adults learn best when learning occurs collaboratively. Encourage learners to share their expertise and experiences with others.

Tell me about a time when you had low blood glucose and what you did to raise it.

What level of blood glucose do you consider to be too low (hypoglycemic)?

Has your provider recommended a range of blood glucose for you?

Have you ever experienced an episode of low blood glucose (hypoglycemia)? What do you think caused it? What did you do to correct it?

What concerns you most about low blood glucose (hypoglycemia)?

What do you think you can do to prevent low blood glucose from happening?

Adults learn best when their learning is self-directed and meaningful to them. Asking questions like, "What do you want to learn today about . . .?" involves learners in deciding on the content that will be covered.

Adults learn best when they feel valued and respected for the experiences and perspectives they bring. **Use probing questions to elicit learners' experiences and perspectives.**

Hypoglycemia Defined: Know Your Target Survival Skill

Hypoglycemia is defined as a blood glucose level that is lower than normal. The lower end of normal blood glucose is 70 mg/dL (3.9 mmol/L). It's important to know the range of blood glucose that's safe for you. Discuss target blood glucose levels with your provider.

If you have certain conditions, your provider may make adjustments to the target to keep you safe. For example, if you are unable to recognize when your blood glucose is dropping too low, your provider may recommend a slightly higher target. Young children with diabetes may also require higher targets.

Signs of Hypoglycemia: Know Your Symptoms Survival Skill

Every person is unique. It's important that you recognize the early warning signs and symptoms that occur when *your* blood glucose begins to drop too low. Two people may have the same low blood glucose level but experience very different symptoms. You may find that your hypoglycemic symptoms vary from episode to episode. Your symptoms may begin at different glucose levels on different occasions. Common signs and symptoms of hypoglycemia include:

- Shaking/trembling
- Dizziness/light-headedness
- Weakness
- Sleepiness
- Nervous feeling
- Trouble concentrating
- Headache
- Sweaty, clammy skin
- Intense hunger
- Blurred vision
- Fast pulse/heart "skips a beat"
- Nausea/queasiness
- Tingling in hands/feet/lips

What are the symptoms that tell you that your blood glucose may be dropping?

Nocturnal Hypoglycemia

Episodes of hypoglycemia occurring during the night are not uncommon, especially for individuals with type 1 diabetes. During the Diabetes Control and Complications Trial (DCCT), 43% of all hypoglycemic episodes and 55% of severe episodes reported occurred during sleep.[12] Incidence rates vary from 12% to 56%[13]; however, because 49% to 100%[13] of episodes occur without symptoms, the actual incidence may be much higher. Patients with type 2 diabetes who were treated with long-acting sulfonylureas, insulin,[14] or insulin combined with oral antidiabetes drugs (OADs) are also susceptible.[15,16] Use of alcohol in the evening may increase the risk for nocturnal hypoglycemia.[13] If you have hypoglycemia during sleep, you may sleep through it. Common symptoms of nocturnal hypoglycemia include:

- Nightmares
- Night sweats
- Seizure/thrashing (observed by a bed partner)
- Bed partner cannot arouse you from sleep
- Unexplained headache upon waking

Treatment of Hypoglycemia: Know Your Plan Survival Skill
Self-Treatment of Hypoglycemia

Following the "Rule of 15" will help you properly treat hypoglycemia. *As soon as* you suspect hypoglycemia, check your blood glucose level. Do not delay! If your blood glucose is below target, promptly eat or drink 15 g of a fast-acting carbohydrate. Wait 15 minutes, then recheck your glucose level.

American Association of Diabetes Educators©

224 Diabetes Education Curriculum

Examples of 15 g of fast-acting carbohydrate[17(p534)]:

- Glucose tablets (3 or 4 tablets, depending on brand)
- Fruit juice (4 to 6 ounces)
- Milk (8 ounces low fat or nonfat)
- Non-diet soft drink (4 to 6 ounces)
- Sugar (3 to 4 teaspoons/packets)
- Hard candy (3 or 4 pieces, depending on size)
- Lifesavers® (5 or 6 pieces)
- Raisins (2 tablespoons)

Being prepared in case of hypoglycemia is the best policy:

- Carry fast-acting carbohydrate with you at all times.
- Have your blood glucose monitor on hand so you can use the Rule of 15.

What to Do at Recheck

- If your glucose level is still below target, repeat the carbohydrate treatment (even if your symptoms have resolved).
- If your glucose level is within target, don't eat or drink any more carbohydrates (even if you still have symptoms).
- After treating hypoglycemia, monitor your blood glucose periodically over the next hour to check for a relapse.

Overtreating Hypoglycemia

A lot of people tend to keep treating their low blood sugar, even after hypoglycemia has resolved. Has that been your experience?

If yes, then ask participant: Describe what happened. How did your blood sugar respond?

A very common response to hypoglycemia is *overtreatment*. The symptoms of hypoglycemia can cause such discomfort that it's tempting to go overboard. The idea that "if 15 g of carbohydrate will correct my blood sugar in 15 minutes, then more carbohydrate will correct it sooner" is not really true.

It is important not to overtreat hypoglycemia in pregnancy because the excess blood glucose can travel through the bloodstream and to the baby.

In most cases, your blood glucose will correct within 15 minutes after treatment. Eating or drinking too much carbohydrate will cause your glucose level to be too high later on. In essence, one problem will have been replaced with another.

While it's very important to recognize and respond to symptoms of low glucose, let your glucose *readings* drive your actions, not just your *symptoms*. Symptoms may persist for a while, even after the glucose level has corrected. Give your body time to readjust to the change in glucose level.

Table 6.2 lists general guidelines for treating hypoglycemia.

Can I treat hypoglycemia with chocolate?

Module 6 *Problem Solving* 225

TABLE 6.2 General Guidelines for Treating Hypoglycemia

- Do not keep eating after the initial treatment; wait 15–20 minutes and then test blood glucose level to determine whether further treatment is needed.
- Do not keep eating until symptoms disappear.
- Avoid using high-fat foods for treatment.
- Always carry some type of carbohydrate.
- Keep something at your bedside to treat nocturnal hypoglycemia.
- Keep something in the car at all times to treat episodes of hypoglycemia that might occur while driving.
- Always wear diabetes identification.

Source: EM Sisson, DL Dixon, "Pharmacotherapy for Glucose Management," in C Mensing, ed, *The Art and Science of Diabetes Self-Management Education: A Desk Reference for Healthcare Professionals*, 3rd ed (Chicago: American Association of Diabetes Educators, 2014), 534-5.

Chocolate is a high-fat food and while it does contain carbohydrate, the fat component will delay absorption of the carbohydrate into the bloodstream. For this reason, chocolate is not a good choice for treating hypoglycemia. On the other hand, if chocolate is the *only* available option, go ahead and take it.

To Treat or Not to Treat?

If you're in a situation where checking your glucose level is not possible or practical, go ahead and take the 15 g of carbohydrate. In this case, based on symptoms, you must assume that you have hypoglycemia. There is the chance, though, that you do not really have hypoglycemia. But if you have to guess, and you make an error in treatment, it is always better to err on the side of safety.

If you take a carbohydrate treatment that you don't need, you will probably have a high glucose level for a few hours. If you withhold treatment when you actually do have hypoglycemia, it could progress to a more severe level. The first option is always the safest.

If You Can't Treat Yourself, Someone Else Will Need to Help You

It's good to have a backup plan involving treatment of hypoglycemia. Decide who you will inform of your diabetes—family, friends, teachers, coworkers, etc—and teach them to recognize the signs of hypoglycemia. Teach them—ahead of time—what to do if you are having hypoglycemia and need help.

Medical Identification (ID)

Always carry a wallet card that states you have diabetes and describes proper treatment of hypoglycemia. This card should also include the name of your diabetes medication(s) as well as the name and number of an emergency contact person.

Medical ID jewelry is an important option, especially for those who take insulin. Jewelry choices include a necklace medallion, bracelet, or slider on the watch band. Medical ID is also available as a medallion on a key chain. This is particularly useful in the case of driving incidents related to hypoglycemia.

Prevention of Hypoglycemia: Know Your Risk Survival Skill

You may have heard the old saying "An ounce of prevention is worth a pound of cure." That is very true when it comes to hypoglycemia. There are actions you can take to prevent blood glucose from dropping too low.

Studies show that just 1 episode of hypoglycemia can lead to fewer warning symptoms if another episode occurs within the next 24 hours. As a result, you could develop hypoglycemia and not know it until it becomes severe. This is a very dangerous situation, especially if no one else is around to help you treat it. If you do experience hypoglycemia, monitor your glucose level more closely for the next several hours to detect whether glucose levels fall again.[17(p534)]

Table 6.3 lists common causes of hypoglycemia and strategies to prevent them.

American Association of Diabetes Educators©

226   Diabetes Education Curriculum

Advanced Detail

Individuals Who Take Insulin

Glucagon Injection

People who experience frequent and severe hypoglycemia should discuss glucagon injection with their provider. Glucagon is a hormone secreted by the adrenal gland. It is normally released into the bloodstream in response to hypoglycemia. Glucagon causes the liver to release stored glucose back into the bloodstream, which helps correct the blood glucose level.

In some people who have had diabetes for a very long time, this process is impaired. Their bodies can't self-regulate when the glucose level begins to drop. The usual early warning symptoms of hypoglycemia don't occur. This condition is known as *hypoglycemia unawareness*. In hypoglycemia unawareness, the first obvious sign may be a loss of consciousness.

It is unsafe to give liquids or food to a person who cannot safely swallow or who is unconscious. For people at high risk for severe hypoglycemia, the provider can prescribe a glucagon emergency kit. An injection of glucagon must be given by someone else.

How to Give a Glucagon Injection

The glucagon emergency kit includes a vial of glucagon in white powder form and a syringe that has been preloaded with a sterile diluting solution. To administer the glucagon, follow these steps:

1. Remove the plastic cap from the top of the vial.
2. Remove the needle cover and inject the diluting solution into the vial of powdered glucagon.
3. Withdraw the needle from the vial, then mix the solution by swirling it until the powder dissolves.
4. Draw the mixed glucagon solution back into the syringe.
5. Inject it into the leg or abdomen. Adults and larger children will need the entire amount in the syringe; small children will need half the amount.

After injection with glucagon, the person should be rolled onto his or her side to protect the airway in case of vomiting. When the person regains consciousness and can safely swallow, oral treatment can then take place. Persons who keep a glucagon emergency kit should be aware of the expiration date.

TABLE 6.3   Common Causes of Hypoglycemia and Preventive Strategies

Common Causes of Hypoglycemia	Preventive Strategies
• Delaying or skipping meals or snacks	• Eat meals and snacks on time. During your waking hours, don't go more than 5 hours without some nutrition. If you take insulin that peaks during your sleeping hours, be sure to eat a bedtime snack; otherwise, no bedtime snack is required.
• Taking too much diabetes medication, or taking it at the wrong time with regard to meals	• Take your diabetes medication as prescribed—the right dose at the right time. If you take rapid-acting insulin, be sure to eat within 15 minutes of the injection. If hypoglycemia persists, even if you are taking your medication as prescribed, inform your provider. He or she may consider adjusting your medication.
• Increased physical activity	• Balance increased activity with increased carbohydrate food intake.
• Drinking too much alcohol, especially without eating	• If you drink alcoholic beverages, use in moderation. Don't drink on an empty stomach.

American Association of Diabetes Educators©

Identifying Barriers to Hypoglycemia Management

Even if you understand the causes and treatment of hypoglycemia, there may be barriers that prevent you from taking the right steps to prevent or properly treat hypoglycemia. For every barrier there may be many possible solutions.

 What might work to overcome this barrier? Let's brainstorm together and learn from one another's experiences.

Reality Scenario for Hypoglycemia	Problem Solving to Manage Hypoglycemia Possible Solutions/What Would *You* Do?
Emotional	
I'm afraid of going low at night. I don't want to go to sleep and never wake up!	• Check your blood glucose before going to sleep. If it is less than 100 mg/dL (5.55 mmol/L), eat a snack of 15 g of carbohydrate, such as a glass of milk. • Some patients on insulin routinely include a bedtime snack incorporated into their daily calorie count. • If you want assurance about your glucose level during the night, every now and then set your alarm for 3 AM. Check your glucose level. If it is low at this time, consult your provider about the possible need for medication adjustment.
I don't want to embarrass myself by having a hypoglycemic reaction in front of other people. So I keep myself "a little on the sweet side."	• Pay attention to your early symptoms of hypoglycemia. At the first symptom, check your glucose level. • Regular glucose monitoring can let you know if you are trending downward. Be prepared to treat low glucose by keeping glucose tablets, hard candy, or other fast-acting carbohydrate options with you at all times. See list under the "Sick-Day Management" section later in this chapter. • Consider letting your close associates know about your diabetes, and educate them on any early signs of low glucose that you may display. Let them know what to do to help you avoid a severe reaction. • Practice prevention—eat your meals and take your medications on time, and balance exercise with food intake.
Environmental	
At work, it's hard for me to eat lunch on time, so I tend to have a lot of lows.	• Discuss reasonable accommodations with your employer so you can eat at a regular time if this will prevent low blood glucose. • If you are allowed to drink liquids during your work duties, consider liquid meal replacement for lunch or as a mid-morning snack. • Visit the American Diabetes Association's Web site to learn about employee rights: http://www.diabetes.org/living-with-diabetes/know-your-rights/discrimination/employment-discrimination/your-rights-on-the-job.html. • Read the American Diabetes Association's position paper *Diabetes and Employment*.* • You may be undereating carbohydrate at breakfast. Check your blood glucose 2–3 hours after breakfast to see if you've eaten enough. You may need to do this on a non-workday.

*American Diabetes Association, "Diabetes and employment," *Diabetes Care* 37, Suppl 1 (2014): S112-7.

Identifying Facilitators for Managing Hypoglycemia

As important as it is to identify barriers to hypoglycemia management, it's just as important to consider the positives, or facilitators, in your situation. Looking deeper, you may find that there are more positives than you thought.

What resources already exist that can help you manage or prevent hypoglycemia?

- Social support—family members, coworkers, friends.
- Community resources—American Diabetes Association, Know Your Rights (http://www.diabetes.org/living-with-diabetes/know-your-rights/) and Employment Discrimination (http://www.diabetes.org/living-with-diabetes/know-your-rights/discrimination/employment-discrimination/). Information about educating employers about making reasonable accommodations for people with diabetes in the workplace (allowing for regularly scheduled mealtimes, and the time and space to check glucose level and take medication at work). Effective January 1, 2009, the amended Americans with Disabilities Act took effect. This act broadens the scope to include people with diabetes and makes it easier for their rights at work to be protected (http://www.ada.gov).
- Reminders and cues—notes, entries on a calendar, or alarms to remember to monitor glucose, eat a meal, or take medication(s) on time.
- Rewards—incentives to maintain motivation.
- Log or journal—by keeping a record (either on paper or on your computer or phone) of your blood glucose, food intake, and treatment of lows, you can look for blood glucose patterns and then make changes in your routine.

Hyperglycemia Management

Identifying Participant Thoughts and Priorities About Hyperglycemia

Adults learn best when they feel valued and respected for the experiences and perspectives they bring. **Use probing questions to elicit learners' experiences and perspectives.**

Tell us about a time when you had high blood glucose and what you did to lower it.

What level of blood glucose do you consider to be too high (hyperglycemic)?

Has your provider recommended a range of blood glucose for you?

How do you feel when your blood glucose is above target?

What do you typically do to treat a blood glucose level that is above target?

Do you do anything differently in your diabetes care when you get sick (a cold, the "flu," or any illness when you can't eat normally)?

What concerns you most about high blood glucose (hyperglycemia)?

At what level of blood glucose would you notify your provider?

What do you want to learn today about dealing with high blood glucose (hyperglycemia)?

Hyperglycemia Defined: Know Your Target `Survival Skill`

Hyperglycemia is any blood glucose level that is above normal. Studies have shown that keeping blood glucose close to normal helps lower the risk of health complications in the long run.[18,19] In the short term, keeping your blood glucose level close to normal can help you feel better. In pregnancy, keeping your blood glucose level close to normal will benefit both you and your baby.

For most nonpregnant adults with diabetes, a target fasting level of 70 to 130 mg/dL (3.9 to 7.2 mmol/L) is recommended (first thing upon waking, before eating); a target of under 180 mg/dL (<10 mmol/L) is recommended for 1 to 2 hours after meals.[20]

- ◆ Goals should be individualized based on[20]:
  - —duration of diabetes
  - —age/life expectancy
  - —comorbid conditions
  - —known cardiovascular disease or advanced microvascular complications
  - —hypoglycemia unawareness
  - —individual patient considerations
- ◆ More or less stringent glycemic goals may be appropriate for individual patients
- ◆ Postprandial glucose may be targeted if A1C goals are not met despite reaching preprandial glucose goals

Some providers recommend even tighter glucose control using targets of <110 mg/dL (6.11 mmol/L) before meals and <140 mg/dL (7.77 mmol/L) 2 hours after meals.[21] Discuss target blood glucose levels with your provider. Your routine self-care and your provider's treatment recommendations are meant to help you achieve these targets and avoid hyperglycemia.

Causes of Hyperglycemia `Survival Skill`

There are a number of factors that can drive your glucose to a high level. Some things may cause glucose to creep up slowly:

- ◆ Not taking enough diabetes medication
- ◆ Eating too many carbohydrates
- ◆ Gaining weight
- ◆ Not engaging in enough physical activity

Other things can cause glucose to rise very quickly to a dangerous level:

- ◆ Becoming ill, especially with an infection
- ◆ Forgetting or skipping diabetes medication
- ◆ Relying on "how you feel" to assess glucose levels

Signs of Hyperglycemia: Know Your Symptoms `Survival Skill`

Possible physical signs include:

- ◆ Frequent urination
- ◆ Thirst
- ◆ Blurred vision
- ◆ Excessive hunger

Blood test:

- ◆ Glucose above 250 mg/dL (13.87 mmol/L)

American Association of Diabetes Educators©

Advanced Detail

For Insulin-Using Participants

My blood glucose was higher after I exercised than before. Why is that?

Possible explanations:

- If you had a pre-exercise snack, it may have contained too many carbohydrates.
- If you had a hypoglycemic (low blood glucose) event during activity, it would have prompted your liver to release extra glucose into your blood.
- Your activity may not have used up enough of the stored glucose that was released from your liver or muscles. This commonly happens with power activities like weightlifting or high-intensity activities like sprinting.
- If you were in a competitive situation, you might have had an adrenalin rush that prompted your liver to release extra glucose into your blood.

Prevention and Treatment of Hyperglycemia: Know Your Plan `Survival Skill`

Generally speaking, physical activity will lower the blood glucose level. This could be any type of physical activity, such as walking or even chair exercises. That's why regular physical activity is one of the main treatments for managing diabetes. For many people, diabetes medication is also needed to prevent and treat hyperglycemia. Taking the right medication at the right time is crucial. As time goes by, the natural progression of diabetes will cause you to need more or different types of medication.

Identifying Barriers to Hyperglycemia Management

Even if you understand the causes and treatment of hyperglycemia, there may be barriers that prevent you from taking the right steps to prevent or properly treat hyperglycemia. For every barrier there may be many possible solutions.

What might work to overcome this barrier? Let's brainstorm together and learn from one another's experiences.

Reality Scenario for Hyperglycemia	Problem Solving to Manage Hyperglycemia Possible Solutions/What Would *You* Do?
Financial *My money situation is tight. I can't afford my medication, so my blood sugar is out of control.*	• Patient assistance programs may be able to help if you qualify for assistance. See Resources at the end of this chapter, which can be copied and used as patient handouts. • Ask your provider for samples to tide you over until you can afford to buy your prescription.

American Association of Diabetes Educators©

Reality Scenario for Hyperglycemia	Problem Solving to Manage Hyperglycemia Possible Solutions/What Would *You* Do?
Sick day—lack of knowledge *I'm sick today and not eating, so I shouldn't take my insulin. If I take my insulin without food, I'll go low.*	Normally, insulin without food will cause your glucose level to decrease. But, remember that illness, especially an infection, usually raises the blood glucose level. Illness also makes you even more resistant to insulin. • You should continue taking your insulin on a sick day, even if you are not eating as usual. • Keep track of your glucose level. Let your provider know if your glucose is consistently out of target during times of illness. • Put together a "sick-day box" that includes extra supplies, instructions from your provider, your provider's phone number, and a list of sick-day rules to remind you what you need to know and do when you get sick.
Lack of organization Gets distracted and often misses insulin dose or diabetes medication. Takes diabetes medication(s) at the wrong time, due to poor organization.	• Organize all your diabetes supplies in one central place so you have everything you need when it comes to injection time. Include the following supplies: insulin or insulin pen, syringes or pen needles, alcohol wipes, meter, lancets, strips, and logbook. If your insulin dose is due during work hours, keep a small kit with supplies at your workplace. Many, but not all, opened insulin pens or vials can be kept at room temperature for at least 28 days. Check with your provider, educator, or pharmacist. If you don't have a safe, temperature-controlled area at work and you need one, carry a portable kit with you. A variety of zippered kits can be purchased online. Your local pharmacy may also carry kits. • Set an alarm (on your watch, clock, or cell phone) to remind you when your insulin injection is due. • Until you get a firm habit in place, post little reminder notes to help you remember when your insulin is due.
Emotional/social *It's embarrassing to have to take my insulin when I'm out with other people, so I just skip it sometimes.*	Discuss patient's agenda.* • If you use a syringe and vial, consider switching to an insulin pen, which is more discreet. • Remind yourself why you want to control your blood glucose. When you are feeling motivated to live a longer, healthier life, you'll find a way to take it.
Insulin makes me gain weight.	Discuss patient's agenda.* • Avoid overtreating hypoglycemia. It amounts to consuming excess calories. • Decide if some weight gain is worth it in exchange for improved glycemic control and the benefits that brings. Delaying starting insulin or increasing the dose can cause a greater weight increase than if insulin was initiated in a timely manner.† • When insulin is inadequate, there is weight loss. Then taking insulin to restore previous levels also results in weight returning to previous levels. • Consult a registered dietitian for help in avoiding or minimizing weight gain. • Realize that there is a strong link between diabetic ketoacidosis and omitted insulin if you have type 1 diabetes. This is a big risk to take.‡ Consider other parts of your self-care plan that affect weight, like your meal plan and your activity level. Are you taking in too many calories? Are you regularly active? Making needed adjustments in these areas may help you avoid, or at least limit, weight gain.

American Association of Diabetes Educators©

Reality Scenario for Hyperglycemia	Problem Solving to Manage Hyperglycemia Possible Solutions/What Would *You* Do?
I'm afraid I'll go too low, so I keep myself a little on the high side just to be safe. This scenario may play out more when the patient is home alone or during very active workdays.	Discuss patient's agenda.* • On days when you are very active, consider adjusting your meal plan to include more carbohydrates. These extra calories will help match the glucose-lowering effect of the insulin PLUS the increased activity. • Talk to your provider about guidelines for adjusting your insulin dose on days when you are going to be more active. • Monitor your glucose level frequently to know where you stand. If you see your glucose level decreasing, you can be prepared to treat it before it gets too low. If the level is low on a regular basis, notify your provider. You may need an adjustment in your insulin dose. • Decide if the increased risk for complications that comes with being chronically high is worth it. It may take more effort to implement a different strategy to prevent going too low, but isn't it worth it in the long run?

*The patient's problem-solving efforts for the scenarios *involving intentional omission of insulin* may uncover his/her attitudes and beliefs about having diabetes, as well as potential emotional problems, such as depression, anxiety, or alcohol and drug abuse. These must be investigated and addressed first in order to successfully resolve the secondary problem of omitting insulin. Consult the AADE *Desk Reference* 3rd edition for strategies for individuals with mental health issues.

†J Freeman, MJ Franz, "Nutrition Therapy," in C Mensing, ed, *The Art and Science of Diabetes Self-Management Education Desk Reference*, 3rd ed (Chicago: American Association of Diabetes Educators, 2014), 442.

‡MA Charfen, M Fernandez-Frackelton, "Diabetic ketoacidosis," *Emerg Med Clin N Am* 23 (2005): 609-28; RC Peveler, KS Bryden, HA Neil, et al, "The relationship of disordered eating habits and attitudes to clinical outcomes in young adult females with type 1 diabetes," *Diabetes Care* 28 (2005): 84-8; D Neumark-Sztainer, J Patterson, A Mellin, et al, "Weight control practices and disordered eating behaviors among adolescent females and males with type 1 diabetes," *Diabetes Care* 25 (2002): 1289-96.

Identifying Facilitators for Managing Hyperglycemia

As important as it is to identify barriers to hyperglycemia management, it's just as important to consider the positives, or facilitators, in your situation. Looking deeper, you may find that there are more positives than you thought.

 What resources already exist that can help you manage or prevent hyperglycemia?

- Social support—family members, coworkers, friends.
- Community resources—pharmacies that carry products which can help you organize your diabetes supplies.
- Reminders and cues—calendar or an alarm to remind you to monitor glucose, eat a meal, or take medication(s) on time.
- Rewards—incentives to maintain motivation.
- Log or journal—by keeping a record (either on paper or on your computer or phone) of your blood glucose, food intake, and treatment of lows, you can look for blood glucose patterns and then make changes in your routine.

Sick-Day Management

Sick-Day Guidelines

Why does my blood glucose rise when I'm sick and can hardly eat?

When you become ill or experience physical trauma, your body responds to those stressors in a predictable way. The stress of infection, severe pain, surgery, or injury causes the release of stress hormones. These hormones in turn cause the liver to release glucose into the bloodstream. This response is your body's way of providing a quick source of energy to the cells to give you the energy to fight infection and activate the healing process. This is called the *stress response*.

Because you have diabetes, this extra glucose becomes a problem. Since your body cannot make enough insulin, or you are resistant to the insulin you have, you may develop severe hyperglycemia when you are sick. In fact, infection leads to more severe insulin resistance.

Knowing what to do on a sick day is important to help you avoid a crisis. These guidelines are called *sick-day rules*. By following these rules, you may be able to avoid a visit to the emergency room or a hospital stay.

Stay hydrated.

- A high blood glucose level causes you to urinate more, and fever causes sweating. If you are vomiting or have diarrhea, even more body fluids are being lost. One of the most important things you can do on a sick day is to stay hydrated.
- Drink at least 8 ounces of calorie-free liquids each hour while you are awake. If you are nauseated, sip a little at a time. Examples of calorie-free liquids include water, sugar-free Kool-Aid®, diet soft drinks, broth, sugar-free Jell-O®, and sugar-free popsicles.
- Caffeine has a mild diuretic effect, so go easy on coffee or consider having only caffeine-free liquids. Liquids that contain salt, such as bouillon, should be included every 3 hours or so to replace the electrolytes lost from urination, sweating, or vomiting. If nausea is a problem, ask your provider about anti-nausea medication.

Check your glucose level every 2 to 4 hours while you are awake.

Because your glucose level may be rising quickly, you should monitor it frequently during a sick day. If you wait until the next day to check it, it could have already risen to an unsafe level. If you use insulin, be sure to monitor your blood glucose prior to taking your injection(s). Check every 2 to 4 hours while blood glucose is elevated or until symptoms subside.[22(p639)]

If you are unable to eat your usual meals, get your nutrition from liquids or soft foods.

On a sick day, your appetite may be affected. You may not be able to eat normally because of nausea. Your body still needs nutrition, however, which would include about 150 to 200 g of carbohydrate every day in divided doses. This amounts to 3 or 4 carbohydrate choices every 4 hours while you are awake. Each choice should contain 15 g of carbohydrate.

Examples of 15-g Sick-Day Carbohydrate Choices[17]

- Glucose tablets (3 or 4 tablets, depending on brand)
- Fruit juice (4 to 6 ounces)
- Milk (8 ounces low fat or nonfat)
- Non-diet soft drink (4 to 6 ounces)
- Sugar (3 to 4 teaspoons/packets)
- Hard candy (3 or 4 pieces, depending on size)

American Association of Diabetes Educators©

234   Diabetes Education Curriculum

♦ Lifesavers® (5 or 6 pieces)

♦ Raisins (2 tablespoons)

Continue to take your usual medications unless advised otherwise by your provider.

Stopping your diabetes medication without consulting your provider is a mistake. This is especially true on a sick day, because even if you aren't eating, your glucose level rises when your body is stressed by an illness.

Not taking your medication will cause your glucose level to rise even higher. If in doubt, contact your provider. Your provider may opt to adjust your medication, depending on the severity of your illness and your glucose levels.

If you take oral diabetes medication:

♦ If you take metformin (Glucophage®, Riomet®, Fortamet®), your provider may temporarily switch you to insulin if you become severely ill. Metformin can be dangerous if your illness causes your blood pressure to drop extremely low.[22]

♦ Call your provider if you cannot hold down oral medication because of vomiting. Temporary insulin treatment may be needed.

If you take insulin:

♦ For people who already use insulin to manage their diabetes, sick days usually call for an *increase* in the usual dose. Skipping your insulin can lead to a life-threatening condition called diabetic ketoacidosis (DKA). If you haven't been given guidelines from your provider for adjusting insulin on a sick day, call for instructions on how much extra insulin to take.

If you use insulin, check your ketone level every 4 hours while you are awake or until negative results are obtained.

Ketones are the substances that form in the bloodstream when you use fat for energy. When there is not enough insulin to move glucose into the muscle cells, the cells are starved for energy. At this point, fat begins to be used for energy. If ketones build up to a high level, they become toxic, and DKA can develop. Diabetic ketoacidosis can be a life-threatening condition.

The signs and symptoms of DKA include:

♦ Nausea and vomiting

♦ Abdominal pain

♦ Fruity-smelling breath

♦ Fast, labored breathing

♦ A change in the level of consciousness

In a state of DKA, the blood glucose level is usually above 250 mg/dL (13.9 mmol/L). Because of hyperglycemia, there is excessive urination. This can lead to rapid dehydration, which can cause your blood pressure to be too low. Notify your provider right away if you ever have signs and symptoms of DKA.

Home Monitoring for Ketones

♦ **Urine Ketone Monitoring** (if your provider so instructed)—To check for ketones in the urine, you will need urine testing strips. These are purchased over the counter (OTC) at most pharmacies. The cost is generally between $10 and $15 for a vial of 50 test strips. Note that test strips do expire. Online pharmacies may offer them at a lower price. To use, dip the testing end of the strip into your urine. Wait as instructed on the label (usually about 15 seconds), then compare the color of the test strip with the color chart on the product label. If the color change is equal to a *moderate* or *large* amount of ketones, call your provider.

American Association of Diabetes Educators©

- **Blood Ketone Monitoring**—Ketones show up in the blood sooner than in the urine. A special strip is required to check the blood for ketones. Meters include the AbbotPrecision Xtra®, novaMax®Plus™, and the FreeStyle Optium®.

Avoid OTC medications and products that can affect the glucose level.

Some OTC medications can raise your glucose level. Read the label to find out if the active ingredients include *phenylephrine* or *pseudoephedrine*. These ingredients are often used in decongestants and antihistamines, and they can raise your blood pressure as well. Some OTC medications contain sugar and alcohol, which can also have negative effects on your glucose level.

OTC products to avoid include:

- Cough syrups or cough drops/throat lozenges that contain sugar (eg, dextrose)
- Sudafed® products that contain *phenylephrine* or *pseudoephedrine*[23]
- Tylenol® Cold products that contain *phenylephrine* or *pseudoephedrine*[24]

Call your provider on a "sick day" if you . . . **Survival Skill**

- Have persistent vomiting (vomited more than once) and cannot keep fluids or oral medications down
- Have persistent diarrhea, more than 5 times or for longer than 6 hours
- Have a persistent fever of 101°F or higher
- Have blood glucose levels above 300 mg/dL (16.65 mmol/L) on 2 consecutive measurements and you are unable to get your blood glucose down below 250 mg/dL (13.87 mmol/L) despite increased insulin and fluids
- Have moderate or large urine ketones or blood ketones

Keep a record of your insulin intake, glucose, and ketone results to report to the provider.

Your provider will be able to make better decisions about your care if you share the results of glucose and ketone monitoring. With complete information, your condition may be manageable with advice over the telephone. Write down all of your results with the time and date, as well as any symptoms you were having at the time. If you take insulin, also keep a record of the dose and what time you took it.

Table 6.4 can be used as a handout for patients.

Sharing of personal experiences has more relevance for patients than passively listening to educational content. Hearing others' suggestions to problems can encourage the development of improved problem-solving skills.

Setting a SMART Goal for Problem Solving for Hypoglycemia, Hyperglycemia, and Sick Days

- **S**— Specific: not vague
- **M**—Measurable: you can measure it (how much, how often, etc)
- **A**— Attainable: challenging but not out of reach
- **R**— Relevant: you have a good reason to want to manage your blood glucose and keep it under control.
- **T**— Timely: short term, for next week or two

TABLE 6.4 Sick-Day Management

	Type 1 Diabetes	Type 2 Diabetes
Hydration	8 ounces fluid per hour	Same
	Every third hour, consume this 8 ounces as a sodium-rich choice such as bouillon	
Self-monitoring of blood glucose	Test every 2–4 hours while blood glucose is elevated or until symptoms subside	Same
Ketones	Test every 4 hours or until negative	Determine for the individual
Medication adjustments	Continue as able	Same
	Adjust insulin doses to correct hyperglycemia, but do not stop or hold insulin if diagnosed as having type 1 diabetes mellitus	
	Hold metformin during serious illness	
	Instruct patients to call their healthcare provider for specific instructions if they have not previously received them	
Food and beverage selections	Guide patients to consume 150–200 g carbohydrates daily, in divided doses	Same
	Switch to soft foods or liquids as tolerated	
	Provide patients a list of foods and beverages in portion sizes containing 15 g carbohydrates	
Contact healthcare professionals	Provide guidelines on conditions that require the patient to call: • Vomiting more than once • Diarrhea more than 5 times or for longer than 6 hours • Blood glucose levels >300 mg/dL (16.65 mmol/L) on 2 consecutive measurements that are not responsive to increased insulin and fluids • Moderate or large urine ketones or blood ketones >10.8 mg/dL (>0.6 mmol/L)	Same

The participant sets individual goals for hypoglycemia, hyperglycemia, and sick-day management. The educator and the participant schedule a date on which to evaluate progress with behavior change.

 Using a mnemonic like SMART to help remember an idea can be a useful teaching tool, especially for those with verbal/auditory intelligence.

Follow-up/Outcomes Measurement

Per the Standards for Outcomes Measurement of Diabetes Self-Management Education, the **first follow-up should be conducted within 2 to 4 weeks** after the initial teaching session on problem solving for hypoglycemia, hyperglycemia, and sick days. **Subsequent follow-up is recommended at 3- to 6-month intervals thereafter**. Use the following table as a guide for identifying outcomes measures and how to measure them. Measurement of these outcomes may be objective or subjective.[25] The exception to this schedule would be during pregnancy. The first follow-up should be conducted within 1 week and subsequent visits at 2 to 4 weeks.

Module 6 *Problem Solving* 237

Self-Care Behavior: Problem Solving Outcomes Measures	Self-Care Behavior: Problem Solving Methods of Measurement
Immediate outcome: Learning Immediate outcomes of learning can be assessed right away after the educational encounter. Immediate outcomes include: K: Acquiring *knowledge* (*what to do*) S: Acquiring *skills* (*how to do it*) CM: Developing *confidence and motivation* (*want to do it*) PS: Developing *problem-solving/coping skills* to overcome barrier (*can do it*)	Immediate outcomes of learning can be measured by patient knowledge testing (paper-and-pen testing, or questioning to determine that the patient understands the information taught, or a questionnaire online). Immediate outcomes for acquiring a skill can be measured by the patient's demonstration of that skill. Following are various methods of measuring immediate outcomes for the self-care behavior of *problem solving.*
Problem solving (K,S)	<u>Subjective:</u> Patient lists the steps in solving problems. <u>Objective:</u> Patient demonstrates problem-solving steps in a real-life situation involving diabetes self-care.
Target blood glucose levels (K)	<u>Subjective:</u> Patient states his or her own recommended target blood glucose levels. <u>Objective:</u> Patient states the blood glucose levels recommended by the American Diabetes Association.
Signs and symptoms of hypoglycemia (K)	<u>Subjective:</u> Patient describes his or her own signs of hypoglycemia. <u>Objective:</u> Patient states the common signs and symptoms of hypoglycemia
Signs and symptoms of hyperglycemia (K)	<u>Subjective:</u> Patient describes his or her own signs of hyperglycemia <u>Objective:</u> Patient describes signs and symptoms of hyperglycemia and DKA.
Prevention and treatment of hypoglycemia (K,S)	<u>Subjective:</u> Patient states his or her plan to prevent and treat hypoglycemia. <u>Objective:</u> Patient explains the signs and symptoms of hypoglycemia and the "Rule of 15."
Prevention and treatment of hyperglycemia (K,S)	<u>Subjective:</u> Patient states his or her own plan to prevent and treat hyperglycemia. <u>Objective:</u> Patient explains the effect of physical activity on blood glucose.
Potential barriers and facilitators to hypoglycemia management (PS)	<u>Subjective:</u> Patient lists his or her own barriers and facilitators for hypoglycemic management. <u>Objective:</u> Patient explains what are potential barriers and facilitators to hypoglycemic management.
Potential barriers and facilitators to hyperglycemia management, including sick-day management (PS)	<u>Subjective:</u> Patient lists his or her own barriers and facilitators for hyperglycemic management and sick days. <u>Objective:</u> Patient explains what are potential barriers and facilitators to hyperglycemic management and sick-day rules.
Strategy to overcome potential barriers to hypoglycemia management (PS)	<u>Subjective:</u> Patient identifies his or her own potential barriers and facilitators to hypoglycemia management.
Strategy to overcome potential barriers to hyperglycemia management, including sick-day management (PS)	<u>Subjective:</u> Patient develops a plan to deal with anticipated obstacle(s) to hypoglycemia management <u>Objective:</u> Patient describes 2 strategies to overcome barriers or obtain facilitators for hypoglycemic management. <u>Subjective:</u> Patient identifies his or her own potential barriers and facilitators to hyperglycemia management, including sick-day management. <u>Subjective:</u> Patient develops a plan to deal with anticipated obstacle(s) to hyperglycemia management, including sick-day management. <u>Objective:</u> Patient describes 2 strategies to overcome barriers or obtain facilitators for hyperglycemic management and sick-day management.

American Association of Diabetes Educators©

Self-Care Behavior: Problem Solving Outcomes Measures	Self-Care Behavior: Problem Solving Methods of Measurement
Intermediate outcome: Behavior change	Intermediate outcomes measures can be assessed over time: after the educational encounter and once the patient has had adequate time to implement new behavior(s) in a real-life setting. *Behavior change* is an intermediate outcomes measure. It is the ultimate outcome of DSME/T. At follow-up intervals, knowledge and skills (discussed above) should be reassessed, as well as behavior change.
Potential barriers and strategies for barrier resolution (PS)	<u>Subjective:</u> Patient self-report of barriers faced, facilitators, and strategies used, as patient made efforts to implement behaviors to prevent and treat hypoglycemia and hyperglycemia.
Plan for problem solving and future behavior change (PS)	<u>Subjective:</u> Patient self-report of problem solving and behavior strategies going forward for a specific AADE7 behavior.

REFERENCES

1. Hill-Briggs F, Gemmell L. Problem solving in diabetes self-management and control: a systematic review of the literature. Diabetes Educ. 2007;33(6):1032-50.

2. Kanzer-Lewis G. Problem solving. In: Mensing C, ed. The Art and Science of Diabetes Self-Management Education Desk Reference. 3rd ed. Chicago: American Association of Diabetes Educators; 2014:247-64.

3. Tang TS, Funnell MM, Anderson RM. Group education strategies for diabetes self-management. Diabetes Spectr. 2006;19(2):99-105.

4. Hill-Briggs F, Gary TL, Yeh HC, et al. Association of social problem solving with glycemic control in a sample of urban African Americans with type 2 diabetes. J Behav Med. 2006;29(1):69-78.

5. Executive Agency for Health and Consumers. Take action to prevent diabetes: a toolkit for the prevention of type 2 diabetes in Europe. On the Internet at: http://www.idf.org/sites/default/files/IMAGEToolkit.pdf.

6. Lindstrom J, Neumann A, Sheppard KE, et al. Take action to prevent diabetes—the IMAGE toolkit for the prevention of type 2 diabetes in Europe. Horm Metab Res. 2010;42 Suppl 1:S37-55.

7. Rosengren, DB. Building Motivational Interviewing Skills: A Practitioner Workbook. New York: Guilford Press; 2009.

8. Schreiner B. The diabetes self-management education process. In: Mensing C, ed. The Art and Science of Diabetes Self-Management Education Desk Reference. 3rd ed. Chicago: American Association of Diabetes Educators; 2014: 31-87.

9. Anderson RM, Funnell MM, Burkhart N, Gillard ML, Nwankwo R. 101 Tips for Behavior Change in Diabetes Education. Alexandria, Va: American Diabetes Association; 2002.

10. Choices & Changes: Clinician Influence & Patient Action in Diabetes Self-Management. Houston, Tex: Bayer Institute for Health Care Communication, Inc; 2004:60-6.

11. Miller WR, Rollnick S. Motivational Interviewing: Preparing People to Change Addictive Behavior. 3rd ed. New York: The Guilford Press; 2013.

12. Allen KV, Frier BM. Nocturnal hypoglycemia: clinical manifestations and therapeutic strategies toward prevention. Endocr Pract. 2003;9:530-43.

13. The DCCT Research Group. Epidemiology of severe hypoglycemia in the diabetes control and complications trial. Am J Med. 1991 Apr;90(4):450-9.

14. Yki-Järvinen H. Insulin therapy in type 2 diabetes: role of the long-acting insulin glargine analogue. Eur J Clin Invest. 2004 Jun;34(6):410-6.

American Association of Diabetes Educators©

15. Davis RE, Morrissey M, Peters JR, Wittrup-Jensen K, Kennedy-Martin T, Currie CJ. Impact of hypoglycaemia on quality of life and productivity in type 1 and type 2 diabetes. Curr Med Res Opin. 2005 Sep;21(9):1477-83.

16. Malone JK, Beattie SD, Campaigne BN, Johnson PA, Howard AS, Milicevic Z. Therapy after single oral agent failure: adding a second oral agent or an insulin mixture? Diabetes Res Clin Pract. 2003;62(3):187-95.

17. Sisson EM, Dixon DL. Pharmacotherapy for glucose management. In: Mensing C, ed. The Art and Science of Diabetes Self-Management Education Desk Reference. 3rd ed. Chicago: American Association of Diabetes Educators; 2014:491-540.

18. The Diabetes Control and Complications Trial Research Group. The effect of intensive treatment of diabetes on the development and progression of long-term complications in insulin-dependent diabetes mellitus. N Engl J Med. 1993;329:977-86.

19. UK Prospective Diabetes Study Group. Intensive blood glucose control with sulphonylureas or insulin compared with conventional treatment and risk of complications in patients with type 2 diabetes (UKPDS 38). Lancet. 1998;352:837-53.

20. American Diabetes Association. Standards of medical care in diabetes—2014. Diabetes Care. 2014;37 Suppl 1: S14-80.

21. Handelsman Y, Mechanick JI, Blonde L, et al. American Association of Clinical Endocrinologists Medical Guidelines for clinical practice for developing a diabetes mellitus comprehensive care plan. Endocr Pract. 2011;17 Suppl 2:1-53.

22. Trence DL. Hyperglycemia. In: Mensing C, ed. The Art and Science of Diabetes Self-Management Education Desk Reference. 3rd ed. Chicago: American Association of Diabetes Educators; 2014:635-61.

23. Sudafed. How our products work (cited 2015 July 15). On the Internet at: http://www.sudafed.com/know/sinus-pressure-congestion-treatment.

24. Tylenol (cited 2015 July 15). On the Internet at: http://www.tylenol.com.

25. Mulcahy K, Maryniuk M, Peeples M, et al. Diabetes self-management education core outcomes measures: technical review. Diabetes Educ. 2003;29(5):768-803.

PROBLEM SOLVING: RESOURCES

Behavior Chain Templates... 239

Problem Solving Activity (English) 240

Problem Solving Activity (Spanish) 242

Problem-Solving Activity Script....................................... 244

Goal-Setting Activity Script... 245

Behavioral Chain Analysis of Problem Behavior Worksheet................ 246

Behavior Chain Templates

For an example of using the behavior chain tool, see Julie Corliss, Executive Editor, Harvard Heart Letter, Harvard Medical School, Harvard Health Publication.
http://www.health.harvard.edu/blog/bridge-the-intention-behavior-gap-to-lose-weight-and-keep-it-off-201103101729

For another example of a behavior chain template, see the following link from Brigham and Women's Hospital:
http://www.brighamandwomens.org/Patients_Visitors/pcs/nutrition/services/healtheweightforwomen/success/behavior_chain.aspx

American Association of Diabetes Educators©

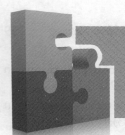

AADE7™ SELF-CARE BEHAVIORS
PROBLEM SOLVING

What do you do when you have a problem like low blood sugar (hypoglycemia)? Do you know what caused it? How can you help reduce the risk of it happening in the future?

Everyone encounters problems with their diabetes control; you can't plan for every situation you may face. However, there are some problem-solving skills that can help you prepare for the unexpected—and make a plan for dealing with similar problems in the future.

Some of the most important problem-solving skills for diabetes self-care are learning how to recognize and react to high and low blood sugar levels and learning how to manage on days when you are sick.

Your diabetes educator can help you develop the skills to identify situations that could upset your diabetes control.

DID YOU KNOW?

Skipping meals and snacks, taking too much diabetes medication, engaging in physical activity and drinking too much alcohol can all cause you to experience low blood sugar problems.

TRUE OR FALSE?

Nobody has perfect diabetes management.

TRUE. You are not perfect—no one is. There WILL be problems and challenges. The important thing is to learn from each situation—what caused your blood sugar to go above or below target, and what you can do to improve your diabetes self-care.

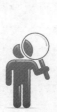 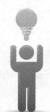

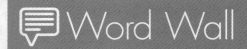

HYPOGLYCEMIA:
Low blood sugar

HYPERGLYCEMIA:
High blood sugar

GOAL SETTING:
Choosing a specific task or activity that you want to achieve and making a plan to get there

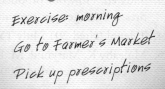

Exercise: morning
Go to Farmer's Market
Pick up prescriptions

QUICK TIPS

Do not go more than 5 hours without eating during your waking hours.

Limit your alcohol consumption. Learn how it interacts with your medications and how it affects your blood sugar. When you do drink alcoholic beverages, don't drink on an empty stomach.

If you do have a problem with your diabetes control, don't beat yourself up over it—solve it and learn from it! Talk to your healthcare provider—they can help you come up with solutions.

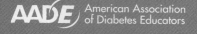

Supported by an educational grant from Eli Lilly and Company.

ACTIVITIES

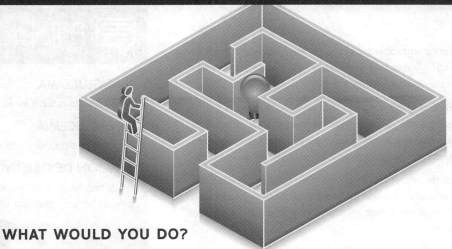

WHAT WOULD YOU DO?

Think about how the following situations may affect you—and about what steps you could take to maintain proper control of your diabetes in similar situations.

You get the flu and notice that your blood sugar levels are higher than normal. What do you do?

_____

While on vacation, you don't have easy access to a gym or time for exercise. How will you handle this?

_____

You have a hard time finding healthy food choices within your family's cultural or taste preferences. What steps can you take?

_____

Is there something you've been struggling with in your diabetes care? What is it?

_____

Why do you think this is a problem? When does it occur?

_____
_____

Name two things you can do to fix it.

_____
_____

What can you do to prevent it from happening in the future?

_____

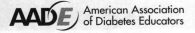

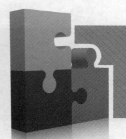

CONDUCTAS PARA EL CUIDADO PERSONA DE AADE7™

RESOLUCIÓN DE PROBLEMAS

¿Qué haces cuando tienes un problema, como un nivel bajo de azúcar en la sangre (hipoglucemia)? ¿Sabes qué lo provocó? ¿Cómo puedes ayudar a reducir el riesgo de que esto suceda en el futuro?

Todos tienen problemas con el control de su diabetes; no puedes planificar cada situación que pueda surgir. Sin embargo, existen algunas técnicas de resolución de problemas que te pueden ayudar a estar preparado para lo inesperado y elaborar un plan para tratar problemas similares en el futuro.

Algunas de las técnicas de resolución de problemas más importantes para la atención personal de la diabetes son aprender a reconocer y reaccionar ante los niveles altos y bajos de azúcar en la sangre y aprender qué hacer los días que estás enfermo.

Tu educador en diabetes te puede ayudar a desarrollar técnicas para identificar situaciones que podrían alterar el control de tu diabetes.

¿LO SABÍAS?

Saltear comidas y refrigerios, tomar demasiados medicamentos para la diabetes, realizar actividad física y beber demasiado alcohol pueden hacer que tengas problemas de bajo nivel de azúcar en la sangre.

¿VERDADERO O FALSO?

Nadie tiene un control perfecto de la diabetes.

VERDADERO. No eres perfecto; nadie lo es. SIEMPRE habrá problemas y desafíos. Lo importante es aprender de cada situación; qué hizo que el nivel de azúcar en la sangre subiera o bajara más de los valores previstos, y qué puedes hacer para mejorar la atención personal de tu diabetes.

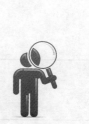
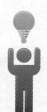

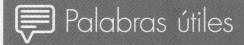

Palabras útiles

HIPOGLUCEMIA:
Bajo nivel de azúcar en la sangre.

HIPERGLUCEMIA:
Alto nivel de azúcar en la sangre.

FIJACIÓN DE OBJETIVOS:
Elegir una tarea o actividad específica que deseas hacer y elaborar un plan para lograrlo.

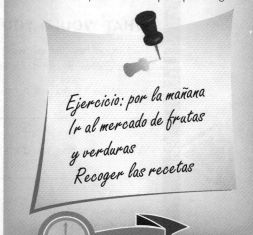

Ejercicio: por la mañana
Ir al mercado de frutas y verduras
Recoger las recetas

CONSEJOS RÁPIDOS

No estés más de 5 horas sin comer durante las horas en que estás despierto.

Limita tu consumo de alcohol. Aprende cómo el alcohol interactúa con tus medicamentos y cómo afecta tus niveles de azúcar en la sangre.

Cuando consumas bebidas alcohólicas, no lo hagas con el estómago vacío.

Si tienes un problema para controlar tu diabetes, no te culpes por esto; ¡resuélvelo y aprende de ello! Habla con tu proveedor de atención médica; te puede ayudar a encontrar soluciones.

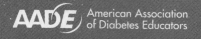

Supported by an educational grant from Lilly USA, LLC.

ACTIVIDADES

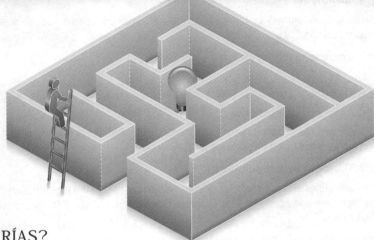

¿QUÉ HARÍAS?

Piensa cómo te pueden afectar las siguientes situaciones y los pasos que podrías dar para mantener el control apropiado de tu diabetes en situaciones similares.

Contraes la gripe y notas que tus niveles de azúcar en la sangre son más elevados que lo normal.
¿Qué haces?

_____

Mientras estás de vacaciones, no tienes un fácil acceso a un gimnasio ni tiempo para hacer ejercicios.
¿Cómo manejas esto?

_____

Te ha sido difícil encontrar opciones de alimentos saludables dentro de las preferencias culturales o los gustos de tu familia. ¿Qué medidas puedes tomar?

_____

¿Hay algo que te esté dando dificultad en la atención de tu diabetes? ¿Qué es?

_____

¿Por qué piensas que esto es un problema? ¿Cuándo ocurre?

_____

Nombra dos cosas que puedes hacer para solucionarlo.

_____

¿Qué puedes hacer para evitar que esto suceda en el futuro?

_____

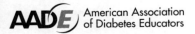

243

Problem-Solving Activity Script

Guide:	**Step 1: Identify the problem** "Describe the problem you are facing. Be very specific. The more specific you can be, the more likely you are to find a solution that works."
Person with diabetes:	"I can't remember to take my meds."
Guide:	"This is a start, but it's too vague. It's important to drill down to the 'sticking point,' the one area of taking your medication that has tripped you up over and over again."
Person with diabetes:	"I do pretty well remembering the morning meds. It's the medicine before dinner that I keep forgetting. I'm so busy getting dinner ready that it just slips my mind every time."
Guide:	**Step 2: Think of possible solutions** "Brainstorm things that you can do to help you remember to take the pre-dinner meds. Keep in mind similar situations you've faced when you came up with a solution that worked. Perhaps that solution will work this time, too. Build on any prior successes. "
Diabetes educator:	Ask participants to share their successes: "Who has faced a similar problem and found a workable solution? What did you do?" Other possible solutions to share with the group: (1) Place the bottle of meds where you eat dinner, next to the salt and pepper shakers; (2) set the alarm on your cell phone for 5 PM; (3) buy a medication reminder alarm from the pharmacy, and set it for 5 PM; (4) place a note in the kitchen to remind you to take the meds.
Guide:	**Step 3: Identify thoughts/attitudes that come with the problem** "Recall the thoughts or attitudes you have experienced when this problem happened before, and what happened then."
Person with diabetes:	"I'll realize after dinner that I forgot my diabetes medicine. Now, it's too late to take it. I feel so stupid! Why can't I get it right? Diabetes is too hard to deal with! No way am I going to check my blood sugar tonight; I know it'll be high because I forgot the medicine again. So I figure why bother? I get so discouraged, I just want to forget it all."
Guide:	"Practice more positive thoughts. This is a skill that you can learn to do. You'll get better with practice. Focus on any progress you've made, even if it's a little thing. Focus on something you can feel good about."
Person with diabetes:	"Well, at least I'm watching my food portions. I do pretty well with that. I haven't gained any weight since I started paying attention to my diet. I guess I'm not a complete failure after all."
Diabetes educator:	Studies show that thinking positive thoughts can lead to more constructive behaviors. It doesn't come naturally. You have to make yourself think about the positives. Give yourself a "pat on the back." It may feel silly at first, but with practice, it'll come more naturally. Negative expectations may discourage you from trying to cope with diabetes-related problems in the future. Negative thoughts about your ability to manage diabetes can easily lead to negative actions in the future. When you feel discouraged, you might slip into actions that will make your blood glucose go even higher. In this example, the person stops monitoring in the evening. That could lead to less monitoring the next day, the day after that, and so on. It's a slippery slope.
Guide:	**Step 4: Choose a solution, try it, see how it works out** "If your solution doesn't work out, don't give up! Try the next option on your list of possible solutions. Remind yourself that trying is worth the effort. Try to view any failure as an opportunity to learn what doesn't work."

Goal-Setting Activity Script

Educator:	"What area of diabetes self-care do you feel you need to improve on the most? There may be lots of areas, but try to prioritize."
Patient:	"Afternoon snacking is a problem for me. I get really hungry around 3 o'clock, so I usually buy chips or a candy bar from the employee lounge."
Educator:	"On a scale of 0 to 10, how convinced are you that it's important to make this change?"
Patient:	"I'd have to give it an 8. I know it's important to do something about this, because once I feel I've already blown my diet, I tend to overeat for the rest of the evening."
Educator:	"What would you have to do differently (or give up) to make this change?"
Patient:	"I'd need to find something different to snack on. There's a vending machine in the lounge, but there's nothing but junk food in there. Also, nearly every day, people bring doughnuts or something sweet to the lounge. I could eat my snack at my desk or outside in the covered area next to the building. That way, I wouldn't be tempted by the stuff in the employee lounge."
Educator:	"How will this change help you?"
Patient:	"If I eat a healthier snack in the afternoon, I'll feel better about myself. When I've done the 'right thing' earlier in the day, it helps me want to keep it up into the evening. If I do that, I'll be in a better frame of mind to stick to my meal plan at dinner. Having a piece of fresh fruit instead of high-fat junk food will help me manage my blood sugar level. In the long run, it might help me lose weight, or at least not gain any more weight."
Educator:	"Are you willing and able to make the changes? On a scale of 0 to 10, how confident are you that you can make this change?"
Patient:	"As far as the confidence to do this, I think I'm a 7 or 8. I am willing to try it. I think my coworker would do it with me, too. She's always talking about eating better, and she needs to lose weight also."
Educator:	"What change can you start with right away?"
Patient:	"I could buy a bag of apples and oranges over the weekend and take them to work with me on Monday."

Behavioral Chain Analysis of Problem Behavior Worksheet

1. **Describe the specific PROBLEM BEHAVIOR (eg, unable to control snacking, no time to exercise).**

   A. Be very specific and detailed. No vague terms.

   B. Identify exactly what you did, said, thought, or felt (if feelings are the targeted problem behavior).

   C. Describe the intensity of the behavior and other characteristics of the behavior that are important.

   D. Describe the problem behavior in enough detail that an actor in a play or movie could re-create the behavior exactly.

2. **Describe the specific PRECIPITATING EVENT that started the whole chain of behavior.**

   Start with the environmental event that started the chain. Always start with some event in your environment, even if it doesn't seem to you that the environmental event "caused" the problem behavior. Possible questions to get at this are:

   - What exact event precipitated the start of the chain reaction?
   - When did the sequence of events that led to the problem behavior begin? When did the problem start?
   - What was going on the moment the problem started?
   - What were you doing, thinking, feeling, imagining at that time?
   - Why did the problem behavior happen on that day instead of the day before?

3. **Describe in general VULNERABILITY FACTORS happening before the precipitating event. What factors or events made you more vulnerable to a problematic chain? Areas to examine are:**

   - Physical illness, unbalanced eating or sleeping, injury
   - Use of drugs or alcohol, misuse of prescription drugs
   - Stressful events in the environment (either positive or negative)
   - Intense emotions, such as sadness, anger, fear, loneliness
   - Previous behaviors of your own that you found stressful

246

4. **Describe in excruciating detail THE CHAIN OF EVENTS that led up to the problem behavior.**

What next? Imagine that your problem behavior is chained to the precipitating event in the environment. How long is the chain? Where does it go? What are the links? Write out all links in the chain of events, no matter how small. Be very specific, as if you are writing a script for a play.

A. What exact thought (or belief), feeling, or action followed the precipitating event? What thought, feeling, or action followed that? What next?

B. Look at each link in the chain after you write it. Was there another thought, feeling, or action that could have occurred? Could someone else have thought, felt, or acted differently at that point? If so, explain how that specific thought, feeling, or action came to be.

C. For each link in the chain, ask yourself if there is a smaller link you could describe.

The links can be thoughts, emotions, sensations, and behaviors.

5. **What are the CONSEQUENCES of this behavior? Be specific.**

A. How did other people react immediately and later?

B. How did you feel immediately following the behavior? Later?

C. What effect did the behavior have on you and your environment?

6. **Describe in detail different SOLUTIONS to the problem.**

A. Go back to the chain of your behaviors following the prompting event. Circle each point or link indicating that if you had done something different, you would have avoided the problem behavior.

B. What could you have done differently at each link in the chain of events to avoid the problem behavior? What coping behaviors or skillful behaviors could you have used?

7. Describe in detail the PREVENTION STRATEGY for how you could have kept the chain from starting by reducing your vulnerability to the chain.

8. Describe what you are going to do to REPAIR important or significant consequences of the problem behavior.

MODULE 7

Healthy Coping

Table of Contents

HEALTHY COPING: AN EDUCATOR'S OVERVIEW..250

    AADE Systematic Review of the Literature 250

    Background Information and Instructions for the Educator 250

        What Is Coping? 250

        Influences on Coping..250

        Diabetes Coping Skills Training 251

        Potential Components of Diabetes Coping Skills Training..........................251

    Learning Objectives 253

        Knowledge 253

        Skill 253

        Barriers and Facilitators 253

    Behavioral Objectives 254

        Coping Skills for People Living With Diabetes..254

        Depression 254

HEALTHY COPING: INSTRUCTIONAL PLAN 254

    Identifying Participant Thoughts and Feelings About Living With Diabetes 254

    Responses to Participants' Feelings About Diabetes 255

        Shock/Denial 255

        Anger/Resentment 255

        Guilt/Self-Blame 256

        Sadness/Worry/Depression 256

    Depression and Anxiety 256

        Depression 256

        Anxiety 256

    Exploring Feelings and Attitudes About Diabetes: Exploration Activity 257

    Problem-Solving Skill 257

    Motivation Skill: Costs Versus Benefits Analysis 259

250   Diabetes Education Curriculum

  Decision-Making Skill: Motivating Yourself to Change 259
    Costs Versus Benefits Learning Activity 260
  Relapse Prevention Skills 260
    Preventing Lapses Skill 261
    Getting Over a Lapse Skill or Preventing Relapse 261
  Obtaining Support Skill: Getting the Support You Need 262
    Support From Family and Friends 262
    Support From Healthcare Providers 265
    Support From Community Resources 266
    Read Diabetes Publications 267
    Visit Reputable Diabetes Web Sites 268
    Consult Patient Assistance Programs 268
    Connect With Your Insurance Companies 268
  Stress Management Skill 269
    Managing Stress 270
  Follow-up/Outcomes Measurement 271
REFERENCES 274
HEALTHY COPING: RESOURCES 276

HEALTHY COPING: AN EDUCATOR'S OVERVIEW

AADE Systematic Review of the Literature

A systematic review of the literature was conducted by the American Association of Diabetes Educators (AADE) "to assess the literature pertinent to healthy coping in diabetes management and to identify effective or promising interventions and areas needing further investigation. Psychological, emotional, related behavioral factors, and quality of life are important in diabetes management, are worthy of attention in their own right, and influence metabolic control."[1]

Background Information and Instructions for the Educator

What Is Coping?

Coping is the psychologic attempt to restore order after a disruption has occurred in one's life. A diagnosis of diabetes and the subsequent challenges of living with this condition are disruptive. As shown in the DAWN (Diabetes Attitudes, Wishes, and Needs) study, the relentless demands of diabetes can lead to a variety of coping problems that influence self-care behavior and are a barrier to achieving metabolic control.[2]

Coping with diabetes does not simply occur within the patient's mind. It takes place within the broad context of his or her life—social support system (or lack thereof), living environment, and personal identity or sense of self.[3] According to Maslow's Hierarchy of Needs, basic physiologic and safety needs must be satisfied before higher-level psychologic needs can be pursued.[4] With this hierarchy in mind, the educator should assess whether any deficits in the patient's basic needs are interfering with his or her motivation for self-care.

Influences on Coping

Efforts to cope with diabetes are affected by health beliefs, which may be influenced by cultural identity, family traditions, spiritual foundation, and social affiliations.[5] Patients' past experiences, the experiences of others

American Association of Diabetes Educators©

with diabetes, and media reports about diabetes can shape attitudes and beliefs.[6] In order to individualize education, diabetes educators should assess the patient's framework for coping with diabetes.[7] Explorative questions are included in this curriculum.

Providers should assess and acknowledge the role of spirituality, religion, and prayer in patients' efforts to cope with illness. Individuals who measure high in spirituality have a stronger coping style and more positive thoughts.[8] Prayer was found to be a primary coping mechanism for African-American women with diabetes.[9] Educators should actively encourage patients who regard spirituality as central to their individual self to draw on it as a coping tool in diabetes management.

The healthcare providers' approach influences how patients cope with diabetes. When instructing patients, diabetes educators should attempt to take a direct but balanced approach. On the one hand, they should avoid minimizing the seriousness of diabetes; on the other hand, educators should avoid using scare tactics when describing potential complications.[10(p221)]

Diabetes Coping Skills Training

Specific training that focuses on coping skills helps patients in several ways to overcome barriers. With strong coping skills, patients can successfully apply self-care knowledge and skills that lead to improved metabolic parameters. As coping skills improve, there is:

- Better application of knowledge
- Better self-care management skills
- More confidence and diabetes self-efficacy
- More hope for a healthy future[11(p112)]

Healthy coping by patients can lessen the release of counter-regulatory hormones in response to perceived stressful situations.[12]

Potential Components of Diabetes Coping Skills Training

There are several different strategies and skills one can employ for coping. The diabetes educator should work with the patient to find alternative behaviors that will relieve the patient's intense emotional response that may have led to avoiding the problem by getting distracted or even by disengaging from diabetes self-care.

Problem-Solving Skills: Better Application of Self-Care Knowledge and Management Skills

Identify the Problem

The first intervention in coping skills training is helping the patient identify his or her "sticking points," or barriers. Educators should ask questions to help patients drill down, to describe the barrier with as much specificity as possible. The more fully the problem is understood, the more likely the patient will eventually find a workable solution.

Generate Alternative Solutions

Once the problem has been identified and described, the educator should encourage the patient to brainstorm solutions. The intent is to generate as many solutions as possible for the problem. Social Cognitive Theory of Behavior Change asserts that individuals learn from observing others.[13] In group diabetes education settings, the educator can call on other participants to share "what worked for them" in similar situations.

Identify Thoughts and Attitudes[14,15(pp21-2)]

- *In the Past.* Ask the patient to recall thoughts and attitudes that he or she experienced when encountering the same problem in the past. This may help the patient discover that one's view of a given situation typically determines one's response: that nonconstructive behavior is often triggered by negative thoughts or attitudes, and constructive behavior is often preceded by more positive thoughts and attitudes.

American Association of Diabetes Educators©

252   Diabetes Education Curriculum

♦ *In the Present.* Actively pursuing more positive thoughts is a skill that comes with practice. To that end, the educator should encourage the patient to focus on any positive progress made (no matter how small) and to repeat the thoughts and behavior that led to the resolution.

♦ *In the Future.* The educator should explain that negative expectations may discourage a person from continuing to try to cope with diabetes-related problems in the future.

Select, Enact, and Evaluate Solutions

At follow-up, the educator should inquire about the patient's experience coping with diabetes-related problems. The educator should ask the patient to describe what he or she believes contributed to the outcome.

Stress Management Skills: Better Application of Self-Care Knowledge and Management Skills

Diabetes educators can integrate stress management content into coping skills training. Studies illustrate that stress management is related to reductions in A1C.[16,17] See the "Resources" section at the end of this module for "Psychological Assessment and Screening Tools," a list of validated tools to screen for stress and quality of life.

Certain mind-body techniques for stress management have proven to be effective.[18-22] Mind-body techniques such as yoga (focus on paced breathing) and Tai Chi require specialized skills. Educators should counsel participants to seek qualified practitioners if they are interested in engaging in yoga or Tai Chi. These techniques are helpful with other negative emotions, not just stress. Some people find physical activity or exercise to be mood lifting.

A woman may become stressed if she is concerned about how diabetes may affect her pregnancy. A referral to childbirth education classes may help the expectant mother learn about the physical and emotional changes that occur during pregnancy.

Stress reduction is also accomplished through distraction, touch, and sound. Focusing on work can distract from the stress for a while. Petting a cat or dog can be calming. Listening to water sounds, waves crashing on a beach, or music can reduce stress too.

Depression Screening: More Hope for the Future

The effect of depression on diabetes outcomes should be included as part of a comprehensive diabetes education curriculum. Diabetes and depression have a bidirectional link. Those living with diabetes are 2 to 3 times more likely to be depressed than those without diabetes, while those with depression are at greater risk for the development of type 2 diabetes.[23,24]

Diabetes educators should teach patients which symptoms should be reported to their healthcare provider.

As recommended by the US Preventive Services Task Force, screening for depression in adults should take place if the local healthcare system has the means to "assure accurate diagnosis, effective treatment and follow-up."[25]

Diabetes educators can play an important role in the assessment of patients for the presence of depressive symptoms. This may be accomplished by including specific questions in the diabetes assessment.

Assessment Questions

♦ In the past 2 weeks, have you had little interest or pleasure in doing things?[26]

♦ In the past 2 weeks, have you been feeling consistently depressed, down, or hopeless?[26]

♦ Has your mood interfered with taking care of your diabetes?[27]

Alternatively, there are a variety of validated screening tools that may be used to screen for depression. Pertinent results should be communicated to the healthcare provider. See the "Resources" section at the end of this module for "Psychological Assessment and Screening Tools" for a list of validated tools to screen for depression.

American Association of Diabetes Educators©

Obtaining Social Support Skills: More Confidence and Diabetes Self-Efficacy

Numerous studies reiterate that social support is a powerful predictor of diabetes self-efficacy, adherence, and positive health outcomes, particularly for regimen-specific support.[28-32] Each person's perception of "support" will naturally vary, depending on his or her life experience, including cultural identification. To maximize support systems, diabetes educators should integrate the following into practice[33(p103),34]:

- Assess patients' need for, and perception of, social support.
- Consider the impact of both supportive and nonsupportive behaviors of support person(s) on patients' self-care.
- Avoid judgmental attitudes about how culturally different groups provide support.
- Build in time for support persons to express their concerns.
- Teach support persons how to help the patient manage his or her diabetes without becoming the "diabetes police."
- Help connect patients and their support persons to culturally sensitive community resources.

Communication Skills: Social Situations That Affect Diabetes Self-Care

Communication skills training involves thinking through how to handle a social problem and then testing out in role play concrete instructions regarding what to say and how to speak up in a group setting so your words are effective and appropriate.[35]

Learning Objectives

Knowledge

The participant will:

- recognize that managing chronic disease requires ongoing adaptation and that this is normal
- identify symptoms of psychologic problems (eg, depression, anxiety) that should be reported to the provider
- state the benefits of treatment and self-care

Skill

The participant will demonstrate one potential coping skill by identifying a barrier and planning a strategy to overcome it.

Barriers and Facilitators

Coping Skills

The participant will:

- identify potential barriers and facilitators that may affect his or her ability to successfully cope with chronic disease
- state his or her feelings about having diabetes and ways to cope with any negative feelings
- develop strategies for overcoming the barriers and increasing the facilitators

Depression—if present

The participant will develop a step-by-step strategy for coping with depression.

Depression prevents the application and maintenance of self-care knowledge and skills. These depressed feelings are a barrier to the patient doing what is required. Depressed patients need a referral to a healthcare professional. The educator can help the patient plan the steps for consulting a mental health professional.

254   Diabetes Education Curriculum

Behavioral Objectives

The participant will:

- develop solutions to triggers that can lead to relapse and make plans to prevent lapses
- set a realistic, measurable, timely behavior change goal
- demonstrate motivation, empowerment, and self-efficacy in self-care by implementing coping skills

Coping Skills for People Living With Diabetes

The participant will apply situational coping skills (eg, problem solving with behavior chain analysis, stress reduction, obtaining support) to diabetes self-care.

Depression

The participant will develop cognitive strategies to psychologically cope with the daily demands of living with a chronic disease.

HEALTHY COPING: INSTRUCTIONAL PLAN

N ▶ This module covers 7 different coping skills. They are not intended to all be taught in one session. The coping skills that participants most frequently use are problem solving, cost-benefit analysis, obtaining support, stress management, and relapse prevention. Choose at most 2 (a short one and a long one) to teach the participants. The behavior chain analysis for problem solving, described in Module 6, complements the problem-solving module and can be taught then or now.

Identifying Participant Thoughts and Feelings About Living With Diabetes

Q ▶ **Survival Skill** *What are your feelings about living with diabetes?*

How did you feel when you were first diagnosed with diabetes? How are you feeling about it now?

What does having diabetes mean to you?

How are you currently handling your concerns about diabetes self-care?

How do you see your future living with diabetes?

Do you believe that diabetes is a condition that can be managed?

Do you have any close friends or relatives with diabetes? How are they doing/ How did they do?

Do you feel there's anything you can do to affect the outcome of your diabetes?

Do you think the effort of trying to manage diabetes is worth the hassles?

How much input do you think you should have in making decisions about your diabetes care?

How do you think diabetes will affect the rest of your pregnancy?

American Association of Diabetes Educators©

Responses to Participants' Feelings About Diabetes

Everybody responds differently to diabetes. A list of feelings about living with a chronic disease would include shock, anger, guilt, worry, shame, fear, and many others. Rest assured, your experience is normal. Your feelings and thoughts will change over time. To adapt to diabetes, it's important for you to acknowledge whatever you are feeling. Bottled-up emotions sometimes have a way of coming out later in destructive ways. Allow yourself some time to feel whatever you are feeling.

Adults learn best when they feel valued and respected for the experiences and perspectives they bring. Use probing questions to elicit learners' experiences and perspectives and reflective responses to validate their feelings.

Shock/Denial

When bad things happen, a first response can be shock. It's hard to believe that it's really true. Denial is a way of protecting yourself against bad news. A new diagnosis of diabetes is certainly an unwanted event. If you've known people who have experienced awful diabetes-related problems, your shock may be linked to fear that the same will happen to you. With type 2 diabetes, people sometimes question their diagnosis. There may be no symptoms, which makes it easy to believe that it's not really happening.

If you've had diabetes for a long time, managing it can be overwhelming. You might even feel burned out. It's times like these that short-term denial provides some relief from reality. But denial becomes a big problem if it continues as your main way of coping with diabetes.

Help foster a more positive attitude about the learning situation by:
- Providing a safe, supportive environment in which patients can express emotions
- Addressing common negative emotions about diabetes up front
- Helping patients realize the universality of their responses, that they are not alone

What You Can Do

- Talk about how you are feeling.
- Realize that what you're feeling is normal.
- Focus on the positives. Learn about the things that are within your power to manage.

Anger/Resentment

Some people feel angry about having diabetes. You may believe that having diabetes means a lifetime of restriction. You may feel like you've been betrayed by your own body. Anger is understandable. This is especially true if you've worked hard to do the "right" things, like exercising and eating well. In this case, you may feel resentment that all your hard work was for nothing. It's not fair! "Why me?" is a common question, especially at the time of diagnosis.

What You Can Do

- Realize that it's OK to feel angry or resentful. It helps to share these thoughts with someone you trust. Just getting it out in the open can help dilute negative feelings, clear the air, and help you take steps to move forward.

American Association of Diabetes Educators©

256   Diabetes Education Curriculum

♦ Try not to let resentment overtake you. Unfortunately, there are no guarantees that doing everything "right" will prevent all diabetes problems. Have realistic expectations of yourself. Understand that diabetes can't be managed perfectly. Instead, focus on what you can do to help improve your situation, and feel good about the positive efforts you have made, no matter how small.

Guilt/Self-Blame

People often believe that diabetes was brought on through their own actions. Maybe the doctor even warned them that if they didn't lose weight, change their diet, and start exercising they'd end up with diabetes. While certain lifestyle choices may help *delay* type 2 diabetes in some cases, no one is responsible for his or her heredity (genetics). Because of this link to lifestyle, though, people often feel guilt. In type 1 diabetes, lifestyle choices are not a factor at all.

For those who have had diabetes complications, guilt is a common response. They may regret that they didn't do enough to prevent the complications from developing.

What You Can Do

♦ If you are newly diagnosed, don't play the blame game! You did not give yourself diabetes.

♦ Realize that you can't change the past but you *can* learn from it. You can't *undo* lifestyle choices that may have contributed to your risk for type 2 diabetes, but you can make different choices going forward.

♦ Focus on what you *can* do in the *future* to improve your situation. Give yourself credit for your efforts to manage diabetes now. Accentuate the positive.

Sadness/Worry/Depression

Sadness about having diabetes is a common response. If you've lost someone to diabetes, the diagnosis may cause you to relive the sadness of this loss. You may worry that you, too, may have a bad outcome. If you have complications that limit your ability to do the things you've always done, sadness is a natural response. You may worry that you'll get worse.

What You Can Do

♦ Realize that sadness and worry are normal emotions.

♦ Talk to your provider if feelings of depression, sadness, or hopelessness are prolonged.

♦ Be involved in regular physical activity for its antidepressant effects. One study showed that a 30-minute brisk walk was just as effective as antidepressant medication.[36]

Depression and Anxiety

Depression

Clinical depression is more than just feeling down when things aren't going well. Depression is a serious condition. A 2011 study found that 12.5% of people with diabetes have major depression, and 20% may have less severe but clinically significant depressive symptoms.[37] Untreated depression makes managing diabetes a lot harder than it is already. Fortunately, depression is treatable. Know the warning signs of depression and let your provider know if you experience them:

♦ Feeling sad, depressed, down, or blue consistently for the past 2 weeks.

♦ Loss of interest or pleasure in things that you used to enjoy, for a period of 2 weeks or longer.

♦ Your mood has interfered with taking care of your diabetes.

Anxiety

Excessive worry, whether it is about a specific thing or a general feeling, can be a sign of an anxiety disorder. Let your provider know if you experience excessive worry, especially if it goes hand-in-hand with these symptoms:

American Association of Diabetes Educators©

- Irritability
- Restlessness
- Poor memory
- Trouble concentrating or making decisions
- Weakness/dizziness/sweating/shaking

The symptoms of anxiety often look like hypoglycemia (low blood glucose). Monitoring your blood glucose level can help you tell the difference.[27]

Exploring Feelings and Attitudes About Diabetes: Exploration Activity[38(p43)]

This activity is intended to help participants explore their attitudes and feelings about diabetes. It is also meant to help them examine the effect their attitude has on diabetes self-care behavior.

- Make a list of words that are often used to describe diabetes. Make sure the list is a balance of words with a positive connotation and words with a negative connotation, eg, *burden, challenge, opportunity, problem, disaster, depressing*.
- Ask participants to pick the word that best fits how they view their diabetes.
- Ask participants to explain why they picked that word, and describe how the feeling affects their diabetes self-care (helps or hinders).

Those with intrapersonal intelligence learn best when allowed to reflect. This activity urges patients to become more aware of their own thoughts. It also works for those with interpersonal/social intelligence because it requires learners to relate to others and sense feelings.

Educators should avoid trying to get participants to change their attitudes. Instead, help them make the connection between their feelings and the self-care behaviors that follow. This would be a good time to ask an open question such as:

How does your blood sugar or diabetes self-care management change when you are feeling negatively or positively?

How can you direct all your emotional energy toward the job of caring for yourself and your diabetes?

Problem-Solving Skill

Problem-solving skill is covered in Module 6: Problem Solving. You may consider using the "Behavioral Chain Analysis" activity as described in that module, or you can teach a variation. In the variation, have the patient focus *less* on his or her thoughts and feelings in the context of the problem behavior and focus *more* on identifying the antecedents to the problem behavior and all possible solutions to the problem.

- Guide participants through an example of problem solving using the "Behavioral Chain Analysis" handout before having them commence solving a problem of their own.

258   Diabetes Education Curriculum

Coping with diabetes involves actively dealing with the problems that come up every day. There may be lots of areas in your diabetes care that need attention—physical activity, eating, taking medication, monitoring your blood glucose, etc. If you try to address them all at once, it can be overwhelming.

Start with the one area in your diabetes care that you feel is a *challenge right now*. Think of a challenge that you feel ready and able to take on at this time. Once you have found some success solving problems in a small area, take on a bigger challenge. The old saying "Nothing succeeds like success" is true. Choose something achievable to try first, and then build on that accomplishment. The steps in problem solving can guide you as you take on each challenge. Let's go through an example of problem solving together.

Step 1: Describe the PROBLEM BEHAVIOR

Tell what you did, said, thought, and felt.

Problem:

"I do pretty well remembering the morning meds. It's the medicine before dinner that I keep forgetting. I'm so busy getting dinner ready that it just slips my mind every time."

Step 2: Describe a typical day when you did the problem behavior, and create a detailed CHAIN OF EVENTS that culminates in the problem behavior

Write out all links in the chain of events that occurred. You can work backward from the time of the behavior or forward from the start of your day.

◆ Recall the thoughts or attitudes that you experienced when this problem happened before, and what happened then.

> Example: "I'll realize after dinner that I forgot my diabetes medicine. Now it's too late to take it. I feel so stupid! Why can't I get it right? This diabetes is too hard to deal with! No way am I going to check my blood sugar tonight; I know it'll be high because I forgot the medicine again. So why bother? I get so discouraged, I just want to forget it all."

◆ Practice more positive thoughts. This is a skill that you can learn to do and get better at with practice. Focus on any progress you've made, even if it's a little thing. Focus on something you can feel good about.

> In the following example, the person thinks about what she's doing right with her diabetes: "Well, at least I'm watching my food portions. I do pretty well with that. I haven't gained any weight since I started paying attention to my diet. I guess I'm not a complete failure after all."

> Studies show that actively pursuing more positive thoughts tends to lead to more constructive behaviors. It doesn't come naturally. You have to make yourself think about the positives, and give yourself a pat on the back. It may feel corny and artificial at first, but with practice it'll be a more natural response.

◆ Realize that negative expectations may discourage you from trying to cope with diabetes-related problems in the future.

> Negative thoughts about your ability to manage diabetes can easily lead to negative actions in the future. When you feel discouraged, you might slip into behaviors that will make your blood glucose go even higher. In the first example above, the person stops monitoring in the evening. That could lead to less monitoring the next day, the day after that, and so on. It's a slippery slope.

Our greatest weakness lies in giving up. The most certain way to succeed is always to try just one more time.

—Thomas Edison

American Association of Diabetes Educators©

Step 3: Describe in detail different SOLUTIONS to the problem behavior

Check your chain after you write out each link, and think of what you could have done differently at each link in order to prevent the problem behavior. Consider what someone else might have done. If in a group education setting, ask participants to share their successes: *"Who has an idea of something different to do?"*

Other Possible Solutions

1. The link says: Busy making dinner—consider making components of the meal the day before and reducing the amount to make just before dinner
2. The link says: Leave office and commute home—consider buying some ready-to-eat components of the meal on the way home
3. The link says: Forgot to take meds—consider trying one of the following ideas:
   — Place the bottle of meds where you always eat dinner, next to the salt and pepper shakers
   — Set the alarm on your cell phone for 5 PM
   — Buy a medicine reminder alarm from the pharmacy, and set it for 5 PM
   — Place a note in the kitchen to remind you to take the meds

Step 4: Describe in detail the PREVENTION PLAN you will try

How could you have kept the chain from starting? Choose one idea from among the many on your worksheet and try it.

See how it works out. If your solution doesn't work out, don't give up! Try another option on your list of possible solutions. Remind yourself that trying is worth the effort. Try to view any failures as opportunities to learn what *doesn't* work.

Thomas Edison tried thousands of different metals before he found the one that would make the lightbulb glow. He had a great attitude about failure. He said, "I have not failed. I've just found 10,000 ways that won't work."

Motivation Skill: Costs Versus Benefits Analysis

You often hear people say "I'm just not motivated" when talking about the self-care involved in managing diabetes. Motivation is what drives you, from the inside, to do the things you do. Everyone is motivated, though at times it is in the wrong direction. Feeling ambivalent is a normal part of change. Anytime an important decision must be made about one's health, on some level, the individual usually weighs the pros and cons, or in other words does a costs versus benefits analysis.

Decision-Making Skill: Motivating Yourself to Change

There are *costs* and *benefits* involved in any change a person thinks about making. Another way to think about it is this:

"What are the hassles involved?"
"What do I have to <u>do</u> to make this change?"
"What will happen if I <u>don't</u> make this change?"
"What will I <u>get</u> in exchange for the hassle?"
"What's in it for <u>me</u>?"

 Use learning exercises to teach new coping skills. Provide practice to enhance patient learning and self-efficacy.

American Association of Diabetes Educators©

TABLE 7.1 The Costs and Benefits of Exercise

Costs	Benefits
• Gym membership is expensive	• Fun
• May get injured	• Lose weight
• Takes too much time	• Better blood sugar level

Costs Versus Benefits Learning Activity[35]

- Ask the participant: "What's one thing you find really hard for you to do in taking care of your diabetes?"
- Write the participant's choice on the board for all to see (eg, exercise).
- Make 2 columns underneath. Label one column "Costs" and the other column "Benefits."
- Ask the participant to list as many costs and benefits he or she can think of. See Table 7.1 for an example involving the costs and benefits of exercise.
- The educator should avoid making value judgments about the participant's thoughts about the costs and benefits. Let the participant lead this process.
- Ask the participant to think about the list and say what he or she thinks about it. Allowing the participant to say it out loud helps solidify it in his or her mind. If no responses from the participant, prompt with these questions:
  — *"Are there more costs than benefits, or vice versa?"*
  — *"Are the costs/benefits you listed short-term or long-term?"*
  — *"Is there anything that can be done to reduce costs or increase benefits so that making this change is more doable?"*

The educator can ask the participant to expound on his or her choices of costs and benefits. This can help raise awareness of the participant's deeper values that motivate him or her. For example, the participant lists a benefit of "live longer." The educator can ask the participant, "Why is living longer important to you?" The participant may then respond with his or her reason, for example, "I want to see my kids grow up."

You are the expert on your own life. Only *you* can decide whether the costs are worth the benefits. You have the right to make a decision to change or *not* to change. With either choice, though, you have to live with the consequences of that decision. Educating yourself about the benefits can help you make more informed decisions.

Relapse Prevention[39] Skills

Describe situations that cause you to slip up with your diabetes self-care.

What are your thoughts when you don't follow through with your diabetes plan?

Can you think of things that trigger a lapse in self-care?

How did you deal with the lapse? Were you able to get back on your plan? If yes, how did you do it?

Adults learn best when the content is meaningful to their experience and fills a perceived need. Slipups are universal, so discussions on relapse prevention are valuable.

No one can manage diabetes perfectly 100% of the time. Everyone slips up. It's expected that things will sometimes happen that make it hard to stick with your plan. That's the nature of living with a chronic condition like diabetes. Temporary lapses of a day or two are to be expected from time to time.

Fortunately, there are things you can do to help deal with lapses and prevent them from becoming a full-blown *relapse* when you ignore your self-care for an extended period of time. A relapse in diabetes self-care can lead to serious consequences.

Preventing Lapses Skill

- As the old saying goes, "Forewarned is forearmed." That means it's always best to think ahead about the future, about what might happen. Then you can plan and be more prepared when it happens. Anticipate what might occur that could threaten your diabetes self-care.
  —Example: For someone planning to walk regularly, bad weather can throw off his or her plan.

For an important part of your diabetes self-care (eg, activity, monitoring, meal planning), what kinds of things are likely to happen to sideline your routine or your intentions?

- Avoid known triggers that can lead to a lapse. Triggers are situations that cause you anxiety, stress, loneliness, boredom, anger, or other **uncomfortable emotions**. Certain **positive emotions** can be a trigger, such as pleasurable feelings during a celebration. A trigger can be social pressure, like wanting to fit in with other people and their plans. A relationship conflict, like an argument with someone, can trigger a lapse. Even **people**, **places**, and **things** can be a trigger for you to give up on your plan.
  —Examples of triggers for an ex-smoker: being around smokers (people), locations where you used to go to smoke (places), and the cigarette machine you pass on your way to work (thing).
  —Example of a trigger for someone trying to cut down on junk food: the smell of cinnamon buns (thing).
- Think about a time you recognized a high-risk situation and were able to avoid a lapse. Think about how that made you feel capable and resourceful. Keeping these positive thoughts in mind can help us repeat the same positive actions.
- Develop solutions ahead of time for situations that threaten your plan; have "plan B" ready.

Getting Over a Lapse Skill or Preventing Relapse

Fortunately, a lapse can be an opportunity for you. You can always get back on track and try again. Here are a few ideas of how to do that.

- Practice self-forgiveness. Acknowledge your lapse but try not to dwell on feelings of guilt and worthlessness afterward. These thoughts often lead to even more negative actions. So avoid overly harsh judgment of yourself when you slip up. If you beat yourself up emotionally for every lapse, it's easy to give up altogether. That kind of response could lead to an all-out relapse. Instead, try to figure out what may have triggered the lapse. Try to identify the various "links in the behavior chain" that eventually led to the behavior you wanted to avoid.
- Practice positive "self-talk," concentrating on what you learned from the lapse.
- Focus your energy on getting back on track. Use your support network.

American Association of Diabetes Educators©

Obtaining Support Skill: Getting the Support You Need

Who can you call on to help when you've slipped up?
Who can help you get back in the right frame of mind to keep going?

Be sensitive to the setting in which these questions are posed to participants. If their significant other (SO) is present, they may be reluctant to answer candidly. You may need to rephrase the questions so that the SO does not feel attacked, manipulated, or put on the spot. Or, you may need to wait until you can address this topic with the participant privately.

Support From Family and Friends

Describe the kind of support from others that will help you with your diabetes self-care.

Describe the things other people (family, friends, coworkers) do that hinder your efforts to take care of your diabetes.

In what way does your diabetes affect your relationships with family and friends?

How do the relationships with those close to you affect how you manage your diabetes?

How does your role in the family or relationship affect your ability to care for yourself?

Diabetes affects the whole family. When one person in the family has diabetes, the other members of the family will inevitably have an effect on that person's self-care. Every family is different. Let's broaden the word *family* to include *any person* who has an important impact on your day-to-day living experience. It could refer to your roommate, your coworker, or your boyfriend or girlfriend.

Identify the Feelings of Family

You will experience a wide range of feelings and emotions and responses to your diabetes, and so will your family. Learning what your diabetes means *to them* can deepen your understanding of one another. And if you understand each other better, you and your family can face diabetes in a more united way.

- One obvious way that diabetes affects the family is the hereditary link. It's important for you and your family to realize that no one gene causes diabetes. And no one person is responsible for causing someone else to get diabetes. No one needs to feel **guilty** about passing on the tendency to develop diabetes.

- It's common for families to be **fearful** when a member has diabetes. Fear is often attached to things that are misunderstood. Your family may fear that you'll develop complications later on. They may be afraid that you'll have a hypoglycemic reaction (low blood sugar) and they won't know what to do. To help allay their fear, educate your family about diabetes and your self-care. Let them know what you are doing to prevent problems, and inform them of ways you want them to be involved. If you know you should be doing more, ask for the help you need to improve your self-care.

American Association of Diabetes Educators©

Module 7 *Healthy Coping* 263

◆ Sometimes families **have unrealistic expectations** about a person's ability to control diabetes. They may expect you to perfectly manage diabetes all of the time by "just following your diet, exercising, and taking your medicine." They may equate high blood glucose levels with a lack of willpower or laziness on your part. You can help your family have realistic expectations by explaining your medical and self-care goals. But also be sure to explain that your diabetes cannot be managed perfectly all of the time.

Even when you follow your plan very carefully, blood glucose levels don't always respond as you would expect. When family members understand this, they are less likely to criticize you or place blame whenever your glucose level falls outside your target range. Let them know what they can do to help you stick with your self-care plan.

◆ Adults generally want to make their own decisions. As an adult, you have the right to make informed self-care decisions that may or may not be good for your diabetes. Your family will, naturally, be concerned when they believe your decisions are bad for your health. Their concern may lead them to **become pushy** or **controlling**. They become the "diabetes police."

But what happens when someone else tries to control you? It creates a power struggle. In a power struggle over your diabetes care, the focus quickly becomes "who's in control?" rather than the original issue (food, exercise, monitoring, etc). And when a person wants to prove that they're in control, they often go to the opposite extreme, even if it hurts them.

An example: The concerned wife tells her husband, "You don't need another slice of pizza. It'll raise your blood sugar too high." The husband then proceeds to eat the rest of the pizza, thinking, *I'll show her who's in charge here!*

Why do families become controlling? Sometimes, they **feel they are responsible** for your health. That's a tall order, and one that family members don't need to take on. Reassure your family that your choices are your own and that they are not responsible. At the same time, realize that you will be the one to live with the consequences of your decisions. Also consider that some consequences will no doubt affect them, too (eg, disability).

Your family can't read your mind. They want to help, but sometimes their attempts to help you can feel more like **nagging**. So you need to let them know what you need—and don't need—from them. Let them know what's helpful and what's not. Be clear and up front. Try to communicate in a way that helps others hear what you have to say. The following 3 steps can help when you ask others to treat you differently.

Asking for Support From Family

Everyone is different. The amount of support individuals need varies, and so too does the number of times an individual asks for support. Sometimes, past experience can make a potential support person reluctant to help you. Plus, it may not be as easy as it sounds for the support person to do. You may want the support person to stop bringing certain foods into the house or stop eating certain snacks around you. The best strategy to obtain support is to turn it into a win-win situation by offering to do something for your support person.

Step 1: Use "I" statements

It helps to use "I" statements when your family does something you don't like. This approach will probably be better received than a "you" statement, which just focuses on the negative thing they are doing. "I" statements show that you are taking responsibility for your own feelings. Here's the difference between an "I" statement and a "you" statement:

◆ "I" statement: "I feel annoyed when you say I shouldn't eat this or that."

◆ "You" statement: "You make me annoyed when you tell me I shouldn't eat this or that."

American Association of Diabetes Educators©

Even if you followed the "you" statement with a request that they do things differently, they would probably not even hear it. A "you" statement puts people on the defensive. Defensive people naturally feel the need to deny or refute what you said.

Step 2: Acknowledge family's concern

Most of the time, people close to you have your best interests at heart. If you acknowledge their concern, this helps them feel valued. When you recognize this concern *before* you make an "I" statement, it helps to soften any hint of criticism. When people feel valued, they more easily accept your request to treat you differently.

An example of acknowledging concern might sound something like this: "I know you care about me when you say I shouldn't eat this or that, but I feel annoyed when you do that."

Step 3: Say what you need, offer to do something in return, and set a time limit

Follow up with a request for what you need. Be specific in what you want people to do differently. If you don't say what would be helpful, they may simply replace their old behavior with something just as unhelpful. Here's an example of a request, along with the acknowledgment of concern and the "I" statement:

> "I know you care about me when you say I shouldn't eat this or that, but I feel annoyed when you do that. It would help me a lot more if you'd just comment when you think I'm doing something good for myself."

> "I know you care about me when you say I shouldn't eat this or that, but I feel annoyed when you do that. It would help me if you just don't comment at all about what I am eating.

> I know you care about me when you say I shouldn't eat this or that, but I feel annoyed when you do that. It would help me if you said 'Are you sure?'"

> "If you would agree to do what I ask, then I will try to do something you want. For instance, you can choose all the TV shows and movies we see for the next week. Are you willing to try this for a week?"

Step 4: Thank your support person for listening (if they don't agree) or for being willing to do what is hard for them (if they do agree)

Step 5: Review the plan at the end of the time limit and renegotiate for more time if you have found the support to be helpful

Getting Support: Participant Activity

For this activity, make sure participants have paper to write on.

Sharing of personal experiences has more relevance for patients than passively listening to educational content. Hearing others' suggestions to problems can encourage the development of improved problem-solving skills.

Let's practice obtaining support by using the 5 steps just discussed. In this activity, you will *rewrite a scene* you've already experienced. This exercise will help you when you enter new scenes in the future.

- Think of a situation where others' attempts to help were not helpful, and how you felt in that situation.
- Create an "I" statement about how you felt.
- Add on an acknowledgment of the support person's concern.
- Ask for a specific action from the person.
- Offer to do something for your support person.
- Set a time limit.
- Reach an agreement.

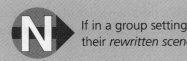

If in a group setting, invite one or more volunteers to share their *rewritten scene* with the group.

Support From Healthcare Providers[40(pp108-9)]

Going to the provider's office can sometimes be intimidating. A lot of people say that their mind goes blank, and they end up leaving the office without discussing their concerns with the provider. Perhaps you feel like a child going to the principal's office, afraid of what's going to happen. There are several things you can do to get what you need from healthcare providers.

- Before your appointment, decide what *you* want to accomplish during the visit. Write down questions you want answered. Make sure to take this list with you to the visit.
- When the provider comes in, speak up. Let him or her know that you have some questions and want to discuss them. Don't wait until the end of the appointment.
- Bring information to the visit that you think will help the provider make decisions about your care. This could include your blood glucose record or your list of current medications.
- Ask for an explanation if you don't understand what the provider is saying. Medical terms are confusing. Providers often need to be reminded to explain things in a way that's clear to someone not in the medical profession.
- When the provider prescribes tests or treatments, be sure to ask why they were ordered. Ask for the results and find out what they mean.
- If you're having difficulty sticking with your diabetes self-care plan, let your doctor know. Work with your provider to find solutions. Pretending that everything is OK (when it's not) not only wastes your time but can complicate your health later on.
- If you've set some goals for your health, let your provider know. Ask if those goals are reasonable and if your current treatment plan will help you reach them. If your treatment is at odds with your goals, ask about options and alternatives.
- If you intend to discuss a current medical topic you read about online or in the newspaper, bring in the clipping.

My doctor doesn't listen to me. I want to change doctors, but I don't want to hurt his feelings. I've been going to him for years. What should I do?

Changing providers can be an uncomfortable task, especially if you've had a long-standing relationship with him or her. Naturally, you don't want to offend or insult.

- **It may help if you think of the doctor/patient relationship as a business contract, which it really is.** In a business relationship, one party can terminate the contract if the requirements haven't been met. The bottom line is this: Your well-being should be the first concern, not the feelings of the provider. Providers are your consultants. You can hire them and you can fire them.

- **Health care, and especially diabetes care, is best approached as a team effort.** You are the captain of the team, so to speak. You bring your lifetime of experience; the professionals—doctors, nurses, dietitians, pharmacists, etc—bring their various medical skills to the team. The professional owns the knowledge of diabetes and the different ways it can be managed; *you* own the knowledge of your situation. *You* know best whether certain approaches to your diabetes care are realistic, based on the details of your life (your culture, your values, your beliefs).

- **Every patient has the right to question what his or her provider recommends.** You have the right to offer your own ideas for alternative treatment. It's true that some providers may become defensive if their patients challenge their advice. They may have the attitude that they know best (eg, "After all, who went to medical school—you or I?"). One key aspect of an effective doctor/patient partnership is that you are listened to and your concerns are addressed.

    If your expertise on the team is not being respected, then the partnership is lopsided. If you feel that the other members of your team don't listen to your concerns, then your needs are not being met.

- **Sometimes, it's just a matter of better communication on your part.** Maybe you need to try a different approach. Perhaps being more assertive would help you be better understood by your provider. Sometimes, though, finding another provider is ultimately the answer. Only *you* can make this decision.

Support From Community Resources

There may be resources within your community that can offer some of the support you need. Examples are support groups (in person or online), diabetes publications (magazines, blogs, and informational Web sites), and patient assistance programs.

Joining a Support Group

Support group formats can vary greatly from group to group. Many support groups begin with a short educational presentation, followed by a question-and-answer session. It may be run by a health professional or even a volunteer who has diabetes. In some support groups, the discussion is focused on coping with the emotional side of diabetes. Participants can share their personal experiences with the group—what worked for them, and how they solved problems related to their diabetes self-care. Other support groups are a combination of these 2 formats.

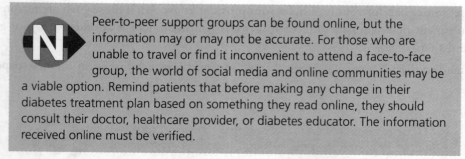

N ▶ Peer-to-peer support groups can be found online, but the information may or may not be accurate. For those who are unable to travel or find it inconvenient to attend a face-to-face group, the world of social media and online communities may be a viable option. Remind patients that before making any change in their diabetes treatment plan based on something they read online, they should consult their doctor, healthcare provider, or diabetes educator. The information received online must be verified.

The best way to find out about groups in your community is to call the support group contact person or try out a session. Support groups can be a big help if you feel isolated by your diabetes. Finding other people who understand what you're going through can be a great relief. If speaking in front of other people intimidates you, online support groups may be more your style. Just be aware that support groups can *add* to your knowledge of diabetes self-care, but they don't take the place of diabetes education with your healthcare team.

Talking Circle Activity

In some American Indian populations, talking circles are traditionally used to facilitate sharing and communication. In the Robert Wood Johnson Diabetes Initiative, talking circles were incorporated into diabetes self-management education programs in some sites with large American Indian populations. Talking circles helped reduce feelings of isolation and promoted healthy coping in these groups.[15(p49)]

The Indian Health Service advocates the use of talking circles as *best practice* when providing diabetes care to American Indians.[41]

Talking circles provide an opportunity for people to talk freely about their diabetes and to find support to manage their condition. They have proven to be a useful format for teaching health education and promotion.[42-44]

Table 7.2 describes the experience of using a talking circle in a class on type 2 diabetes.

Read Diabetes Publications

See the Diabetes Resources Appendix for a list of diabetes publications. Use for a patient handout.

There are a number of reputable magazines that cater to the needs of people living with diabetes. Some are available by subscription only, while others can be purchased in grocery stores and pharmacies. Reading a diabetes magazine can give you a boost every month as you learn new information and skills.

Online "chat rooms" or "blogs" can be found on the Internet. It's important to keep in mind that the information found there may or may not be factual. You will read about other people's experiences, which may or may not

TABLE 7.2 Excerpt From a 2003 *Qualitative Health Research* Article
During a diabetes wellness Talking Circle, the Talking Circle participants, who numbered between 5 and 20, sat in chairs placed in a circle. The Talking Circle facilitator led, guided, and maintained the group process by first creating a comfortable environment that emphasized safety and confidentiality. Next, the Talking Circle facilitator welcomed everyone and asked someone in the group to offer a prayer to the Creator (higher being). The facilitator then delivered information on a specific type 2 diabetes topic from the curriculum.
The Talking Circle was opened to all; each participant was given the opportunity to speak, and many told traditional stories and/or a story about their experiences. A Talking Circle participant, when speaking, may hold a feather, rock, or other symbolic item. During this time, the speaker takes the lead in sharing experiences, stories, and information with the group.
While one person speaks, the facilitator and the other Talking Circle members respect and support the speaker by honoring them, being present, and attending to their words. After each person has had a chance to contribute, the facilitator summarizes the events, and the Talking Circle is closed.

Source: R Struthers, FS Hodge, B Geishirt-Cantrell, L De Cora, "Participant experiences of talking circles on type 2 diabetes in two Northern Plains American Indian tribes," *Qual Health Res* 13, no. 8 (2003): 1094-115.

work for you. Always turn to your healthcare team for specific guidance pertaining to managing your diabetes. For many people, the online experience is a good outlet for coping with the daily frustrations of diabetes.

Visit Reputable Diabetes Web Sites

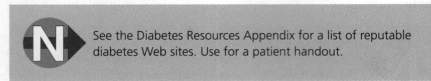

There are many diabetes Web sites, but it's not always easy to know which ones you can trust. You can have some assurance that the information found on government, university, and drug company Web sites is factual. Government Web site addresses end in *.gov*; university Web site addresses end in *.edu*. Any drug company whose product is approved by the US Food and Drug Administration (FDA) must have all its claims approved by the FDA before posting online.

Nonprofit healthcare associations also generally have accurate information. Four well-known reputable associations are:

- American Association of Diabetes Educators: http://www.diabeteseducator.org
- American Diabetes Association: http://www.diabetes.org
- American College of Obstetricians and Gynecologists: http://www.acog.org
- JDRF: http://www.jdrf.org

Consult Patient Assistance Programs

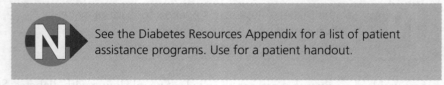

- **Medication Assistance**—RxAssist (http://www.RxAssist.org) offers an updated directory of all patient assistance programs in the United States. You can search for a medication by name or by drug company. Call 401-729-3284.
- **Community Health Centers**—Community health centers that are regulated by the federal government exist in many communities. They are required by law to provide care to those without health insurance. These centers have sliding fee scales based on a person's income. Many of these clinics have a pharmacy or contract with local pharmacies. To get medication from these clinics, you must be enrolled as a patient. For the nearest community health center, call 1-888-ASK-HRSA (275-4772) or visit http://findahealthcenter.hrsa.gov.
- **Free Clinics**—http://www.rxassist.org/patients/res-free-clinics offers a listing of free clinics, listed by state.
- **Social Service Agencies**—http://www.uw.org/211/ is the United Way referral service; http://www.safetynetcenter.org is a directory of public and private community resources and services.

Connect With Your Insurance Companies

There are some insurance companies that have telehealth services. If your insurance offers diabetes management, you may find the counselors supportive and informative and only a phone call away. Some insurance companies have reputable information on their Web sites.

Stress Management Skill

 What situations in your life currently cause you a lot of stress? In what way does your diabetes self-care change when you feel stressed, depressed, or upset?

Stress is a fact of life. The word *stress* has become common in our everyday vocabulary. People often say things like "I'm stressed out" or "There's a lot of stress at work." For this discussion, let's define stress, the effects it can have, and, most importantly, how you can manage it.

Situations or events that cause you to have an emotional and physical response are called *stressors*. Stressors can be either positive or negative events. For example, conflict with another person, money troubles, or a death in the family can be a negative stressor. Welcoming a new baby or planning a wedding can be a positive stressor. With either of these stressors, there is an emotional response and a physical response. This response is called *stress*.

The stress response is your body's way of helping you survive in situations that call for immediate action. Can you think of a time when your "survival instinct" kicked in? Have you ever just barely escaped a car accident? Have you ever been chased by a mean dog? Have you ever had to quickly move a heavy object to save someone from being trapped underneath?

In extreme cases like these, your body automatically reacts to the life-threatening situation. Hormones and brain chemicals are released that prepare you for action. Your mind becomes very alert so you can react immediately. Your heart beats faster and your blood pressure rises to pump blood to your arms and legs so you can use your muscles to fight or to escape. The glucose level in your blood instantly rises so there is fuel available to your muscles.

The everyday situations you face at home or work with family or coworkers can also cause the stress response to occur. If you experience stress but don't take some kind of action to deal with it, physical problems can result. If it's prolonged, it can be very harmful to your health.

The physical symptoms of unrelieved stress can include:

- Headache, caused by unconsciously tensing the muscles in the neck, forehead, or shoulders
- Trouble sleeping
- Fatigue
- High blood pressure
- Nervousness
- Excessive sweating
- Hair loss
- Ulcers

The emotional and mental symptoms of unrelieved stress can include:

- Anxiety
- Anger
- Depression
- Irritability
- Frustration
- Overreaction to everyday problems
- Memory problems
- Trouble concentrating

270   Diabetes Education Curriculum

Managing Stress

Managing stress basically involves either reducing the stressors in your life or reducing your stress response. Some stressors cannot be eliminated altogether; they're out of your control to change. But your response to stress is something you *can* change if you learn certain skills and get the support you need. This brings to mind the serenity prayer that many people rely on when facing difficult events[45]:

> *Grant me the serenity to accept the things I cannot change,*
>
> *the courage to change the things I can,*
>
> *and the wisdom to know the difference.*

Read through the following suggestions to find a tactic you can use to manage your stress. It pays to have a plan on hand and even a backup plan or two when things are really tough for you.

- **Take inventory** of the stressors in your life, especially those in the past year.[46]
  - —*Major life events*—retirement, job change or job loss, death, marriage, birth, change of school
  - —*Chronic stressors*—everyday demands of jobs, family, and finances
  - —*Diabetes-related stressors*—keeping up with the recommended self-care, feeling deprived of food, not meeting treatment goals

- **Be aware** of any counterproductive ways you currently use to manage stress: smoking, drugs, alcohol, over-eating, or engaging in high-risk "thrill" activities. These things may help you feel better in the short term. But long-term they can be harmful to your health and actually worsen your stress.

- **Engage in regular physical activity**—Regular activity helps lower the production of stress hormones. It may also help you sleep better.

- **Eat healthfully**—Good nutrition can help equip your body to ward off the negative physical effects of stress.

- **Get enough sleep**—When you are chronically sleep-deprived, the stress response can be even worse. Turning off the TV, creating a quiet atmosphere in the bedroom, avoiding alcohol or caffeine late in the evening, and taking a bath before bed may help you relax and fall asleep.

- **Reach out** to your support system—Talking to people about your stress and asking for help is one way to de-stress.

- **Take a break**—Even short breaks away from your stressors can help, such as taking a walk during your lunch break—but don't talk about work! Schedule some time during the week to just "do nothing."

- **Create predictability**—One of the most upsetting forms of stress is the kind that is unexpected. No one can completely prevent the unexpected from happening. But when day-to-day life is structured as much as possible, it helps you feel more solid when the unexpected occurs.

- **Use positive affirmations**—Developing a more positive mind-set is one strategy for dealing with stress. Affirmations are positive statements that are repeated over and over. Affirmations can help reprogram the way we normally think. They may feel, at first, like a "great big lie." You may even feel silly saying affirmations at first. The human mind, though, tends to eventually believe repeated thoughts as *truth*.

  Thoughts that affirm how we want to see ourselves (eg, "I am capable of change," "I handle stress well") can help us change our actions over time. Research shows that repeated affirmations help people cope with daily stressors and can actually lower the release of stress hormones.[46]

  Saying affirmations aloud (with feeling!) while looking at yourself in the mirror helps the new thoughts take root even more firmly in your mind. Writing your affirmations on paper and posting them in places where you will see them throughout the day increases the chances of success with this technique.

American Association of Diabetes Educators©

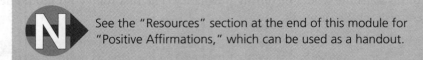

See the "Resources" section at the end of this module for "Positive Affirmations," which can be used as a handout.

- **Practice mind-body techniques**—There is a definite link between the mind and the body. For thousands of years, people in the Far East have practiced mind-body techniques as part of their spirituality. In Western culture, mind-body techniques are typically used to address physical problems or to support relaxation. Numerous studies show that by doing certain physical actions, one's mental state can be altered. The opposite is also true. When the mental state changes, it can bring about changes in one's physical state. To combat stress, consider trying these mind-body techniques. With repetition, they become easier and feel more natural.
  - **Progressive muscle relaxation** is a technique that involves tightening and then relaxing different muscle groups. It helps you be aware of the difference between relaxed and tensed muscles. This is an important distinction to make because people are often unaware that their neck or shoulders are tensed. During times of stress, try to consciously relax your muscles. This will reduce muscle tension and lower your physical stress response.[21]
  - **Deep breathing** can lower the stress response. Take several slow, deep breaths. Inhale slowly and exhale slowly.[47]
  - **Imagery** is a mental technique that uses the power of your imagination. Close your eyes and imagine a peaceful nature scene until you feel less stressed. Or picture yourself as you *want* to be—strong, in control, peaceful, calm, etc. Imagery is a popular technique among athletes who want to improve their performance. They imagine, in great detail, every movement they will make in their next game. Imagery can be a powerful tool to help you manage stress. You can do it at the time you are feeling stressed or anxious. You can also practice imagery at any time to reinforce your desired image of yourself.[47]
  - **Meditation** includes a variety of practices that are intended to quiet the mind. When meditating, your attention is focused on a single thing, such as the rhythm of your breathing, an image you are looking at or thinking of, or a sound. This intense concentration on one thing, while tuning out everything else, can bring about physical and mental calmness. Find a quiet place, away from distractions. Get in a comfortable position, preferably sitting down. Give yourself 20 to 30 minutes to meditate.[21,48]
  - **Yoga** is a series of physical postures that are practiced along with breathing techniques. As muscles are slowly stretched and breathing is controlled, a sense of physical and mental calm can result.[16]
  - **Tai Chi** (*tai chi chuan*) is a traditional Chinese practice. It combines deep breathing and relaxation with gentle movements. The movements of Tai Chi are deliberately slow and resemble a dance. The body is in constant slow motion. Like yoga, Tai Chi can induce a state of relaxation as the mind is concentrated on the body motion and breathing.[19]

    If you decide to try yoga or Tai Chi, be sure to find a trained instructor. Also, consult your provider before starting these or any other physical activity programs.
  - **Spirituality** is the search for meaning and appreciation of life.[49] This quest for meaning may involve organized religion, faith, and belief in a higher power. Belonging to a group that shares your core beliefs can be a powerful source of spiritual support. For many, prayer is a powerful tool in managing stress and coping with life's problems, including diabetes.

Follow-up/Outcomes Measurement

Per the Standards for Outcomes Measurement of Diabetes Self-Management Education, the **first follow-up should be conducted within 2 to 4 weeks** after the initial teaching session on healthy coping. **Subsequent follow-up is recommended at 3- to 6-month intervals thereafter.** Use the following table as a guide for identifying outcomes measures and how to measure them. Measurement of these outcomes may be objective or subjective.[50]

272 Diabetes Education Curriculum

The exception to this schedule would be during pregnancy. The first follow-up should be conducted within 1 week and subsequent visits at 2 to 4 weeks.

> **N** ▶ In a randomized study that tracked 164 participants' outcomes for 24 months, relapses in diabetes self-care and resultant elevation in A1C were less likely to occur in patients with *quarterly telephone follow-up* (21% relapse rate) as compared with those with routine follow-up (27% relapse rate) and those with monthly follow-up (31% relapse rate). It was postulated that the frequency of monthly follow-up may have actually *fatigued* participants.[51]

Self-Care Behavior: Healthy Coping Outcomes Measures	Self-Care Behavior: Healthy Coping Methods of Measurement
Psychosocial factors are outcomes and should be measured. Psychosocial factors include depression, stress, quality of life, and self-efficacy. Psychosocial factors affect motivation, confidence, and the ability to resolve barriers to self-care.*	Immediate outcomes of learning can be measured by patient knowledge testing (paper-and-pen testing, or questioning to determine that the patient understands the information taught, or a questionnaire online). Immediate outcomes for acquiring a skill can be measured by the patient's demonstration of that skill. Following are various methods of measuring immediate outcomes for the self-care behavior of *healthy coping*.
Immediate outcome: Learning Immediate outcomes of learning can be assessed right away after the educational encounter. Immediate outcomes include: K: Acquiring *knowledge* (*what to do*) S: Acquiring *skills* (*how to do it*) CM: Developing *confidence and motivation* (*want to do it*) PS: Developing *problem-solving/coping skills* to overcome barrier (*can do it*)	
Problem solving (K,S,PS)	<u>Subjective:</u> Patient lists the 4 steps in solving problems, or the patient explains how to do a behavior chain analysis for problem solving. <u>Objective:</u> Patient describes a behavior chain for a personal problem behavior in diabetes self-care and possible solutions to solve the problem.
Goal setting for healthy coping (S)	<u>Subjective:</u> Patient defines a SMART goal. <u>Objective:</u> Patient describes a SMART goal for implementing a healthy coping skill for behavior change.
Potential barriers (lack of support, emotional) and facilitators to healthy coping (PS)	<u>Subjective:</u> Considering his/her individual situation, patient identifies anticipated obstacle(s) that may limit the ability to adequately cope with the demands of diabetes self-care. Patient describes facilitators which may help him or her cope in a healthy manner. <u>Objective:</u> Patient demonstrates healthy coping by developing a plan to overcome a barrier or enlist a facilitator in order to change behavior.
Intermediate outcome: Behavior change	Intermediate outcomes measures can be assessed over time: after the educational encounter and once the patient has had adequate time to implement new behavior(s) in a real-life setting. *Behavior change* is an intermediate outcomes measure. It is the ultimate outcome of DSME/T. At follow-up intervals, knowledge and skills (discussed above) should be reassessed, as well as behavior change.

American Association of Diabetes Educators©

Self-Care Behavior: Healthy Coping Outcomes Measures	Self-Care Behavior: Healthy Coping Methods of Measurement
Coping behavior	<u>Subjective:</u> Patient self-report of how he or she is coping with the demands of diabetes self-care and solving problems.
	<u>Objective:</u> Patient demonstrates use of the steps in problem solving in real-life situations involving his or her diabetes self-care or describes the behavior chain for a problem behavior. Patient's responses on diabetes-specific problem-solving measurement tool (eg, Test of Diabetes Knowledge: Problem Solving, Social Problem Solving for Diabetic Youth Interview [SPSDY], Diabetes Problem-Solving Measure for Adolescents [DPSMA], Diabetes Problem-Solving Inventory [DPSI], and Diabetes Problem-Solving Scale, Self-Report [DPSS-SR]).
	N See the "Resources" section at end of this chapter for "Psychological Assessment and Screening Tools."
Stress management	<u>Subjective:</u> Patient self-report of how he or she is managing perceived stress.
	<u>Objective:</u> Patient's responses on stress/distress measurement tool (eg, Problem Areas in Diabetes Scale [PAID], Diabetes Distress Scale [DDS], Questionnaire on Stress in Patients with Diabetes [QSD-R], Appraisal of Diabetes [ADS], and Perceived Stress Scale [PSS-10]. Patient explains a plan for reducing stress (eg, physical activity, obtaining support, mind-body techniques, spirituality).
	N See the "Resources" section at end of this chapter for "Psychological Assessment and Screening Tools."
Depression	<u>Subjective:</u> Patient self-report on perceived feelings of depression.
	<u>Objective:</u> Patient's responses on depression screening tool (eg, Patient Health Questionnaire [PHQ], Patient Health Questionnaire-9 [PHQ-9], Beck Depression Inventory [BDI], Center for Epidemiological Studies Depression [CES-D], Zung Self-Assessment Depression Scale, Geriatric Depression Scale [GDS]). Patient states plan to seek help from a mental health professional.
	N See the "Resources" section at end of this chapter for "Psychological Assessment and Screening Tools."
Quality of life	<u>Subjective:</u> Patient self-report on perceived quality of life.
	<u>Objective:</u> Patient's responses on quality of life measurement tool (eg, SF-36, SF-12, and Diabetes 39).
	N See the "Resources" section at end of this chapter for "Psychological Assessment and Screening Tools."
Barrier identification and resolution (PS)	<u>Subjective:</u> Patient self-report of barriers faced, facilitators and strategies used, as patient made efforts to implement healthy coping behaviors.
	<u>Objective:</u> Patient set a SMART goal for implementing a healthy coping skill for behavior change.
Plan for future behavior change (PS)	<u>Subjective:</u> Patient self-report of healthy coping goals and behavior change strategies going forward.
	<u>Objective:</u> Patient describes a plan for coping with a lapse and preventing a relapse.

*K Mulcahy, M Maryniuk, M Peeples, et al, "Diabetes self-management education core outcomes measures: technical review," *Diabetes Educ* 29, no. 5 (2003): 768-803.

American Association of Diabetes Educators©

REFERENCES

1. Fisher EB, Thorpe CT, DeVellis BM, DeVellis RF. Healthy coping, negative emotions, and diabetes management: a systematic review and appraisal. Diabetes Educ. 2007;33(6):1080-103.

2. Funnell MM. Beyond the data: moving towards a new DAWN in diabetes. Diabet Med. 2013;30:765-6.

3. Nelson JB, Nelson Ward KI. Healthy coping. In: Mensing C, ed. The Art and Science of Diabetes Self-Management Education Desk Reference. 3rd ed. Chicago: AADE; 2014:265-85.

4. Maslow AH. A theory of human motivation. Psychological Review. 1943;50:370-96.

5. Leininger M. What is transcultural nursing and culturally competent care? J Transcult Nurs.1999;10(1):9.

6. American Association of Diabetes Educators. AADE position statement: individualization of diabetes self-management education. Diabetes Educ. 2007;33(1):45-9.

7. Anderson RM, Fitzgerald JT, Funnell MM, Gruppen LD. The third version of the Diabetes Attitude Scale. Diabetes Care. 1998;21(9):1403-7.

8. Rowe M, Allen RG. Spirituality as a means of coping. Am J Health Studies. 2004;19(1):62-7.

9. Penckofer S, Estwing Ferrans C, Velsor-Friedrich B, Savoy S. The psychological impact of living with diabetes: women's day-to-day experience. Diabetes Educ. 2007;33(4):680-90.

10. Rubin RR, Peyrot M. Psychological adjustment to diabetes and critical periods of psychological risk. In: Young-Hyman D, Peytor M, eds. Psychological Care for People With Diabetes. Alexandria, Va: American Diabetes Association; 2012:219-28.

11. Monti PM, Kadden RM, Rohsenow DJ, Cooney NL, Abrams DB. Alcohol Dependence: A Coping Skills Training Guide. 2nd ed. New York: Guilford Press; 2002.

12. Peyrot M, McMurry JF. Psychosocial factors in diabetes control: adjustment of insulin-treated adults. Psychosom Med. 1985;47:542-7.

13. Rimer BK, Glanz K. Theory at a Glance: A Guide for Health Promotion Practice. 2nd ed. Bethesda, Md: National Institutes of Health; 2005. NIH publication no. 05-3896.

14. Rubin RR, Peyrot M, Saudek CD. The effect of a diabetes education program incorporating coping skills training on emotional well-being and diabetes self-efficacy. Diabetes Educ. 1993;19(3):210-4.

15. Fisher EB, Thorpe C, Brownson CA, et al. Healthy Coping Guide in Diabetes: A Guide for Program Development and Implementation. St Louis, Mo: Diabetes Initiative National Program Office; 2008.

16. Attari A, Sartippour M, Amini M, Haghighi S. Effect of stress management training on glycemic control in patients with type 1 diabetes. Diabetes Res Clin Prac. 2006;73(1):23-8.

17. Surwit RS, van Tilburg MA, Zucker N, et al. Stress management improves long-term glycemic control in type 2 diabetes. Diabetes Care. 2002;25(1):30-4.

18. Barrows KA, Jacobs BP. Mind-body medicine: an introduction and review of the literature. Med Clin North Am. 2002;86(1):11-31.

19. National Center for Complementary and Alternative Medicine. Tai Chi and Qi Gong (cited 2008 Nov 30). On the Internet at: http://nccam.nih.gov/health/taichi/#3.

20. National Center for Complementary and Alternative Medicine. Complementary, alternative, or integrative health: what's in a name? (cited 2008 Nov 30). On the Internet at: http://nccam.nih.gov/health/backgrounds/mindbody.htm.

21. Astin JA, Shapiro SL, Eisenberg DM, Forys KL. Mind-body medicine: state of the science, implications for practice. J Am Board Fam Pract. 2003;16(2):131-47.

22. Whitebird R, Kreitzer M, Vazquez-Benitez G, et al. A2-2: Improving diabetes management with mindfulness-based stress reduction. Clin Med Res. 2014 Sept;12(1-2):84.

23. Lloyd CE, Roy T, Nouwen A, et al. Epidemiology of depression in diabetes: international and cross-cultural issues. J Affect Disord. 2012 Oct;142 Suppl:S22-9.

24. Nash J. Diabetes and Wellbeing: Managing the Psychological and Emotional Challenges of Diabetes Types 1 and 2. 2nd ed. West Sussex, UK: John Wiley & Sons; 2013.

25. US Preventive Services Task Force. Screening for depression: recommendations and rationale. Ann Intern Med. 2002;136(10):760-4.

26. Kroenke K, Spitzer R, Williams J. The PHQ-9: validity of a brief depression severity measure. J Gen Intern Med. 2001;16(9):606-13.

27. Ruggerio L, Wagner J, de Groot M. Understanding the individual: emotional and psychological challenges. In: Mensing C, ed. The Art and Science of Diabetes Self-Management Education: A Desk Reference for Healthcare Professionals. Chicago: American Association of Diabetes Educators; 2006: 59-89.

28. Wilson W, Ary DV, Bigland A, et al. Psychosocial predictors of self-care behaviors and glycemic control in NIDDM. Diabetes Care. 1986;9:614-22.

29. Sherbourne CD, Hays RD, Ordway L, et al. Antecedents of adherence to medical recommendations: results from the Medical Outcomes Study. J Behav Med. 1992;32 Suppl:S5-20.

30. Lloyd CE, Wing RR, Orchard TJ, Becker DJ. Psychosocial correlates of glycemic control: the Pittsburgh Epidemiology of Diabetes Complications (EDC) Study. Diabetes Res Clin Pract. 1993;21:187-95.

31. Tillotson LM, Smith MS. Locus of control, social support, and adherence to the diabetes regimen. Diabetes Educ. 1996;22:133-9.

32. Ruggerio L, Spirito A, Coustan D, et al. Self-reported compliance with diabetes self-management during pregnancy. Int J Psychiatry Med. 1993;23:195-207.

33. Skelly AH, Burns D. Social support: conceptualization, issues, and complexities. In: Mensing C, ed. The Art and Science of Diabetes Self-Management Education: A Desk Reference for Healthcare Professionals. Chicago: American Association of Diabetes Educators; 2006.

34. Anderson B. Involving family members in diabetes treatment. In: Anderson BJ, Rubin RR, eds. Practical Psychology for Diabetes Clinicians. 2nd ed. Alexandria, Va: American Diabetes Association; 2002:199-207.

35. Grey M. Coping skills training for youth with diabetes. Diabetes Spectr. 2011 spring;24(2):70.

36. Blumenthal JA, Babyak MA, Moore KA, et al. Effects of exercise training on older patients with major depression. Arch Intern Med. 1999;159:2349-56.

37. Ciechanowski P. Diapression: an integrated model for understanding the experience of individuals with co-occurring diabetes and depression. Clin Diabetes. 2011 Apr;29(2):43-9.

38. Anderson RM, Funnell MM, Burkhart N, Gillard ML, Nwankwo R. Attitudes, beliefs, and values. In: Raynor J, ed. 101 Tips for Behavior Change in Diabetes Education. Alexandria, Va: American Diabetes Association; 2002.

39. Larimer ME, Palmer RS, Marlatt GA. Relapse prevention: an overview of Marlatt's cognitive-behavioral model. Alcohol Res Health. 1999;23(2):151-60.

40. Anderson RM, Funnell MM, Burkhart N, Gillard ML, Nwankwo R. Help from other professionals. In: Raynor J, ed. 101 Tips for Behavior Change in Diabetes Education. Alexandria, Va: American Diabetes Association; 2002: 108-12.

41. Indian Health Service. Indian Health Diabetes Best Practices: community advocacy and diabetes. 2006 Jun (cited 2009 Feb 18). On the Internet at: http://www.ihs.gov/medicalprograms/diabetes.

42. Hodge FS, Pasqua A, Marquez CA, et al. Utilizing traditional storytelling to promote wellness in American Indian communities. J Transcult Nurs. 2002;13(1):6-11.

43. Struthers R. Storytelling as a healing tool. In: Snyder M, Lindquist R, eds. Complementary/Alternative Therapies in Nursing. 4th ed. New York: Springer; 2006:124-34.

44. Struthers R, Hodge FS, Geishirt-Cantrell B, De Cora L. Participant experiences of talking circles on type 2 diabetes in two Northern Plains American Indian tribes. Qual Health Res. 2003;13(8):1094-115.

45. Shapiro FR. Who wrote the Serenity Prayer? The Chronicle Review. 2014 Apr 28.

46. Creswell JD, Welch WT, Taylor SE, et al. Affirmation of personal values buffers neuroendocrine and psychological stress responses. Psychol Sci. 2005;16(11):846-51.

American Association of Diabetes Educators©

276   Diabetes Education Curriculum

47. Seaward B. Managing Stress: Principles and Strategies for Health and Well-being. 5th ed. Sudbury, Mass: Jones and Bartlett; 2006.

48. National Center for Complementary and Alternative Medicine. Meditation: what you need to know. On the Internet at: https://nccih.nih.gov/health/meditation/overview.htm.

49. Shreve-Neiger A, Edelstein B. Religion and anxiety: a critical review of the literature. Clin Psychol Rev. 2004; 24(4):379-97.

50. Mulcahy K, Maryniuk M, Peeples M, et al. Diabetes self-management education core outcomes measures: technical review. Diabetes Educ. 2003;29(5):768-803.

51. Huizinga MM, Ulen CG, Gebrestadik T, et al. Glycemic Relapse Prevention Study: a randomized controlled trial. Abstract no. 119-OR. Alexandria, Va: American Diabetes Association; 2008.

HEALTHY COPING: RESOURCES

Behavior Chain Templates. 276

Healthy Coping Activity (English) 277

Healthy Coping Activity (Spanish) 279

Diabetes Online Community 281

Problem-Solving Activity Script 283

Motivation Cost Versus Benefit Worksheet 284

Positive Affirmations 285

Psychological Assessment and Screening Tools. 286

Behavior Chain Templates

For an example of using the behavior chain tool, see Julie Corliss, Executive Editor, *Harvard Heart Letter*, Harvard Medical School, Harvard Health Publication: http://www.health.harvard.edu/blog/bridge-the-intention-behavior-gap-to-lose-weight-and-keep-it-off-201103101729

For another example of a behavior chain template, see the following link from Brigham and Women's Hospital: http://www.brighamandwomens.org/Patients_Visitors/pcs/nutrition/services/healtheweightforwomen/success/behavior_chain.aspx

American Association of Diabetes Educators©

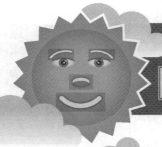

AADE7™ SELF-CARE BEHAVIORS
HEALTHY COPING

Did You Know?

Diabetes can affect you physically and emotionally. Living with it every day can make you feel discouraged, stressed or even depressed. It is natural to have mixed feelings about your diabetes management and experience highs and lows. The important thing is to recognize these emotions as normal. Take steps to reduce the negative impact they could have on your self-care.

The way you deal with your emotional lows is called "coping." There are lots of ways to cope with the upsets in your life—and not all of them are good for your health (smoking, overeating, not finding time for activity, or avoiding people and social situations).

However, there are healthy coping methods that you can use to get you through tough times (faith-based activities, exercise, meditation, enjoyable hobbies, joining a support group).

Having a support network is key to healthy coping. Be sure to develop and nurture partnerships in your personal life with your spouse, loved ones and friends. Go to group educational sessions where you can meet and relate to other people going through the same experiences. Build healthy relationships—and remember that you're not alone.

Sometimes, emotional lows can be lengthy and have a more serious impact on your life, health, and relationships. This can be a sign of depression. Tell your diabetes educator if you:

» Don't have interest or find pleasure in your activities.
» Avoid discussing your diabetes with family and friends.
» Sleep most of the day.
» Don't see the benefit in taking care of yourself.
» Feel like diabetes is conquering you.
» Feel like you can't take care of yourself.

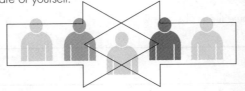

Physical activity can influence your mood. If you are sad, anxious, stressed or upset, go for a walk, stand up and stretch, or take a bicycle ride. Exercise actually increases the chemicals in your brain that help make you feel good!

TRUE OR FALSE?

Nobody wants to hear about your problems. When you are feeling down, you should keep it to yourself.

FALSE. You need to talk about your emotions with friends, family, or your healthcare provider. Sometimes just talking about a problem will help you solve it...and loved ones can help you gain perspective.

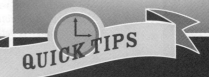

QUICK TIPS

Recognize the power of positive thinking. When you are feeling down, think about your successes and feel good about the progress you've made toward a goal—even if it's just a little bit.

Find time to do something pleasurable every day.

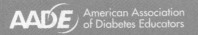
American Association of Diabetes Educators

Supported by an educational grant from Eli Lilly and Company.

ACTIVITIES

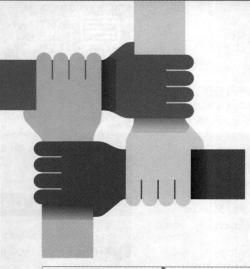

HEALTHY COPING

Name 3 emotions that you feel when you think about your diabetes.			
Who can you talk to when you feel this way?			
Name 3 activities that will help you work through this emotion and feel better.			

What might prevent you from doing these activities?
_____
_____

How can you overcome these obstacles?
_____
_____

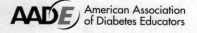
American Association of Diabetes Educators

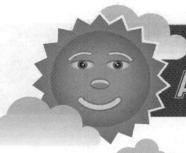

CONDUCTAS PARA EL CUIDADO PERSONA DE AADE7™
AFRONTAMIENTO SALUDABLE

La diabetes puede afectarte física y emocionalmente. Vivir con ella todos los días puede hacerte sentir desanimado, estresado o, incluso, deprimido. Es natural tener sentimientos mezclados sobre el control de tu diabetes y experimentar altibajos. Lo importante es que reconozcas que estas emociones son normales. Toma medidas para reducir el impacto negativo que estas emociones podrían tener en tu cuidado personal.

La manera en que manejas tus bajones emocionales se denomina "afrontamiento". Hay muchas maneras de sobrellevar los disgustos en tu vida y no todas son buenas para tu salud (fumar, comer en exceso, no encontrar tiempo para hacer actividad física o evitar personas y situaciones sociales).

Sin embargo, existen métodos de afrontamiento saludables que puedes utilizar para atravesar los momentos difíciles (actividades basadas en la fe, ejercicio, meditación, pasatiempos agradables, unirte a un grupo de apoyo).

Tener una red de apoyo es esencial para un afrontamiento saludable. Asegúrate de desarrollar y alimentar relaciones en tu vida personal con tu cónyuge, tus seres queridos y tus amigos. Asiste a sesiones educativas grupales donde puedas conocer y relacionarte con otras personas que están atravesando las mismas experiencias que tú. Construye relaciones saludables; y recuerda que no estás solo.

Algunas veces, los bajones emocionales pueden extenderse y tener un impacto más grave en tu vida, tu salud y tus relaciones. Esto puede ser un signo de depresión. Comunícale a tu educador en diabetes si:

» No tienes interés o no encuentras placer en tus actividades.
» Evitas hablar de tu diabetes con familiares y amigos.
» Duermes la mayor parte del día.
» No ves los beneficios de cuidarte a ti mismo.
» Sientes que la diabetes te está ganando.
» Sientes que no puedes cuidarte a ti mismo.

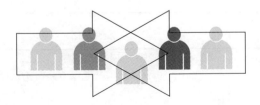

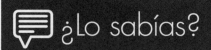
¿Lo sabías?

La actividad física puede influir en tu estado de ánimo. Si estás triste, ansioso, estresado o molesto, puedes salir a caminar, levantarte y estirarte, o dar un paseo en bicicleta. El ejercicio aumenta las sustancias químicas en tu cerebro que te ayudan a sentirte bien.

¿VERDADERO O FALSO?

Nadie quiere escuchar tus problemas. Cuando te sientes desanimado, debes guardarte tu tristeza.

FALSO. Necesitas hablar sobre tus emociones con amigos, familiares o con tu proveedor de atención médica. Algunas veces tan solo con hablar de un problema, te ayuda a resolverlo... y tus seres queridos pueden ayudarte a tener una mejor perspectiva del problema.

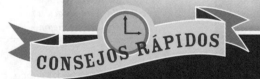
CONSEJOS RÁPIDOS

Reconoce el poder del pensamiento positivo.

Cuando te sientas desanimado, piensa en tus logros y siéntete bien por el progreso que has hecho para alcanzar un objetivo, aunque sólo sea un poquito.

Busca tiempo para hacer algo que te dé placer todos los días.

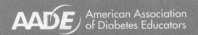

Supported by an educational grant from Lilly USA, LLC.

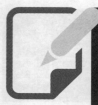

ACTIVIDADES

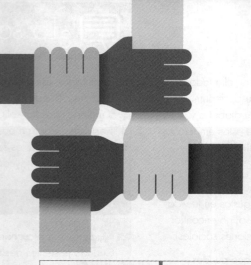

AFRONTAMIENTO SALUDABLE

Nombra 3 emociones que sientes cuando piensas en tu diabetes.			
¿Con quién puedes hablar cuando te sientes de esta manera?			
Nombra 3 actividades que te ayudarán a controlar esta emoción y a sentirte mejor.			

¿Qué podría impedirte hacer estas actividades?
_____
_____
_____

¿Cómo puedes superar estos obstáculos?
_____
_____
_____

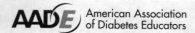

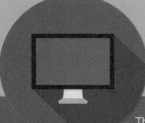

Learn, Connect, Engage
with the Diabetes Online Community

The Diabetes Online Community (for short, the DOC) is a conglomerate of people with diabetes and their caregivers, diabetes health care providers, foundations, organizations, and associations within the global diabetes environment who are engaging online, offering support, and sharing knowledge to improve the lives and health of people with diabetes. Ever-evolving, what was once a small sampling of personal bloggers has grown over the last decade into an engaged support network and platform for patient advocacy. The DOC is an online home for everyone and anyone touched by diabetes.

Why Should I Connect With The DOC?

- Get and Give Support
- Offer practical insights about dealing with diabetes
- Share challenges and stresses
- Minimize the isolation of living with and caring for diabetes
- Stay abreast of diabetes research, technologies, treatments, and more
- Find someone going through the same stage of life with diabetes (college, complications, pregnancy, retirement)
- Advocate for diabetes causes and concerns

How can I connect with the DOC?
There are many places and ways to engage with the DOC. To get started, think about your goals for engaging. Feel free to lurk, tip-toe in, or fully engage. The DOC will welcome you.

Where Do I Find The DOC?

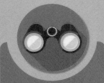

As you start to get more comfortable online you'll start to discover that there are hundreds of websites like these. This list is a good spring board to help you begin that discovery.

Large Active Community Forums:

Children With Diabetes
http://www.ChildrenWithDiabetes.com
for parents

Diabetes Daily
http://www.DiabetesDaily.com
all types of diabetes

Diabetes Sisters
http://www.DiabetesSisters.org
women with diabetes

Glu
http://www.MyGlu.org
access through T1D exchange

TuDiabetes
http://www.TuDiabetes.org
all types of diabetes

EsTuDiabetes
http://www.EsTuDiabetes.org
Spanish language community

Advocacy Organizations:

Diabetes Advocates
http://www.DiabetesAdvocates.org
a program of Diabetes Hands Foundation

Personal Blogs:

Kerri Sparling
http://www.SixUntilMe.com
t1 adult female patient opinion leader

Scott Johnson
http://www.ScottsDiabetes.com
t1 adult male patient opinion leader

Kim Vlasnik
http://www.TextingMyPancreas.com
t1 adult female patient opinion leader

Lorraine Sisto
http://www.ThisIsCaleb.com
parent of a t1 son

Kate Cornell
http://www.Kates-Sweet-Success.blogspot.com
t2 adult female

The Type 2 Experience
http://www.TheType2Experience.com
t2 adult bloggers

Online E-Magazines & News Sources:

DiabetesMine at Healthline
http://www.healthline.com/DiabetesMine

A Sweet Life
http://www.ASweetLife.org

diaTribe
http://www.diaTribe.org

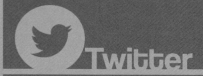 ## Twitter

You can follow #diabetes related hashtags like #diabetes, #doc, #bgnow, #sweatbetes, #vote4dm, #stripsafely

Weekly Twitter Chats:
* Diabetes Social Media Advocacy
    twitter.com/DiabetesSocMed - #DSMA
* Diabetic Connect
    twitter.com/DiabeticConnect - #DCDE
* Health Care Social Media
    twitter.com/HealthSocMed - #hcsm

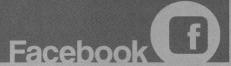 ## Facebook

Find thousands of diabetes groups on Facebook. There are many groups that offer conversations about different things like devices, therapies and geography.

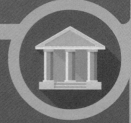

Diabetes Advocacy Online

The DOC has been able to amplify the voice of the diabetes community to support diabetes causes, research, treatment options, state and Federal government actions, and more. Many of these resources offer opportunities to participate in advocacy efforts at every level of engagement - regulatory, educational, and legislative. To learn more, go to DiabetesAdvocates.org - a program of Diabetes Hands Foundation.

Diabetes Organizations Online

AADE - American Association of Diabetes Educators
http://www.diabeteseducator.org
Find an accredited diabetes education program in your area:
http://www.diabeteseducator.org/ProfessionalResources/accred/Programs.html

ADA - American Diabetes Association
http://www.diabetes.org
Find a recognized diabetes education program in your area:
http://professional.diabetes.org/ERP_List.aspx

CDC - Centers for Disease Control and Prevention
http://cdc.gov/diabetes

CDN - College Diabetes Network
http://www.collegediabetesnetwork.org

DCAF – Diabetes Community Advocacy Foundation
http://diabetescaf.org/

IDF - International Diabetes Federation
http://www.idf.org

JDRF - Juvenile Diabetes Research Foundation
http://www.jdrf.org

NDEP - National Diabetes Education Program
http://ndep.nih.gov

NIDDK - National Institute of Diabetes and Digestive and Kidney Diseases
http://niddk.nih.gov

This resource, available in both web-based and PDF version, was developed by a group of people with diabetes and diabetes educators. It's hosted on Diabetes Hands Foundation's website. If you or your organization is interested in making this resource available on your website, please email info@diabeteshf.org. The authors encourage you to share this resource widely and freely to people with diabetes, caregivers, diabetes healthcare providers and educators and others who touch people with diabetes. This resource is not intended to be an exhaustive list of resources. If you are aware of resources that you believe should be included on a future update, please email info@diabeteshf.org for consideration. As people with diabetes and their caregivers engage in the DOC keep in mind that online support and information doesn't replace advice and counsel from your diabetes healthcare providers.

Problem-Solving Activity Script

Guide:	**Step 1: Identify the problem** "Describe the problem you are facing. Be very specific. The more specific you can be, the more likely you are to find a solution that works."
Person with diabetes:	"I can't remember to take my meds."
Guide:	"This is a start, but it's too vague. It's important to drill down to the 'sticking point,' the one area of taking your medication that has tripped you up over and over again."
Person with diabetes:	"I do pretty well remembering the morning meds. It's the medicine before dinner that I keep forgetting. I'm so busy getting dinner ready that it just slips my mind every time."
Guide:	**Step 2: Think of possible solutions** "Brainstorm things that you can do to help you remember to take the pre-dinner meds. Keep in mind similar situations you've faced when you came up with a solution that worked. Perhaps that solution will work this time, too. Build on any prior successes. "
Diabetes educator:	Ask participants to share their successes: "Who has faced a similar problem and found a workable solution? What did you do?" Other possible solutions to share with the group: (1) Place the bottle of meds where you eat dinner, next to the salt and pepper shakers; (2) set the alarm on your cell phone for 5 PM; (3) buy a medication reminder alarm from the pharmacy, and set it for 5 PM; (4) place a note in the kitchen to remind you to take the meds.
Guide:	**Step 3: Identify thoughts/attitudes that come with the problem** "Recall the thoughts or attitudes that you experienced when this problem happened before, and what happened then."
Person with diabetes:	"I'll realize after dinner that I forgot my diabetes medicine. Now, it's too late to take it. I feel so stupid! Why can't I get it right? Diabetes is too hard to deal with! No way am I going to check my blood sugar tonight; I know it'll be high because I forgot the medicine again. So I figure why bother? I get so discouraged, I just want to forget it all."
Guide:	"Practice more positive thoughts. This is a skill that you can learn to do. You'll get better with practice. Focus on any progress you've made, even if it's a little thing. Focus on something you can feel good about."
Person with diabetes:	"Well, at least I'm watching my food portions. I do pretty well with that. I haven't gained any weight since I started paying attention to my diet. I guess I'm not a complete failure after all."
Diabetes educator:	Studies show that thinking positive thoughts can lead to more constructive behaviors. It doesn't come naturally. You have to make yourself think about the positives. Give yourself a "pat on the back." It may feel silly at first, but with practice, it'll come more naturally. Negative expectations may discourage you from trying to cope with diabetes-related problems in the future. Negative thoughts about your ability to manage diabetes can easily lead to negative actions in the future. When you feel discouraged, you might slip into actions that will make your blood glucose go even higher. In this example, the person stops monitoring in the evening. That could lead to less monitoring the next day, the day after that, and so on. It's a slippery slope.
Guide:	**Step 4: Choose a solution, try it, see how it works out** "If your solution doesn't work out, don't give up! Try the next option on your list of possible solutions. Remind yourself that trying is worth the effort. Try to view any failure as an opportunity to learn what doesn't work."

Motivation Cost Versus Benefit Worksheet

Challenge:

Cost	Benefit

Positive Affirmations

I can find balance in my life.	I breathe in peace.
I can find love and support.	Today my intention is for peace.
I can accomplish anything.	I am in charge of my life.
I can handle whatever comes.	I have many options.
I can create inner peace.	I can create positive change.
My intention is for peace.	I am wise.
I am strong.	My happiness comes from within.
Peace is power.	I can start healthy habits.
This too shall pass.	Each moment brings choice.
My intentions create my reality.	I can stay calm under pressure.
Stress is leaving my body.	I choose happiness.
Today I choose joy.	I choose healthy relationships.
I can make healthy choices.	I can find my happy place.
I am doing my best.	

Source: E Scott, "Free positive affirmations for stress relief" (cited 2015 July 17), on the Internet at: http://stress.about.com/od/optimismspirituality/a/freeaffirmation.htm.

Psychological Assessment and Screening Tools

Tools to Measure Overall Emotional Health

Name and Source	Length	Administration	Description
Patient Health Questionnaire (PHQ)	4 pages, 88 items	Self-administered or verbally by a trained administrator	Screens for 8 conditions: major depressive disorder, other depressive disorder, panic disorder, other anxiety disorder, alcohol abuse/dependence, somatoform disorder, bulimia nervosa, and binge eating disorder. Some items can be skipped based on responses to previous items.

R Spitzer, K Kroenke, J Williams, "Validation and utility of a self-report version of PRIME-MD: the PHQ primary care study (Primary Care Evaluation of Mental Disorders, Patient Health Questionnaire)," *JAMA* 282, no. 18 (1999): 1737-44. Patient Health Questionnaire: http://www.integration.samhsa.gov/images/res/PHQ%20-%20Questions.pdf.

Name and Source	Length	Administration	Description
SF-36	36 items	Self-administered	Assesses 8 aspects of health-related quality of life: physical functioning, social functioning, physical role limitations, bodily pain, emotional well-being, emotional role limitations, energy and fatigue, and general health perceptions. A summary measure (the Mental Component Score) can be formed to summarize overall mental health status.

JJ Ware, M Kosinski, M Bayliss, et al, "Comparison of methods for the scoring and statistical analysis of SF-36 health profile and summary measures: summary of results from the Medical Outcomes Study," *Med Care* 33, no. 4 (1995): AS264-79. SF-36: http://www.sf-36.org/tools/SF36.shtml.

Name and Source	Length	Administration	Description
SF-12	12 items	Self-administered	Assesses the same aspects of quality of life as the SF-36, but with fewer items.

JJ Ware, M Kosinski, S Keller, "A 12-item short-form health survey: construction of scales and preliminary tests of reliability and validity," *Med Care* 34, no. 3 (1996): 220-33. SF-12: http://www.sf-36.org/tools/sf12.shtml.

Tools to Measure Depression

Name and Source	Length	Administration	Description
Patient Health Questionnaire-9 (PHQ-9)	9 items	Self-administered or verbally as part of a clinical encounter	Part of the larger PHQ. Copyrighted by Pfizer, but may be printed without permission. In some programs, the first 2 questions serve as a screen; only if the patient responds "yes" to either of the first 2 questions do they need to continue.

R Spitzer, K Kroenke, J Williams, "The PHQ-9: validity of a brief depression severity measure," *J Gen Intern Med* 16, no. 9 (2001): 606-13; *Healthy Coping Guide in Diabetes: A Guide for Program Development and Implementation* (St Louis: Diabetes Initiative National Program Office, 2008). PHQ-9: http://www.phqscreeners.com/pdfs/02_PHQ-9/English.pdf.

Name and Source	Length	Administration	Description
Beck Depression Inventory (BDI)	21 items	5–15 minutes; self-administered or verbally by a trained administrator	The full BDI consists of 21 items and has been revised several times. It assesses general life satisfaction, mood, relations with others, self-esteem, appetite, and libido. Shorter versions (eg, 13 items) are also available.

A Beck, C Ward, M Mendelson, et al, "An inventory for measuring depression," *Arch Gen Psychiatr* 4 (1961): 561-71; AT Beck, RA Steer, MG Garbin, "Psychometric properties of the Beck Depression Inventory: twenty-five years of evaluation," *Clin Psychol Rev* 8, no. 1 (1988): 77-100; P Richter, J Werner, A Heerlein, et al, "On the validity of the Beck Depression Inventory: a review," *Psychopathology* 31, no. 1 (1998): 160-8. BDI: http://www.apa.org/pi/about/publications/caregivers/practice-settings/assessment/tools/beck-depression.aspx.

Tools to Measure Depression *(continued)*

Name and Source	Length	Administration	Description
Center for Epidemiological Studies Depression (CES-D)	20 items	10 minutes; self-administered or verbally as part of a clinical encounter	Assesses 4 dimensions of depressive symptoms: depressed affect, positive affect, somatic complaints, and interpersonal problems.

L Radloff, "The CES-D Scale: a self-report depression scale for research in the general population," *Appl Psychol Meas* 1, no. 3 (1977): 385-401; M Naughton, I Wiklund, "A critical review of dimension-specific measures of health-related quality of life in cross-cultural research," *Qual Life Res* 2, no. 6 (1993): 397-432. CES-D: http://counsellingresource.com/lib/quizzes/depression-testing/cesd/.

Name and Source	Length	Administration	Description
Zung Self-Rating Depression Scale	12 items	10 minutes; self-rating scale	Assesses affective, cognitive, behavioral, and physiological symptoms of depression. Best used in conjunction with the active participation of a healthcare professional or clinician during or immediately following a client interview.

W Zung, "A self-rating depression scale," *Arch Gen Psychiatr* 12 (1965): 63-70; M Naughton, I Wiklund, "A critical review of dimension-specific measures of health-related quality of life in cross-cultural research," *Qual Life Res* 2, no. 6 (1993): 397-432. http://healthnet.umassmed.edu/mhealth/ZungSelfRatedDepressionScale.pdf.

Name and Source	Length	Administration	Description
Geriatric Depression Scale (GDS)	30 items	10–15 minutes; no mental health expertise required to administer	Assesses 5 dimensions of depressive symptoms: sad mood, lack of energy, positive mood, agitation, and social withdrawal.

J Yesavage, T Brink, T Rose, et al, "Development and validation of a geriatric depression screening scale: a preliminary report," *J Psychiatr Res* 17, no. 1 (1982-1983): 37-49; J Sheikh, J Yesavage, "Geriatric Depression Scale (GDS): recent evidence and development of a shorter version," in *Clinical Gerontology: A Guide to Assessment and Intervention* (New York: The Haworth Press, 1986), 165-73; J Sheikh, J Yesavage, J Brooks, et al, "Proposed factor structure of the Geriatric Depression Scale," *Int Psychogeriatr* 3, no. 1 (1991): 23-8; J Wancata, R Alexandrowicz, B Marquart, et al, "The criterion validity of the Geriatric Depression Scale: a systematic review," *Acta Psychiatr Scand* 114, no. 6 (2006): 398-410. http://consultgerirn.org/uploads/File/trythis/try_this_4.pdf.

Name and Source	Length	Administration	Description
Edinburgh Postnatal Depression Scale (EPDS)	10 items	5 minutes; no mental health expertise required to administer	Identifies women at risk for perinatal depression. The EPDS is easy to administer and an effective screening tool.

JL Cox, JM Holden, R Sagovsky, "Detection of postnatal depression: development of the 10-item Edinburgh Postnatal Depression Scale," *Br J Psychiatry* 150 (1987): 782-6. http://www2.aap.org/sections/scan/practicingsafety/toolkit_resources/module2/epds.pdf.

Tool to Measure Stress/Distress

Name and Source	Length	Administration	Description
Perceived Stress Scale (PSS-10)	10 items	Self-administered	Assesses how unpredictable, uncontrollable, or overloaded patients find their lives to be.

S Cohen, T Kamarck, R Mermelstein, "A global measure of perceived stress," *J Health Soc Beh* 24, no. 4 (1983): 385-96; S Cohen, G Williamson, "Perceived stress in a probability sample of the United States," in S Spacapan, S Oskamp, eds, *The Social Psychology of Health* (Newbury Park: Sage, 1988), 31-67. http://www.psy.cmu.edu/~scohen/PSS.html.

(continued)

Tools to Measure Diabetes-Specific Stress/Distress

Name and Source	Length	Administration	Description
Problem Areas in Diabetes Scale (PAID)	20 items	Self-administered or verbally as part of a clinical encounter	Assesses overall diabetes-specific emotional distress.

W Polonsky, B Anderson, P Lohrer, et al, "Assessment of diabetes-related distress," *Diabetes Care* 18, no. 6 (1995): 754-60; G Welch, A Jacobson, W Polonsky, "The Problem Areas in Diabetes Scale: an evaluation of its clinical utility," *Diabetes Care* 20, no. 5 (1997): 760-6; K Watkins, C Connell, "Measurement of health-related QOL in diabetes mellitus," *Pharmacoeconomics* 22, no. 17 (2004): 1109-26. http://care.diabetesjournals.org/content/20/5/760.abstract.

Name and Source	Length	Administration	Description
Diabetes Distress Scale (DDS)	17 items	Self-administered or verbally as part of a clinical encounter	Assesses 4 types of distress: emotional burden, physician-related distress, regimen-related distress, and interpersonal distress.

W Polonsky, L Fisher, J Earles, et al, "Assessing psychosocial distress in diabetes: development of the diabetes distress scale," *Diabetes Care* 28, no. 3 (2005): 626-31; L Fisher, MM Skaff, JT Mullan, et al, "Clinical depression versus distress among patients with type 2 diabetes: not just a question of semantics," *Diabetes Care* 30, no. 3 (2007): 542-8. http://www.diabetesuniversitydmcp.com/uploads/1/0/2/7/10277276/dds_scale_in_english.pdf.

Name and Source	Length	Administration	Description
Questionnaire on Stress in Patients with Diabetes (QSD-R)	45 items	Self-administered	Assesses 8 types/sources of stress: leisure time, depression, fear of failure, hypoglycemia, treatment regimen/diet, physical complaints, work, partner and doctor-patient relationship.

P Herschbach, G Duran, S Waadt, et al, "Psychometric properties of the Questionnaire on Stress in Patients with Diabetes--Revised (QSD-R)," *Health Psychol* 16, no. 2 (1997): 171-4; AM Garratt, L Schmidt, R Fitzpatrick, "Patient-assessed health outcome measures for diabetes: a structured review," *Diabetic Med* 19, no. 1 (2002): 1-11. http://academicdepartments.musc.edu/family_medicine/rcmar/qsdr.htm.

Name and Source	Length	Administration	Description
Appraisal of Diabetes (ADS)	7 items	Self-administered	Assesses individuals' overall appraisal (thoughts and feelings) of their diabetes.

AM Garratt, L Schmidt, R Fitzpatrick, "Patient-assessed health outcome measures for diabetes: a structured review," *Diabetic Med* 19, no. 1 (2002): 1-11; MP Carey, RS Jorgensen, RS Weinstock, et al, "Reliability and validity of the appraisal of diabetes scale," *J Behav Med* 14, no. 1 (1991): 43-51. http://academicdepartments.musc.edu/family_medicine/ResidencyProgram/.

Tool to Measure Diabetes Quality of Life

Name and Source	Length	Administration	Description
Diabetes 39	39 items	Self-administered or verbally as part of a clinical encounter	Assesses 5 aspects of quality of life: energy/mobility, diabetes control, anxiety/worry, social burden, and sexual functioning.

K Watkins, C Connell, "Measurement of health-related QOL in diabetes mellitus," *Pharmacoeconomics* 22, no. 17 (2004): 1109-26; AM Garratt, L Schmidt, R Fitzpatrick, "Patient-assessed health outcome measures for diabetes: a structured review," *Diabetic Med* 19, no. 1 (2002): 1-11; JG Boyer, JA Earp, "The development of an instrument for assessing the quality of life of people with diabetes: Diabetes 39," *Med Care* 35, no. 5 (1997): 440-53. http://www.atsu.edu/research/pdfs/diabetes_outcomes.pdf.

MODULE 8

Reducing Risks

Table of Contents

REDUCING RISKS: AN EDUCATOR'S OVERVIEW 290
    AADE Systematic Review of the Literature 290
    Background Information and Instructions for the Educator 290
    Learning Objectives 291
        Knowledge. 291
        Skills 291
        Barriers and Facilitators 291
    Behavioral Objective 291
REDUCING RISKS: INSTRUCTIONAL PLAN 291
    Identifying Participant Thoughts and Feelings About Diabetes Complications 291
    Reducing Risks to Prevent Diabetes Complications 292
        Personal Care Record 292
        A1C: Measurement of Glucose Control 293
    Cardiovascular Health 294
        The Diabetes–Heart Disease Connection 294
        Blood Pressure 294
    Kidney Health 309
        Reducing Your Risk for Diabetic Kidney Disease 310
    Eye Health 311
        General Vision Examination Versus Diabetic Eye Examination: What's the Difference? 312
    Nerve Health 314
        Peripheral Neuropathy 314
        Reducing Your Risk for Foot Problems 314
        Autonomic Neuropathy 316
    Sleep Health 320
    Dental Health 321
        Reducing Your Risk for Dental Problems 321

290   Diabetes Education Curriculum

    Skin Health 322

        Reducing Your Risk for Skin Problems 322

    Immunizations 324

    Psychosocial Assessment and Care 325

    Reducing Risks Before and During Pregnancy 325

        Preconception Care 325

        For Women With Diabetes WHO ARE NOT PLANNING to Become Pregnant 325

        Identifying Participant Feelings and Concerns About Pregnancy and Diabetes 327

        For Women With Diabetes WHO ARE PLANNING to Become Pregnant 327

        For Women With Diabetes WHO ARE PREGNANT 329

        Postpartum Concerns 336

    Identifying Barriers to Reducing Risks 340

    Identifying Facilitators for Reducing Risks 341

    Setting a SMART Goal to Reduce Risks 342

    Follow-up/Outcomes Measurement 342

REFERENCES 344

REDUCING RISKS: RESOURCES 352

REDUCING RISKS: AN EDUCATOR'S OVERVIEW

AADE Systematic Review of the Literature

A systematic review of the literature on reducing risks was conducted by the American Association of Diabetes Educators (AADE). A variety of interventions were evaluated, including smoking cessation, eye examinations, foot care, oral health, immunizations, and cardiovascular risk reduction. To maximize control of health conditions, patients need to acquire the skills to interpret basic data (blood pressure, A1C, lipids, etc) in order to fully understand the benefits of self-care behaviors to reduce risks. The ability for patients to recognize their risk factors for diabetes complications, as well as understanding what constitutes optimal preventive care, is a vital aspect of managing diabetes. Studies assessed in this review provide evidence that educational interventions for reducing risks in diabetes are beneficial.[1]

Background Information and Instructions for the Educator

This module is largely organized around the American Diabetes Association's Standards of Medical Care in Diabetes.[2] The diabetes educator has a responsibility to help patients learn what to expect as a standard of care, as well as the therapeutic targets that their treatment aims to achieve. Patients who comprehend the standards can better partner with their provider to access the necessary tests, examinations, preventive services, and interventions that can reduce their risk for developing the complications of diabetes.

    The AADE7 Self-Care Behaviors™ provide a framework for addressing the standards of care. It is important that patients acquire knowledge about the various standards in the context of diabetes complications. But more important is that patients adopt the behaviors that will help them avoid those complications. The diabetes educator should help patients develop the skills that will help them reduce their risk for complications. Such skills include self-monitoring of blood glucose level and blood pressure; foot self-examination; getting regular eye, foot, and dental examinations; aspirin use; smoking cessation; and keeping a personal care record.[1] An important role of the diabetes educator is to assist patients in identifying barriers to risk-reduction behaviors and developing strategies to overcome them.

American Association of Diabetes Educators©

Fear of complications is fairly universal among people with diabetes. The belief that complications are inevitable is a common one. Many patients' fears, however, are based on a lack of information while interpreting others' negative experiences with diabetes. Attention to patients' feelings and thoughts about diabetes and its complications can serve as a springboard for fruitful discussion about self-care behaviors that can make a real difference in reducing risks. This module begins with several questions that can help the educator assess what is most relevant to participants. The educator should use as much of the content in this module as needed to meet patients' individual needs and to facilitate adequate risk-reduction behavior.

Learning Objectives

Knowledge

The participant will:

- describe the standards of care—necessary tests and their frequency, eg, dilated eye examination annually
- state the recommended therapeutic goals for tests in the standards of care, eg, blood pressure less than 140/90 mm Hg
- explain proper foot care, as well as findings that should be reported to provider
- explain proper operation of home blood pressure monitor
- explain how to effectively use personal care record

Skills

The participant will:

- demonstrate proper self-examination of feet
- demonstrate proper technique using his or her home monitor (for those individuals for whom home blood pressure monitoring is appropriate)
- set up his or her personal care record (tests/examinations that are due, frequency, therapeutic goals, available current results, etc)

Barriers and Facilitators

The participant will:

- identify potential barriers/facilitators that may affect his or her ability to reduce risks (access preventive care services or perform risk-reduction behaviors)
- develop strategies for reducing barriers and increasing facilitators to successfully reduce risks

Behavioral Objective

The participant will set realistic, measurable individual goals for reducing risks.

REDUCING RISKS: INSTRUCTIONAL PLAN

Identifying Participant Thoughts and Feelings About Diabetes Complications

Adults learn best when they feel valued and respected for their experiences and viewpoints. **Use probing questions to uncover their thoughts about diabetes complications.**

American Association of Diabetes Educators©

What have you heard about diabetes complications?

What is your greatest concern/What worries you the most about diabetes complications?

Do you believe that you will have health problems if you have diabetes, no matter what you do?

Do you think a person can do anything to prevent diabetes complications?

What do you want to learn today about staying healthy with diabetes?

What have you heard about diabetes complications in pregnancy?

Reducing Risks to Prevent Diabetes Complications

For people with diabetes, there is an important set of tests that should be done each year to detect any complications related to diabetes. These tests are referred to as the **Standards of Medical Care in Diabetes**.[2] The importance of following the standards of care is backed up by research.

You and your provider share responsibility regarding these tests and reducing your risk for complications.[3] Your provider's role is to order the tests on time, tell you what the results mean, and discuss treatment options with you. Your role is to do what you can to take care of your diabetes. This means seeing your provider regularly and getting the tests done when ordered.

It's very important that you be informed about these tests and know when they are due. If they are not ordered on time, you should talk with your provider about this.

Personal Care Record

Distribute a personal care record to each participant. If current results of tests and examinations are available, assist the participant with filling in the information.

Keeping track of the tests you need throughout the year is made easier with a personal care record. It includes the names of the tests, how often you should have them done, and target results for each test. At visits to the provider, you can update the record with the help of the office staff. Many people prefer a wallet-size personal care record, since it's more likely to be with them when they go for healthcare visits. Some people prefer to keep their information in a notebook so there's room to write more information about their health. Others use their phones, as there are many apps to help you track your health care.[4(p300)]

See the "Resources" section at the end of this module for information about the free Diabetes Goal Tracker mobile app, available in English and Spanish.

Adults learn best when the learning experience is active and not passive. **Keep participants engaged by having them customize the care record with their results. Assist as needed.**

A1C: Measurement of Glucose Control

The following content about A1C is duplicated in Module 5: Monitoring. More detailed information about A1C, including the comparison with estimated average glucose, is in Module 5: Monitoring.

Consider using a visual teaching aid that can help illustrate the concept of glucose adhering to red blood cells. This approach is especially useful for those who have strong visual/spatial intelligence.

What does the A1C test tell you?
How often should your A1C be measured?
Do you know your target for A1C?
Is the A1C target different in pregnancy?

The A1C blood test tells you your glucose control over the past 2 to 3 months.[5] A1C results will be a number followed by a percent sign. For someone without diabetes, A1C is between 4% to 6%.

Red blood cells are in your bloodstream for 2 to 3 months, then they die. Your body is always making fresh red blood cells. During their lifespan, some of the glucose in your blood gets stuck to the red blood cells. If the glucose levels are normal, then a normal amount of glucose will be found on the red blood cells. If the glucose levels are often higher than normal, there will be a higher amount of glucose found on the red blood cells. By measuring the amount of glucose on the red blood cells, your glucose level for the past 2 to 3 months can be determined.

The Standards of Medical Care in Diabetes provide a comprehensive list of preventive-care practices and how frequently each should be recommended to all people with diabetes. Throughout the remainder of this chapter you will see recommendations that you can share with your patients.

Standard of Medical Care in Diabetes[2]

- If your A1C is within target and your glucose control is stable, you should have an A1C test done at least twice a year.
- If your A1C is above target, or if how you treat your diabetes has changed, you should have an A1C test done every 3 months.
- In pregnancy, A1C levels may need to be monitored more frequently (eg, monthly) because of the alteration in red blood cells.

> **Targets for A1C**
> In general, the target level for A1C for a person with diabetes is as close to normal as possible without undue hypoglycemia.
>
> ❖ The American Diabetes Association (ADA) advocates an A1C target of <7% (some people may need higher or lower goals).[2-7]
>
> ❖ The American Association of Clinical Endocrinologists (AACE) recommends an A1C target of <6.5% (some people may need different A1C goals).[6]
>
> ❖ The ADA advocates an A1C target of <6% in pregnancy without hypoglycemia.

Different professional groups have slightly different opinions about A1C targets. The different groups agree that the attempt to achieve these targets should not put a person at risk for having too many episodes of hypoglycemia (low blood sugar).

Many studies show that keeping A1C near normal most of the time drastically lowers your risk for long-term complications.[7-12] In fact, people who keep glucose levels near normal for an extended time *soon after diagnosis* tend to have more protection against complications years later, even if their glucose levels begin to creep up over time. This shows how important early glucose control is.[13-15]

Both ADA and AACE agree that some people with diabetes may benefit from higher A1C targets. Examples include someone who experiences frequent episodes of severe hypoglycemia or someone with many health problems. The ADA also agrees with AACE that some may benefit from an A1C less than 6.5%. Be sure to discuss your A1C target with your provider.[2,6]

Cardiovascular Health

When we talk about cardiovascular health, we are referring to the heart and the blood vessels. People with diabetes are 2 to 3 times more likely than people without diabetes to have heart disease. But with the right lifestyle and medical treatment, you can keep your heart healthy.

The Diabetes–Heart Disease Connection

There are still many things science cannot answer about the link between diabetes and heart disease. One thing that is known is this: Managing diabetes can help reduce your risk for heart disease. In one large study involving people with type 2 diabetes, it was found that for *every 1% drop in the A1C (such as going from 11% to 10%)*, you are less likely to have a heart attack or stroke.[16]

When there is too much glucose in the bloodstream most of the time, the insides of the blood vessels become sticky. This makes it very easy for cholesterol and other particles to collect on the vessel wall, leading to a buildup called plaque. Plaque can decrease or stop blood flow. When plaque bursts or breaks off, a clot can form in the blood vessel. This clot can block blood flow and prevent oxygen from getting to the heart or brain, which can lead to a heart attack or stroke.

Therefore, it's important to take steps to reduce your risk for cardiovascular disease. This means keeping tabs on your blood glucose level, blood pressure, and a blood test called the lipid profile.

Blood Pressure

Do you know what the numbers in a blood pressure reading mean?

Your heart beats in 2 phases: pumping and relaxing. During the pumping phase, the heart is pushing blood to your lungs and the rest of your body. The pressure inside the heart is higher during the pumping phase because the heart muscle is actively squeezing (contracting). In the relaxation phase, the heart muscle relaxes, and the heart fills up with blood from all parts of your body. The pressure inside the heart during relaxation is lower.

When your blood pressure is taken, it is an indirect measure of the pressures in your heart during the 2 phases. The top number is the *systolic pressure*, and it reflects the pressure in the heart during the pumping phase. The bottom number is the *diastolic pressure*, and it reflects the pressure in the heart when it's relaxing.

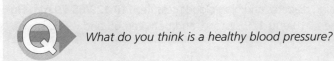

What do you think is a healthy blood pressure?

If you have clogged or stiff blood vessels throughout your body, the passageway for blood to flow through is narrowed. Your heart has to work very hard to push blood through narrowed vessels. This strain on your heart shows up as high blood pressure. Other conditions can cause your blood vessels to constrict (tighten up) more than they should, also resulting in high blood pressure. In either case, high blood pressure should be treated so that the heart does not have to work too hard all the time.

> **Standard of Medical Care in Diabetes[2]**
>
> At every routine visit to your provider, your blood pressure should be taken.

A normal blood pressure is <120/80 mm Hg. The blood pressure target for people with diabetes is based on studies that show better health outcomes if blood pressure is kept below 140/90 mm Hg. For some with diabetes, such as those who are younger or at high risk for having a stroke, a goal of under 130/80 mm Hg may be more desirable—this is something you should talk over with your healthcare provider. Making lifestyle changes and using 1 or more medications to keep your blood pressure under 140/90 mm Hg is one of the most important things you can do to avoid diabetes complications.[17-22]

> **Blood Pressure Target: Nonpregnant Adults[22]**
>
> The blood pressure target for nonpregnant adults with diabetes is **<140/90 mm Hg.**

If your blood pressure is 140/90 mm Hg or higher, your provider should retake it on another day. If it stays higher than 140/90 mm Hg, you have high blood pressure (hypertension) and should be started on blood pressure medication.[22] Healthy lifestyle changes, including more physical activity and healthy eating, should also be put into place.

If your blood pressure is above 120/80 mm Hg and less than 140/90 mm Hg, making some lifestyle changes may help keep your blood pressure at a desirable level.[22]

For Pregnant Women With Diabetes and Hypertension[22,23]

Hypertension in pregnancy is classified into 4 categories based on guidelines by the American College of Obstetricians and Gynecologists (ACOG) Task Force:

- Preeclampsia-eclampsia: hypertension in association with thrombocytopenia, impaired liver function, the new development of renal insufficiency, pulmonary edema, or new-onset cerebral or visual disturbances
- Chronic hypertension: hypertension that predates pregnancy

- Preeclampsia superimposed on chronic hypertension: chronic hypertension in association with preeclampsia
- Gestational hypertension: BP elevation after 20 weeks of gestation in the absence of proteinuria

As a result of poor glycemic control, the incidence of hypertensive disorders in pregnancy is higher in women with diabetes.

Blood Pressure Target: Pregnant Women With Hypertension[21,22]
The blood pressure target is lower for pregnant women who have preexisting diabetes and high blood pressure: **110-129/65-79 mm Hg** (between 110 and 129 systolic, and between 65 and 79 diastolic).

For Children With Diabetes[24,25]

Blood pressure levels for children are based on age, sex, and height. A blood pressure chart for children would show *at what percentile* a child's blood pressure is, much as growth charts show height and weight.

For example, a child with a blood pressure in the 90th percentile means that 90% of other children of the same age, sex, and height have a blood pressure that is the same or lower. If a child's blood pressure is considered high-normal (in the 90th to 95th percentile), then he or she should make lifestyle changes, including healthy eating and physical activity aimed at weight control. If this approach doesn't bring the blood pressure to the target level within 3 to 6 months, then blood pressure medication should be considered.

If a child's blood pressure is consistently at or above the 95th percentile, then he or she should be started on blood pressure medication and lifestyle changes right away.

Blood Pressure Target: Children With Diabetes[24-26]
The target blood pressure in children is below the 90th percentile for age, sex, and height.

Advanced Detail

Ankle/Brachial Index (ABI)

Another blood pressure measurement that may be done is called the *ankle/brachial index*, or ABI. This test involves checking your blood pressure in both arms while you are lying down. Then, blood pressure in both lower legs is checked, placing the cuff just above the ankles. A calculation is done with the results of the systolic (top number) readings from the arm and leg.[27]

The ABI is used to help diagnose a serious circulation problem in the legs called *peripheral arterial disease* (PAD). Diabetes and smoking put a person at the highest risk for PAD.[28] And PAD is linked to strokes, heart attacks, and amputations.

A person with PAD may experience cramping, pain, and aching in the calves, thighs, or buttocks when walking, but this discomfort is relieved with rest. Other symptoms of PAD include a reddish-purple color to the feet when they dangle, but a paler color when the feet are elevated. A loss of foot hair, very thick toenails, and cool dry skin on the feet are also common in PAD. Some people have no symptoms of PAD.

In people who have diabetic nerve disease, though, the pain and cramping are often not evident. Nerve damage keeps them from feeling the pain from reduced blood flow. On the other hand, they may notice that they now walk more slowly than before, and that their legs get tired easily.[29,30] If you have any of the symptoms of PAD, report them to your provider.

> **Standard of Medical Care in Diabetes**[29,30]
>
> ❖ An ADA consensus statement suggests that people with diabetes who are older than 50 years should have the ABI test.
>
> ❖ The ABI should be considered in people younger than 50 who have PAD risk factors (smoking, high blood pressure, high lipids, or diabetes over 10 years).

> *Do you know what your blood pressure is?*
>
> *When you have your blood pressure taken at the doctor's office, do you ask to be told the reading?*
>
> *Do you take your blood pressure at home?*
>
> *Do you know if your blood pressure monitor is accurate?*

When the doctor's office staff takes your blood pressure, you should always ask for the result.

> Evidence shows that self-monitoring of blood pressure may improve blood pressure control by improving compliance, because patients become more involved in their care.[31]

In addition to getting your blood pressure checked at the doctor's office, home blood pressure monitoring is also recommended for many people. Checking your blood pressure at home helps you know if you have "white coat" high blood pressure, a condition where the anxiety of being in the clinic raises your blood pressure.[17,32] It also helps you see if medication and lifestyle changes are helping your blood pressure.

In recent years, numerous studies have shown that blood pressure readings taken at home are often lower than those taken in the doctor's office. The readings taken at home may better predict your risk of developing heart problems.[31,33]

Advanced Detail

Choosing and Using a Home Blood Pressure Monitor

❖ Automatically inflating (*oscillometric*) blood pressure monitors are preferred over the traditional type (requiring pumping up the cuff manually and using a stethoscope) because they are easier to use and less prone to user error.[32]

❖ Monitors with memory allow you to easily look at past readings and see how you are doing.[32]

❖ Make sure the accuracy of the monitor is confirmed according to standard international protocols.[32] Not all of the devices that are currently on the market have passed proper validation tests (eg, Association for the Advancement of Medical Instrumentation and British Hypertension Society protocols). The product information that comes with the monitor should say that the unit was validated against the direct method of measurement.[33]

While the US Food and Drug Administration (FDA) regulates blood pressure devices, it only requires companies to show that new monitors are as good as models already on the market.[34] Foreign-made monitors sold over the Internet are not subject to the FDA regulation, so they may not be up to US standards; they may also not be properly validated. To check whether your monitor is properly validated, see if it appears on the list of validated devices provided by the Web site of the dabl® Educational Trust (http://www.dableducational.org).

- Have your healthcare provider watch while you use your home blood pressure monitor for the first time. He or she can help you use the monitor properly.[33]

- Unless otherwise directed by your provider, check your blood pressure 2 or 3 times during the course of a week. Make sure that you are in a seated position. Take some readings in the morning after you have urinated but before eating or taking any blood pressure medication. Some of your readings should be taken in the evening. Write down your blood pressure results, along with the date and the time of day. Show these results to your provider at your appointments. Your provider will need at least 12 readings in order to make any decisions about your care.[32]

- Cuff placement on your upper arm will give more accurate readings than other styles of blood pressure monitors (eg, wrist and finger). Having the right size and fit of the cuff is the most important thing you can do to get a correct reading.

- Using a monitor that measures blood pressure in the wrist is generally not recommended. Wrist readings will be inaccurate if your arm is not kept at heart level during measurement. The position of your wrist during measurement may also affect accuracy.[35]

- Blood pressure monitors that use a finger cuff are not recommended.[32]

- Blood pressure machines in public places are often not maintained, and so you can't be certain that the blood pressure number is right.

Have you heard about any actions you can take to help control blood pressure? If so, what are they?

Controlling Blood Pressure

Controlling blood pressure is JUST AS IMPORTANT as glucose control to reduce your risk for diabetes complications such as kidney or eye disease, heart attack, or stroke.[36] The current thinking in medicine is to *treat to target*. That means whatever is necessary should reasonably be done to get your blood pressure to the target level.

The blood pressure target for people with diabetes is less than 140/90 mm Hg.[18,29] Your provider may set a different target for your special needs. For example, the initial goal for those aged 60 or over is less than 150/90 mm Hg, and for those with kidney disease and high levels of protein in the urine, a blood pressure of less than 130/80 mm Hg is desirable.[17] There are lots of things you can do to help control blood pressure.

Invite participants who have successfully managed their high blood pressure to share with others in the group how they did it. Adults with social/interpersonal intelligence learn by telling their story; hearing and telling stories helps those with verbal/auditory intelligence learn.

Healthy Eating

The DASH diet has been shown to help lower blood pressure in the general population.[22,28] It involves:

- Eating less salt.[37-42] Avoid salty foods, such as processed meats and snack foods. Don't add salt to your food while cooking or at the table. Instead of salt, use spices, herbs, lemon, or vinegar for flavor.
- Eating more fruit and vegetables (8 to 10 servings a day).
- Choosing 2 to 3 low-fat dairy servings each day.
- Eating whole-grain cereal, rice, and bread.
- Choosing small servings of lean meats, poultry, and fish.
- Eating nuts, seeds, or dried beans at least 3 times per week and having small amounts of fat from vegetable sources each day (corn, olive, or canola oil).
- Limiting alcohol and sugar in the diet.

Being Active[40-43]

Being physically active will help control blood pressure. It may also help you lose weight if you need to.

Reducing Risks

- If you drink alcohol, do so in moderation—up to 1 drink a day for women or up to 2 drinks a day for men (1 drink equals 12 ounces of beer, 5 ounces of wine, or 1½ ounces of alcohol).[42,44]
- Caffeine may affect the blood pressure of some people—talk with your doctor about whether you should limit caffeine.
- If you smoke, stop. While smoking has not been shown conclusively to increase blood pressure, it definitely plays a role in heart disease.[45]
- Maintain a healthy weight. Lose weight if you need to, as weight reduction has been shown to reduce blood pressure.[42]

Taking Medication

Even if you do your best with lifestyle efforts, taking medication is often necessary to get blood pressure under control. But with adequate lifestyle effort, you may not need as much blood pressure medication.

Most people with diabetes require 2 or more types of medication to gain control of their blood pressure.[22] Many people will require 3 or more medications in order to get their blood pressure to the target level.[38] That's because different blood pressure medications work in different ways, to attack the problem from different angles. It is also recommended that you take 1 of your blood pressure meds at bedtime (talk to your provider about this).[22,40,41]

Starting and Staying on Blood Pressure Medication

 The following is an extensive (but not exhaustive) list of blood pressure medications. Share with participants only the information that is relevant to their prescribed medications to facilitate safe and effective medication-taking behavior.

Your provider will start by trying 1 type of blood pressure medication to see how it works for you. If it is not effective, he or she may change the dose. Or, if side effects are a problem, then the provider will need to try a different medication. What medication your provider selects will depend on your race—for black people, calcium channel blockers (CCBs) and some diuretics (thiazides) seem to work best. For others, the first medication used may be a thiazide-type diuretic, CCB, angiotensin-converting enzyme (ACE) inhibitor, or angiotensin receptor blocker (ARB). If you have kidney disease, an ACE or ARB should be part of the initial treatment.[18]

Be patient while your provider figures out the right dose of medication, or the best combination of medications, that will work to control your blood pressure. Be sure to tell your provider if you are having side effects that you don't like. Working with your provider to change when you take the medication or the type of medication may help. High blood pressure may not hurt, but it can cause major problems to your eyes, kidneys, and blood vessels if it is not properly controlled. **Take your blood pressure medication every day, even if you feel good.**

Adults learn best when the content is meaningful to their experience and fills a perceived need. Help each participant identify the blood pressure medication(s) he or she takes. Then, share only the salient points about the medication(s). Don't overwhelm with irrelevant information.

Your doctor may give you an **ACE inhibitor** or **ARB** as the first medication to help control your blood pressure if it is too high.[22,46] Research shows that ACE inhibitors can reduce heart attacks and strokes in people with diabetes.[47] Angiotensin-converting enzyme inhibitors are generally taken 1 hour before a meal, on an empty stomach, at about the same time every day.

Angiotensin-converting enzyme inhibitors are often combined with a diuretic ("water pill") to help better control blood pressure. Your provider should do certain laboratory tests to check the health of your kidneys as well as your potassium level before starting you on an ACE inhibitor, and should repeat these tests periodically for as long as you take it.[2] Pregnant women should not take ACE inhibitors. **After starting therapy with an ACE inhibitor, if you develop a persistent or severe cough that does not go away, notify your doctor.**[48] Angiotensin-converting enzyme inhibitors are listed in Table 8.1.

Angiotensin receptor blockers are a type of blood pressure medication that can be used in place of an ACE inhibitor.[22] They have been shown to help lower the risk of additional heart problems for those with congestive heart failure. Angiotensin receptor blockers may generally be taken with or without food, but it is important to take them at about the same time every day.

Some ARBs are combined with a diuretic ("water pill") to help better control blood pressure. Your provider should do certain laboratory tests to check the health of your kidneys as well as your potassium level before starting you on an ARB, and should repeat these tests periodically for as long as you take it.[22] Pregnant women should not take ARBs.[22,48] Angiotensin receptor blockers are listed in Table 8.2.

TABLE 8.1	Recognizing ACE Inhibitors
Generic Name*	**Trade Name**
Benazepril	Lotensin®
Captopri	Capoten®
Enalapril	Vasotec®
Fosinopril	Monopril®
Lisinopril	Prinivil®, Zestril®
Moexipril	Univasc®
Perindopril	Aceon®
Quinipril	Accupril®
Ramipril	Altace®
Trandolapril	Mavik®

*Generic names end in "pril."

TABLE 8.2	Recognizing ARBs
Generic Name*	**Trade Name**
Azilsartan	Edarbi
Candesartan	Atacand®
Eprosartan	Teveten®
Irbesartan	Avapro®
Losartan	Cozaar®
Olmesartan	Benicar®
Elmisartan	Micardis®
Valsartan	Diovan®

*Generic names end in "sartan."

Beta-blockers are a class of medications that are often added to therapy if the first blood pressure medication along with a diuretic is not effective enough. They are also used in patients with coexisting heart problems. Beta-blockers may generally be taken with or without food, but it is important to take them at about the same time every day.

Your heart rate should be monitored periodically. If your heart rate falls below 50 beats per minute, your provider will need to adjust the dose. Pregnant women generally should not take beta-blockers. Do not stop taking a beta-blocker medication abruptly, unless directed by your provider.[48]

Many people with diabetes experience a fast heart beat if hypoglycemia (low blood glucose) occurs. Beta-blockers may hide this symptom, so you may not realize if your blood glucose level has dropped too low. Other symptoms of hypoglycemia, such as sweating and dizziness, are usually not affected by beta-blockers.[48] Beta-blockers may decrease the amount of insulin released from the pancreas, which may in turn increase blood glucose levels. Glucose monitoring will help you know if beta-blocker therapy is affecting your diabetes control. Share glucose monitoring results with your provider. Beta-blockers are listed in Table 8.3.

Diuretics ("water pills") help control blood pressure by changing how your body uses water, sodium, and potassium. There are 3 types of diuretics, and the thiazide class is often used as one of the first treatment options for high blood pressure. In addition, they are often used with ACE inhibitors or ARBs. Diuretics are listed in Table 8.4.

Diuretics are generally taken once a day. Morning is the best time to take a diuretic because it will increase urination. Taken at bedtime, a diuretic will cause you to get up to go to the bathroom, interrupting your sleep.

Your provider should do laboratory tests to check your kidney function and potassium level before prescribing a diuretic, and should repeat these tests periodically for as long as you take it.[2] Some diuretics may cause your body to lose potassium, while others (potassium-sparing) help your body store potassium. It is dangerous to have potassium levels in your blood that are too high or too low.

If you are taking a diuretic that is not potassium sparing, you may need to include more high-potassium foods (eg, bananas or strawberries) in your diet to replace what is lost in urination. Ask your provider if you need more potassium in your diet. If you develop muscle cramps or tiredness, notify your doctor. This may be a sign of low potassium level.

TABLE 8.3 Recognizing Beta-Blockers	
Generic Name*	**Trade Name**
Acebutolol	Sectral®
Atenolol	Tenormin®
Betaxalol	Kerlone®
Bisoprolol	Zebeta®
Carvedilol	Coreg®
Labetalol	Normodyne®
Metoprolol	Lopressor®, Toprol XL®
Nadolol	Corgard®
Nevebilol	Bystolic®
Penbutolol	Levatol®
Pindolol	Viskin®
Propranolol	Inderal®, Inderal LA®
Ramipril	Blocadren®

*Generic names end in "lol."

TABLE 8.4 Recognizing Diuretics	
Generic Name*	**Trade Name**
Thiazide class:	
Chlorthalidone	Clorpres®
Indapamide	Lozol®
Metolazone	Zaroxolyn®
Loop class:	
Bumetanide	Bumex®
Furosemide	Lasix®
Torsemide	Demedex®
Potassium-sparing class:	
Amiloride	Midamor®
Eplerenone	Inspra®
Spironolactone	Aldactone®
Triamterene	Dyrenium®

*Generic names end in "ide" or "one."

American Association of Diabetes Educators©

Low potassium level in people taking some diuretics increases the risk for stroke.[49,50] Your provider also may prescribe potassium and/or magnesium supplements to replace what you lose in urination.[48] Diuretics are not recommended in pregnancy.

Calcium channel blockers are a class of blood pressure medication that can be tried if you cannot take ACE inhibitors or ARBs. They may work better for black people than other blood pressure medications.[17,22]

Calcium channel blockers should be taken at the same time each day. Taking CCBs with meals will help minimize any stomach side effects, such as nausea or heartburn. Calcium channel blockers are listed in Table 8.5.

Avoid grapefruit juice while taking CCBs, as it can cause the medication to not work.[51] If you develop swelling or have trouble breathing while taking a CCB, notify your provider right away.[48]

High Blood Pressure Medication Use in Pregnancy

The following blood pressure medications have been proven safe and effective for use during pregnancy: methyldopa (Aldomet®), labetalol (Normodyne®), diltiazem (Tiazac®), clonidine (Catapres®), and prazosin (Minipress®).[23]

Angiotensin-converting enzyme inhibitors and ARBs should NOT be used during pregnancy. It is also recommended that pregnant women should not use diuretics long term while pregnant.

Kidney Protection

One of the major reasons that ACE inhibitors and ARBs are chosen as the first medication for blood pressure control in those with diabetes is that they help keep the kidneys healthy and can be taken even if there is no problem with high blood pressure.[52] Preventing problems with the kidneys is extremely important for people with diabetes.

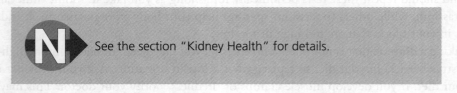

See the section "Kidney Health" for details.

Because people with diabetes often need multiple medications to control their blood pressure, it is important to check on barriers to medication-taking adherence, like cost and medication side effects.

TABLE 8.5	Recognizing CCBs
Generic Name*	**Trade Name**
Amlodipine	Norvasc®
Diltiazem	Cardizem SR®, Cardizem CD®, Cardizem LA®, Tiazac®
Felodipine	Plendil®
Isradipine	DynaCirc CR®
Nicardipine	Cardene SR®
Nifedipine	Adalat CC®, Procardia XL®
Nisoldipine	Sular®
Verapamil	Calan®, Calan SR®, Covera-HS®, Verelan PM®

*Generic names may end in "pine," "mil," or "zem."

Recommended Initial Medication Treatment for Hypertension from JNC8[17]

For the nonblack population, including those with diabetes, beginning treatment for hypertension should include a thiazide-type diuretic, CCB, ACE inhibitor, or ARB.

In the general black population, including those with diabetes, beginning treatment for hypertension should include a thiazide-type diuretic or CCB.

Adults aged 18 or older with chronic kidney disease should have an ACE inhibitor or ARB as an initial or add-on hypertension treatment to protect or improve kidney function. This applies to all races, with or without diabetes.

Lipids

Lipid refers to cholesterol and fat in your blood. Cholesterol is a waxy substance that is found naturally in the body. In fact, the liver regularly produces cholesterol. You need cholesterol for proper body function. Some people make too much cholesterol in their liver, and that is a problem. You also get or make cholesterol from foods you eat.

Not all forms of cholesterol are the same. You've probably heard that there is "good" cholesterol and "bad" cholesterol. Depending on the type of cholesterol, having too much or not enough can cause problems in the body. Let's look at the difference between the types of cholesterol.

Using alliteration can be a useful teaching tool to help remember important facts, especially for those with verbal/auditory intelligence. To help distinguish which lipid reading is healthy and which should be higher than or lower than the target, use these alliterations:

Limit **L**DL, **L**ower **L**DL and **H**ealthy **H**DL, **H**igh **H**DL

LDL Cholesterol

LDL stands for low-density lipoprotein. Particles of LDL cholesterol are considered to be the "bad" form of cholesterol. In the right amount, LDL is not really bad. But if you have too many LDL particles in your blood, they tend to collect in the blood vessel walls. They can build up, forming plaque, which can decrease or block your blood flow. If the plaque bursts or breaks off, a clot can form. If this happens in the blood vessels in the brain, it can lead to a stroke. If it happens in the blood vessels in the heart, it can lead to a heart attack. In the legs, it can lead to circulation problems to your legs and feet. That's why you want to **L**imit **LDL**; a **l**ower number for LDL is better.

HDL Cholesterol

HDL stands for high-density lipoprotein. Particles of HDL cholesterol are considered to be the "good" form of cholesterol. HDL cholesterol particles do good things in the blood vessels. As they circulate through your body, they attract particles of LDL cholesterol. The HDL particles pick up the LDL particles that are within your vessels and take them to the liver, where they drop them off for reprocessing. One way to remember which cholesterol is the "good" form is to think of HDL as the cleaning crew that helps rid your blood vessels of the particles that can lead to plaque formation. That's why it's **H**ealthy to have a **h**igh number for **HDL**.

Triglycerides

Triglycerides are the fats in our blood, such as the fat from our diet that is absorbed during digestion. Other body processes can also add fat to our blood. Too much fat in the blood can build up plaque, which can lead to blockages in our blood vessels.

304   Diabetes Education Curriculum

Standard of Medical Care in Diabetes[2]

For adults with diabetes, a lipid screening at diagnosis and periodically (eg, every 1 to 2 years) thereafter is reasonable.

- ◆ The lipids blood test should be done fasting.
- ◆ High-dose statin therapy is recommended for all adults with diabetes who have cardiovascular disease (CVD), regardless of LDL level.
- ◆ Consider moderate- to high-dose statin and lifestyle therapy for adults with diabetes younger than 40 who have CVD risk factors.
- ◆ For people with diabetes who are aged 40 and over without CVD risk factors, consider using a moderate statin dose and lifestyle therapy.
- ◆ For those aged 40 to 75 with CVD risk factors, consider a high-dose statin and lifestyle therapy.

Standard of Medical Care in Diabetes[24,26]

In children aged 2 and over with type 1 diabetes, measure lipids after diagnosis when blood glucose is controlled. Monitor annually if lipids are abnormal. If LDL is under 100 mg/dL (5.55 mmol/L), repeat screening every 5 years.[24]

All children with type 2 diabetes should have a baseline fasting lipid screening.[24]

Lipid Targets

While lipid levels are important, part of the decision to use a statin drug is based on whether you have heart problems or heart disease risk factors, which include high blood pressure, smoking, overweight/obesity, and LDL cholesterol at 100 mg/dL (5.55 mmol/L) or higher, and your age. All individuals with LDL levels at or above 100 mg/dL should also include lifestyle changes as part of their care.

Statin drugs are recommended for all adults with diabetes who have or have had heart problems. In addition, statins are recommended for all people with diabetes over the age of 40, even if they have no heart problems and no heart disease risk factors. Of course, lifestyle changes are also important.

Statin medications don't work the same way in all people. Keeping the heart healthy is directly linked to the statin's ability to lower LDL cholesterol levels. So you will want to work with your provider to find the type of statin that works best for you. Once you find a statin that works for you and you are on a stable dose, your provider may order cholesterol tests less often.

There are also other drugs that are used to help lower LDL levels. However, there is currently no strong evidence that it is helpful to add another drug to your statin therapy to treat your LDL level.

High triglycerides (at or above 150 mg/dL [8.33 mmol/L] when you have not eaten for more than 8 hours) and/or low HDL (under 40 mg/dL [2.22 mmol/L] for men and less than 50 mg/dL [2.77 mmol/L] for women) may be treated with lifestyle therapy and improved blood glucose control. If fasting triglycerides are equal to or higher than 500 mg/dL (27.77 mmol/L), your provider will check for other causes of the high triglycerides and you may need medication. For triglycerides over 1000 mg/dL (55.55 mmol/L), medications such as fibric acid or fish oil are usually needed right away.

Another time you may take another medication for your cholesterol is when your HDL is under 40 mg/dL (2.22 mmol/L) and your LDL is between 100 mg/dL (5.55 mmol/L) and 125 mg/dL (6.94 mmol/L). Your provider may give you a fibrate or niacin, especially if you cannot take a statin. There was one study that showed niacin

---

American Association of Diabetes Educators©

TABLE 8.6 Recommendations for Statin Treatment in People With Diabetes

Age	Risk Factors	Recommended Statin Dose (in Addition to Lifestyle Therapy)	Schedule to Monitor Lipids
Less than 40 years	None	None	Annually or as needed to check adherence to treatment
	CVD risk factors	Moderate or high	
	Overt CVD	High	
40 to 75 years	None	Moderate	As needed to check adherence to treatment
	CVD risk factors	High	
	Overt CVD	High	
Over 75 years	None	Moderate	As needed to check adherence to treatment
	CVD risk factors	Moderate or high	
	Overt CVD	High	

Sources: PA James, S Oparil, BL Carter, et al, "2014 evidence-based guideline for the management of high blood pressure in adults: report from the panel members appointed to the Eighth Joint National Committee (JNC8)," *JAMA* 311 (2014): 507-20; American Diabetes Association, "Cardiovascular disease and risk management—2015," *Diabetes Care* 38, Suppl 1 (2015): S49-57.

with a statin did not help with preventing heart problems more than just a statin alone. In fact, those given niacin may have had an increase in stroke risk.

Most efforts should focus on lowering your LDL with statins. In addition, those with a history of heart problems and those with heart disease risk factors should be treated with statins, regardless of LDL levels. See Table 8.6 for recommendations for statin treatment in people with diabetes.

Controlling lipids is JUST AS IMPORTANT as glucose control to reduce your risk for complications. There are lots of things you can do to help decrease LDL and triglycerides and raise HDL.

Healthy Eating[53,54]

- Limit foods high in saturated fat—common sources include cheese, pizza, fatty meats, and large servings of meat or chicken.
- Limit cholesterol to less than 200 mg per day—cholesterol is only found in animal products.
- Avoid trans fats—often found in fried foods, fast foods, and store-bought baked goods.
- Include 2 servings per week of fish with omega-3 fatty acids, such as sardines, albacore tuna, salmon, mackerel, cod, or herring.[55,56]
- Eat more fiber, especially from oats, citrus fruits, and dried beans (such as black, lima, navy, or pinto beans).[57-59]
- Choose healthier liquid oils such as canola or olive oil instead of butter, lard, sour cream, or shortening.

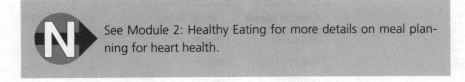

See Module 2: Healthy Eating for more details on meal planning for heart health.

Being Active

Being physically active may help with weight loss and raise HDL levels.[60]

Taking Medication

As mentioned already, most people with diabetes will benefit from taking a moderate- or high-dose statin whether or not they have high cholesterol levels. Most of the effort should focus on lowering LDL cholesterol levels. The statins lower the risk of developing heart problems. For those who already have heart problems, it can help protect them from having further problems. Using additional medications to control LDL has not shown to improve heart health and is generally not recommended.

The following is an extensive (but not exhaustive) list of lipid medications. Share with participants only the information that is relevant to their prescribed medications to facilitate safe and effective medication-taking behavior.

Adults learn best when the content is meaningful to their experience and fills a perceived need. Help each participant identify the lipid medication(s) he or she takes. Then, share only the salient points about the medication(s). Don't overwhelm with information that is not relevant.

Statins are one of the most widely used lipid medications. They *keep your liver from making too much cholesterol, as well as help you clear away LDL cholesterol.* The generic names of these medications end in *statin*. It is generally best to take a statin at supper or bedtime (with or without food), because your liver starts making cholesterol in the nighttime hours.

Your provider should do certain laboratory tests to check the health of your kidneys and liver before starting you on a statin and shortly after you begin taking the statin. You shouldn't need more liver tests unless you have signs of liver problems such as unusual fatigue, loss of appetite, pain in the upper portion of your stomach area, dark urine, or your eyes or skin turns yellow. See Table 8.7 for a list of statins.

If you experience muscle weakness, tenderness, pain, or fever after starting a statin, notify your doctor. Statins should not be taken during pregnancy.[48]

Ezetimibe (Zetia®) keeps you from absorbing too much cholesterol from your intestine. Take this medication with or without food. Your provider should do certain laboratory tests to check the health of your liver before starting you on this medication.[48]

Some lipid medications bind to bile, so less cholesterol is produced (eg, **colesevelam [Welchol®], colestipol [Colestid®],** and **cholestryramine [Questran®]**). Gastrointestinal side effects, including flatulence, bloating, constipation, and a bad taste in the mouth, are common. You should take your other medications either 1 hour before or 4 hours after taking any of these cholesterol medications.[48]

TABLE 8.7	Recognizing Statins
Generic Name	**Trade Name**
Atorvastatin	Lipitor®
Fluvastatin	Lescol®
Lovastatin	Mevacor®
Pravastatin	Pravachol®
Rosuvastatin	Crestor®
Simvastatin	Zocor®

Lipid medications that are mainly used for lowering triglycerides include **fenofibrate (Tricor®)** and **gemfibrozil (Lopid®)**. Take gemfibrozil 30 minutes before a meal. Take fenofibrate with food. Gastrointestinal side effects, including flatulence, diarrhea, indigestion, nausea, and abdominal pain, are common. Your provider should do certain laboratory tests to check the health of your liver before starting you on this medication, and should repeat these tests periodically for as long as you take this medication. *If you experience muscle weakness, tenderness, pain, or fever after starting this medication, notify your doctor.* This type of medication should not be taken by people with gallbladder or liver problems, or severe kidney disease.[48]

Niacin (Niaspan®, Niacin®, Slo-Niacin®) works to increase HDL cholesterol, and to some extent lowers LDL cholesterol and triglycerides.[48] Gastrointestinal side effects of nausea, vomiting, or diarrhea are common. Drinking alcohol or hot beverages can cause facial flushing and itching. Take niacin at bedtime, 30 to 45 minutes after a full-strength aspirin or with a low-fat snack to minimize flushing effects. Niacin in doses >2 g per day also raises blood sugar, which is of course a concern for people with diabetes.

If you get up during the night, be sure to do so slowly to avoid falling. Niacin can cause the blood pressure to drop quickly when changing from a lying to a standing position. Your provider should do certain laboratory tests to check glucose, uric acid, and the health of your liver before starting you on this medication, and should repeat these tests periodically for as long as you take this medication.[48,61]

Omega-3 Fatty Acids (Lovaza® [previously named Omacor®] or over-the-counter fish oil) work mainly to lower triglycerides. Usually fish intake is not adequate for lowering triglycerides. Supplementation with omega-3 therapy is usually necessary when triglycerides are too high.[55,56,62]

Omega-3s also have a beneficial effect on HDL. Take Lovaza® with food to minimize side effects such as nausea, abdominal pain, and heartburn. Your provider should do certain laboratory tests to check the health of your liver before starting you on this medication, and should repeat these tests periodically for as long as you take this medication. If you also take blood-thinning medication while taking Lovaza®, you will need periodic laboratory tests to check your bleeding times. Your provider can advise you if over-the-counter fish oil capsules or liquid will be effective for your needs.

Combination lipid medications include 2 medications in one pill: ezetimibe plus simvastatin (**Vytorin®**) or lovastatin plus niacin (**Advicor®**).

Reducing Risks

- Maintain a healthy weight.
- Stop smoking. See Figure 8.1 and the "Resources" section for tips on quitting smoking.

> **Standard of Medical Care in Diabetes[2]**
>
> All patients should receive counseling to not use tobacco products.
> Smoking cessation counseling and other forms of treatment should be considered as a routine part of diabetes care.

> **If there are smokers in the group, invite any willing participant who has successfully quit smoking to share with others in the group how he or she did it.**
>
> The learning experience is enhanced for adults with social/interpersonal intelligence when they are allowed to "tell their story" to help another learner. Participants in a group setting can draw strength and encouragement from one another, if given the opportunity.

308   Diabetes Education Curriculum

FIGURE 8.1 Tips to Quit Smoking

1. Set a quit date.
2. Let friends and family know that you are planning to quit and let them know how they can help you.
3. Change your environment—get rid of all cigarettes, lighters, and ashtrays at work, home, or in your car. Freshen up your home and car to get rid of the tobacco smell.
4. List reasons why you want to quit (be healthier, protect family from smoke, save money) and remind yourself of those reasons every day. It may also be helpful to write them down and post them somewhere that you will see them often.
5. Identify smoking triggers and make a plan to deal with them.
6. Find ways to cope with the withdrawal from nicotine (meds, nicotine replacement, and behavior modification can help).
7. Know where you can go for help.
   - Friends and family
   - Tell your doctor. Ask for smoking cessation medication and referral to a program or counseling.
   - Plug into a smoking cessation program:
     — Call a quit line such as 1-800-QUIT-NOW (1-800-784-8669).
     — Join an online quit program like the Freedom from Smoking Online from the American Lung Association (ffsonline.org).
     — Sign up for text messaging at smokefree.gov.
     — Download and use a quit-smoking app.
     — Attend a smoking cessation program.

If you slip up, set a new quit date and try again. Some people need several tries before they quit smoking.

North American Quitline Consortium: 1-800-QUIT-NOW, http://www.naquitline.org/indexasp?dbsection=map&dbid=1.

Click on the map to find a smoking cessation program in your state. Find out if the program in your state offers telephone counseling and/or free or discounted smoking cessation medication.

QuitNet: https://quitnet.meyouhealth.com/#/

Smokefree.gov: 1-877-44U-QUIT, http://smokefree.gov

Trained smoking cessation counselors from the National Cancer Institute can help via real-time instant messaging (English) or by telephone (English/Spanish).

Aspirin Therapy

Standard of Medical Care in Diabetes[2]

Aspirin therapy (75 to 162 mg per day) is recommended for those with diabetes who already have cardiovascular disease.

Consider aspirin therapy in those who are at higher cardiovascular risk (includes most men with diabetes over age 50 or women over the age of 60 with at least 1 major CVD risk factor such as smoking, high blood pressure, abnormal lipid levels, abnormal urine protein levels, or family history of cardiovascular disease).

Aspirin is not recommended for CVD prevention for adults with low CVD risk such as men under 50 and women under 60 with no other CVD risk factors.

For people with CVD and aspirin allergy, clopidogrel should be used (75 mg per day).

Two antiplatelet drugs should be given for up to 1 year after a coronary event.

American Association of Diabetes Educators©

Aspirin is an inexpensive form of treatment that can help lower the risk of dying or having additional heart problems in those people who have already had a stroke or heart attack. Aspirin has also been shown to be a reasonable treatment for adults with diabetes who are at higher risk for having heart problems—this includes most men with diabetes who are over the age of 50 and women over the age of 60 who have at least 1 major heart disease risk factor such as family history of heart disease, high blood pressure, smoking, protein in the urine, or abnormal lipid levels.

One baby aspirin is 81 mg. One regular-strength aspirin is 325 mg; if you use a regular-strength aspirin, you should split it and take half to get the 162-mg dose. *If you notice any bleeding or bruising problems while taking aspirin, notify your provider.*

If you do not already take aspirin, ask your provider if aspirin is safe for you. If you are at high risk for heart disease but are allergic to aspirin or have bleeding problems, your provider may consider therapy with an antiplatelet medication (eg, clopidogrel [Plavix®]).[63]

At this time, it is no longer recommended that people with diabetes at lower risk of developing heart disease take aspirin daily; that includes most men under the age of 50 and most women younger than 60 who have no other major heart disease risk factors.[2] Check with your doctor before stopping aspirin, as sudden stopping may have some negative effects. Aspirin is not recommended for people younger than 21 years because of the risk for Reye syndrome.[63]

Kidney Health

Having diabetes increases a person's risk for diabetic kidney disease, also known as *diabetic nephropathy*. Monitoring the health of your kidneys means keeping tabs on your blood glucose, blood pressure, and tests that measure protein in the urine.

The kidneys serve a number of functions in your body, including[64(p531)]:

- Cleaning waste and toxins from the blood
- Managing fluid and electrolytes (eg, sodium, potassium)
- Helping to regulate blood pressure
- Helping to make red blood cells
- Helping to maintain the health of the bones

If a person has high levels of blood glucose (and/or high blood pressure) for a long time, it can slowly damage the kidneys. The parts of the kidney that filter the blood begin to break down. You may not even know this is happening. One of the first signs of kidney disease is too much protein (albumin) in the urine.

One of the tests used to check the health of your kidneys is the urine albumin to creatinine ratio (UACR). Another test checks your blood creatinine level, which your provider can use to tell what your estimated glomerular filtration rate (eGFR) is—this tells you how well your kidneys are cleaning your blood. These tests should be done right away for all with type 2 diabetes and after 5 years for those with type 1 diabetes and then once a year for all after that.

A UACR of 30 to 299 mg/g may mean early kidney disease in those with type 1 diabetes and a possible increased risk of kidney disease in those with type 2 diabetes. It is also linked to an increased risk of heart disease. Many (40%) of those with type 1 diabetes show improvement in UACR, while 30% to 40% of those with diabetes and elevated UACR do not get any worse over the next 5 to 10 years. Those who constantly have protein in their urine are most likely to develop kidney disease.

For patients who feel kidney-related complications are inevitable, help them build a more realistic outlook by:

- Examining beliefs, expectations, and assumptions about their vulnerability to kidney-related complications.
- Presenting evidence that metabolic control can lower risk, and correlating that evidence to their actual situation (eg, their own A1C, blood pressure, and lipid values).

> **Standard of Medical Care in Diabetes[2]**
>
> - Beginning at diagnosis, and repeated each year, adults with type 2 diabetes should be screened for diabetic kidney disease.
> - Adults with type 1 diabetes should begin screening 5 years after diagnosis and then annually.
> - The preferred test is the UACR. A blood creatinine test should also be taken, which is then used to calculate the eGFR.
> - A blood test for creatinine should be done at least annually for all adults with diabetes, regardless of urine protein status.

The target for UACR is <30 mcg/mg (micrograms [mcg] of albumin per milligrams [mg] of creatinine).[2] Your provider may perform the microalbumin-to-creatinine test a number of times within a 3- to 6-month period to be sure of your kidney status. The eGFR will help show how well your kidneys are working. Greater than or equal to 90 means your kidneys are cleaning your blood well. When it gets below 15, your kidneys are not working well, and you will probably need dialysis.

> **Standard of Medical Care in Diabetes[2,65]**
>
> - Children with type 1 diabetes should have urine microalbumin-to-creatinine ratio testing once he or she reaches age 10 and has had diabetes for 5 years. Testing should then be done annually.
> - Children with type 2 diabetes should have annual urine microalbumin-to-creatinine ratio testing.

Reducing Your Risk for Diabetic Kidney Disease

There are many things you can do every day to reduce your risk for getting kidney disease.

- **Control blood glucose as best you can.** Studies show that keeping blood glucose near normal dramatically lowers the risk for kidney disease. In studies involving people with type 1 diabetes, controlling glucose led to a 56% reduction in risk.[7] In type 2 diabetes studies, the risk was lowered 25%.[9-11] This means that your efforts at managing diabetes can go a long way to keeping your kidneys healthy. Even if a person already has diabetic kidney disease, glucose control will help delay further progression. See Table 8.8 for the stages of chronic kidney disease.
- **Control blood pressure by whatever means necessary.**[15,66] If a person already has diabetic kidney disease, blood pressure control will help delay further progression.[66,67]

 See the section "Controlling Blood Pressure" for details.

- Take an ACE inhibitor or ARB if your urinary albumin is greater than 300 mg per day, and it is suggested for those with urinary albumin between 30 and 299 mg per day. Do not take if pregnant. Your provider should also check your blood creatinine and potassium levels if you are taking an ACE, ARB, or diuretic. Angiotensin receptor blockers can help slow down increases in albumin in the urine and protect the kidneys. Angiotensin-converting enzyme inhibitors help with heart protection when urinary albumin levels are high. There is no benefit of taking ACE inhibitors and ARBs together.[2]

TABLE 8.8	Stages of Chronic Kidney Disease	
Stage	Description	GFR 9mL/min/1.73 m²
1	Kidney damage with normal or increased GFR	≥90
2	Kidney damage with slightly decreased GFR	60–89
3	GFR that is moderately decreased	30–59
4	GFR that is severely decreased	15–29
5	Kidney failure	<15 or dialysis

❖ Keep your protein intake around 0.8 g/kg per day (based on ideal body weight) if you already have diabetic kidney disease. A dietitian can customize a meal plan to help you accomplish this goal. This is the amount of daily protein that an average adult needs. Compared with the usual protein intake of most adults, though, *this may seem like a restriction.*[2] Lower amounts of protein are not recommended.

Eye Health

Having diabetes increases a person's risk for diabetic eye disease, also known as *diabetic retinopathy.* Monitoring the health of your eyes means keeping tabs on your blood glucose level[8,9] and blood pressure,[11,17,68] and having regular eye examinations. Also, if you have kidney disease, you are more likely to have eye problems.[2]

At the back of the eye there is a layer of nerve cells that are responsible for vision. This part of the eye is called the retina. Tiny blood vessels bring oxygen and nutrients to the retina. If these vessels are exposed to high levels of glucose (and/or high blood pressure) for a long time, they become weakened.

Weakened vessels allow leakage of fluid into the eye. If leakage gets into a part of the eye called the macula, it can cause problems with the part of the eye that allows for your central vision. This is referred to as *macular edema.*

If eye vessel damage continues, these weakened vessels gradually close up, and blood flow to the retina stops. New vessels grow to replace the damaged ones, so that the retina can still receive oxygen and nutrients. Unfortunately, the new vessels are very fragile and break easily. This causes bleeding in the eye.[69]

In the early and middle stages of retinopathy, there may be no obvious changes in vision. Vision changes typically occur only after there is an extensive amount of vessel damage. This means that even if your vision seems normal, you can't assume that your eyes are OK.

The only way to be assured that your eyes are healthy is to have a dilated eye examination, where the eye doctor puts drops in your eyes. Having this examination regularly allows for early detection of any problems and treatment, which saves vision.

Cataract, glaucoma, and other eye problems are also more common in people with diabetes.[2]

Standard of Medical Care in Diabetes

Adults with type 1 or type 2 diabetes:

❖ Beginning at diagnosis, and repeated each year, adults with type 2 diabetes should have a dilated eye examination.[70]

❖ Adults with type 1 diabetes should have their first dilated eye examination 5 years after diagnosis and then annually.[71]

❖ Less frequent exams may be considered after 1 or more eye examinations with normal results.[2]

❖ If you have already been diagnosed with retinopathy, you may need to have eye examinations more often than each year. In this case, it's important to see if your eye condition is advancing and whether treatment is needed.[72(p766),73]

American Association of Diabetes Educators©

312   Diabetes Education Curriculum

Standard of Medical Care in Diabetes[2]

Pregnant women with type 1 or type 2 diabetes:

- Women with type 1 or type 2 diabetes who are contemplating pregnancy should be informed that there is an increased risk of developing retinopathy during pregnancy. Pregnancy can cause preexisting retinopathy to worsen.

- Women with diabetes who are planning to become pregnant should have a comprehensive diabetic eye examination before conception.

- Pregnant women with preexisting type 1 or type 2 diabetes should have a comprehensive diabetic eye examination in their first trimester.

- Close follow-up during pregnancy and for 1 year after childbirth is important to monitor for retinopathy.

Standard of Medical Care in Diabetes

Children with type 1 or type 2 diabetes:

- Children with type 1 diabetes should have their first diabetic eye examination once they have reached age 10 <u>AND</u> have had diabetes for 3 to 5 years.

- Annual updates are generally recommended, but they may be less frequent on the advice of the ophthalmologist.[2]

- Adolescents with type 2 diabetes should have an eye examination at diagnosis and then annually.[65]

General Vision Examination Versus Diabetic Eye Examination: What's the Difference?

It's important that you understand the difference between an examination for diabetic eye disease and a general examination meant to check your vision and fit you for glasses. These 2 types of examinations are usually covered under different parts of health insurance. The general vision examination is typically part of the vision (optical) plan benefits; the diabetic eye examination is usually under the medical plan benefits.

General Vision Examination

A general vision examination will measure your vision by having you read letters that get smaller, row by row. This determines your visual acuity (eg, 20/20 vision). A refraction test may be done to find the best corrected vision if you need prescription glasses or contacts. A color blindness test is also done, as well as a pressure test to check for glaucoma. A handheld instrument called an ophthalmoscope is used to look into the inside of the eye. The eye may or may not be dilated to allow a wider view of the retina.

Getting Prescription Lenses (Glasses or Contacts)

If you are planning to have a general vision examination to update your lens prescription, do it when your blood glucose is close to normal. If you get prescription lenses made while your vision is blurry, they may not be effective later on when your glucose is normalized.[74(p523)] This will save you time, money, and frustration.

Diabetic Eye Examination

The diabetic eye examination generally includes the tests that are performed in the general examination. The focus is then turned to the internal structure of the eye. The eye specialist will carefully examine your retina, the

American Association of Diabetes Educators©

back of the eye, to look for retinopathy. It is recommended that the diabetic eye examination be performed by an ophthalmologist or an optometrist.

A direct examination with the eye care specialist will require dilation of the pupils. This is done by putting drops of a dilating solution in each eye. After a while, the pupils open wide. You will be sensitive to light during this time, and your vision will be blurry. The examination uses equipment that helps hold your head still. Have a pair of sunglasses to protect your eyes for the ride home. Generally, a report is mailed to your primary care provider to be put in your medical record.

Another acceptable option for visualizing the retina is by way of retinal photography. In retinal photography, a trained technician takes pictures of your retinas using a high-powered camera. The camera is mounted on equipment that helps hold your head still. Your eyes may or may not need dilation, depending on the imaging system used. The photographs are examined and interpreted by specialists. If the photographs show abnormalities, then you are referred for an in-person examination with the ophthalmologist.[75]

Reducing Your Risk for Diabetic Eye Disease

There are things you can do every day to reduce your risk for getting eye disease.

- **Control blood glucose as best you can.** Studies show that keeping blood glucose near normal dramatically lowers the risk for eye disease. In studies involving people with type 1 diabetes, controlling glucose led to a 76% reduction in risk for eye disease.[8] Studies in people with type 2 diabetes also show that lowering blood glucose reduces the risk for eye disease.[9] Efforts at managing diabetes will go a long way to keeping your eyes healthy. And if a person already has diabetic eye disease, diabetes control will help delay further progression.[9]

- **Control blood pressure by whatever means necessary.** Even if a person already has diabetic eye disease, blood pressure control will help delay further progression.[16,68]

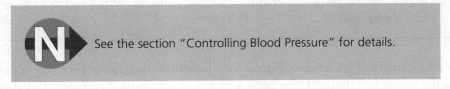

See the section "Controlling Blood Pressure" for details.

If a person is found to have diabetic eye disease, treatment is aimed at maintaining vision and preventing any further damage. Laser surgery is an outpatient procedure that cauterizes the bleeding vessels in the eye. It can also be done to treat macular edema. Laser surgery can help lower the risk for further vision loss, but it can't reverse vision loss that has already happened.[76,77]

Adults learn best when they can relate new information to what they already know. Consider comparing nerve fibers to electrical cords; eg, electricity cannot flow properly through a damaged cord. This technique is particularly helpful for those with visual/spatial intelligence.

See the "Resources" section at the end of this module for "Resources for People With Impaired Vision"—which can be used as a handout for patients with vision loss. Discuss state and local resources available for persons with vision loss, and refer as necessary.

For patients who feel vision-related complications are inevitable, help them build a more realistic outlook by:

- Examining beliefs, expectations, and assumptions about their vulnerability to vision-related complications.
- Presenting evidence that metabolic control can lower risk, and correlating that evidence to their actual situation (eg, their own A1C, blood pressure, and lipid values).

Nerve Health

Having diabetes increases a person's risk for diabetic nerve disease, also known as *diabetic neuropathy*. Monitoring the health of your nerves means keeping tabs on your blood glucose level,[7,10,11,16] being aware of important symptoms to report, and having regular medical examinations.

Nerves are present throughout the body. Some nerves allow for body movement and sensation. These nerves are called *peripheral nerves*. Other nerves allow for automatic functions like heart beat, bowel and bladder function, sweating, and sexual responsiveness. These nerves are called *autonomic nerves*.

Standard of Medical Care in Diabetes

- Beginning at diagnosis, and repeated each year, people with type 2 diabetes should be screened for diabetic peripheral neuropathy.[2,78] Those with type 1 diabetes should begin annual screenings 5 years after diagnosis.
- People with neuropathy should have a visual inspection of the feet at each visit with their provider.[2]

When nerves are exposed to high levels of glucose for a long time, they can begin to break down and "misfire." This changes how the nerves function and may cause a variety of symptoms. Symptoms vary depending on where in the body the affected nerves are located. Symptoms also vary from person to person.

Peripheral Neuropathy

One part of the body where nerve damage can occur is the feet. About half of the people with diabetes who have nerve damage to the feet, called *peripheral neuropathy*, feel no symptoms. Others have burning, tingling, and numbness in their feet, and for some, the pain can be severe.[79-81] If not detected and treated, nerve damage to your feet can lead to serious problems.

Getting a foot exam at least once a year is important. One thing your provider will do to check for nerve damage is touch your feet in different places with a tuning fork or a monofilament (it is sort of like a toothpick that bends). If you can't feel 1 or more of the touches, you are at higher risk for injuring your foot and may not even know it (eg, you could step on a small piece of broken glass or a tack and not feel a thing). That small injury could become infected, and you probably would not feel that, either. If not treated, it could lead to an amputation. The good news is that up to 75% of amputations can be prevented with good foot care and glucose control.[2,79,80]

Some people with diabetes should be referred to a foot care specialist for ongoing preventive care with lifelong follow-up. This group includes those with loss of protective sensation or abnormal foot structure, or those with a history of lower leg complications.[2]

Reducing Your Risk for Foot Problems

There are things you can do to lower your risk for neuropathy and foot problems.

T&L Engage learners in critical thinking activities by asking them to think of a situation (being at the clinic) and what they could do to influence the outcome (ensure the doctor looks at their feet). Those with logical intelligence will especially benefit from this approach to learning.

When you go to the doctor, what can you do to make sure he or she takes a look at your feet?

- **At each visit to the provider, ask that he or she looks at your feet.**[80] This is an opportunity to catch any small problems before they become big problems. Once you get into the examination room, go ahead and take off your socks and shoes and have your feet visible and ready for the provider.
- **Tell your provider about any abnormal feelings in your feet, legs, or hands.** If nerve pain is an ongoing problem, discuss treatment options with your provider. There are medications that can help relieve neuropathic pain. They include amitriptyline (Elavil®, Endep®); nortriptyline (Aventyl®, Pamelor®); imipramine (Tofranil®); gabapentin (Neurontin®), carbamazepine (Tegretol®); pregabalin (Lyrica®); duloxetine (Cymbalta®), and capsaicin cream.
- **Control blood glucose as best you can.** Studies show that keeping blood glucose near normal greatly lowers the risk for nerve disease.[11,17] In studies involving people with type 1 diabetes, controlling glucose led to a 60% reduction in risk.[8] Efforts at managing diabetes will go a long way to keeping your nerves healthy. And if a person already has diabetic nerve disease, diabetes control will help delay further progression.
- **If you smoke, stop.** Smoking constricts your blood vessels. Over time, this decreases the blood flow to your feet, which raises your risk for poor healing if you get a foot injury or infection.[82] The Surgeon General said that "smoking cessation is the most important intervention in the management of peripheral artery occlusive disease."[83]

What have you been told about taking care of your feet?
What can a person do if he or she has trouble seeing his or her feet?
Probe for use of home remedies or alternative therapies: *What kind of home remedies or cures do you use for your feet?*

- **If you drink alcohol, practice moderation.** Excessive alcohol intake can cause nerve damage and/or make existing neuropathy worse.[84] Of course, no drinking alcohol when you are pregnant!
- **Take care of your feet.** Proper foot care guidelines include the following actions[4,85,86]:
  - *Check your feet daily.* Tops, bottoms, sides, and between the toes. Look to see if there are any breaks in the skin, cuts, calluses, or changes in skin color or temperature that might indicate infection. If you can't easily see the bottoms of your feet, use a mirror (or a magnifying mirror). You can also ask someone else to look at your feet. If you can't see your feet, and no one is able to help you, at least feel your feet with your hands to check for any changes in texture or temperature. Notify your provider promptly if you have any problems.
  - *Wear shoes at all times, even when you are indoors.* Make sure your shoes fit well and don't cause skin irritations. Shake your shoes out before putting them on.

American Association of Diabetes Educators©

See the "Resources" section at the end of this module for "Medicare Part B Coverage of Therapeutic Shoes and Inserts." Consider using it as a patient handout.

—*If you wear closed shoes, also wear clean socks that fit well.* Consider the following when choosing socks[87]:
- For healthy feet, choose socks that fit well, are not too tight at the top, and have no lumps or uncomfortable seams.
- For feet at risk for ulcers, densely padded socks are preferred. Studies were done with 100% acrylic socks with nylon and spandex added to make the socks more elastic (cotton socks were not studied).
- For people who jog or do vigorous activities, padded acrylic socks may be best.
- Choosing light-colored socks will help you see any signs of drainage or blood if your foot is injured.

—*Keep your feet clean.* After washing, dry thoroughly, especially between your toes.

—*Keep skin moisturized to prevent cracking.* Cracks in the skin are open doors to germs that can cause infection. Don't put moisturizer *between* the toes, as this may keep skin too wet. Wet skin can lead to fungus or skin sloughing (peeling). Avoid moisturizers that contain alcohol, as this tends to dry the skin.

—*Cut toenails straight across, the nail tip following the shape of the toe.* The best time to trim toenails is after a bath or shower, when they are softer and easier to cut. Avoid cutting into the corners, as this may lead to problems with ingrown nails. File the sharp edges of the nails. If you can't reach your toes easily or you can't see them well, ask a professional to do the trimming.

—*Avoid routine soaking in hot water.* Check the temperature of the water with your elbow to avoid getting scalded by hot water. If your skin wrinkles ("prunes") after being in water, it's a sign that you soaked for too long. During a prolonged soak, moisture is removed from the skin. If you have dry skin to begin with, long soaks will ultimately make it worse. Soaking also softens the skin, which allows any germs in the water to move deeper into your skin. This can increase your risk for infection.

—*Avoid drug-store remedies that contain chemicals to remove warts, corns, and calluses.* These chemicals can cause a skin ulcer. Ask your provider for assistance with warts, corns, or calluses.

—*Avoid using sharp instruments on the skin.* Clipping dead skin off the feet is risky and can lead to injury and skin infection. Soft buffing with a pumice stone can safely remove dead skin cells, but scraping with metal instruments is riskier. If you have neuropathy and cannot feel your feet properly, avoid buffing away dead skin cells. You may not realize it if you are buffing too hard.

Autonomic Neuropathy

It is important to tell your provider about any changes you have noticed. Nerve damage can affect most any part of your body and cause problems with sexual function, your stomach, your bladder, and your intestines. You may also have heart problems that are linked to nerve damage. Your doctor may check you for dangerous drops in your blood pressure or a fast heart rate, which are 2 signs of possible nerve damage to your heart. Also, if you have felt dizzy, fainted, or are much more tired than usual, be sure to tell your provider.

Standard of Medical Care in Diabetes[2,88]

Consider screening for signs and symptoms (eg, drop in blood pressure upon standing, resting elevated heart rate) of cardiovascular autonomic neuropathy (CAN) in those with more advanced disease.

Advanced Detail

Is it safe for a person with diabetes to have a pedicure?

There is always an element of risk when you have a pedicure, whether or not you have diabetes. Risks involve skin or nail infection from unclean water, equipment, or instruments. The technician may accidentally clip your nail too short or cut your skin. Your risk is higher because of diabetes.

- If glucose levels are above target, there is a higher risk for infection.
- If you have poor circulation, you may not heal as well if infection or injury occurs.
- If you have neuropathy in your feet, you may not realize if the water is too hot. You may not feel it if the technician is too aggressive when buffing the skin.

For these reasons, pedicures *cannot be recommended* for people with diabetes. If you choose to have a pedicure despite the risks, advise the technician of your diabetes. Request that any buffing of the skin be done gently, and with a pumice stone, not a metal instrument. Check to make sure the salon sterilizes equipment between customers. Be sure that it sanitizes its pedicure tubs and changes filters appropriately. If you choose to have a pedicure, proceed as an informed consumer, aware of the risks.

Good blood glucose control and avoiding wide swings in glucose levels is the only thing that has been found to work well to prevent or delay nerve damage in those with type 1 diabetes and slow down nerve damage in those with type 2 diabetes.[2] Other specific treatment of nerve damage depends on what body system is affected.

Table 8.9 contains an extensive list of the different types of neuropathy and relevant education points. Share content with participant(s) only as indicated, per individual situation and/or participant inquiry.

TABLE 8.9 Important Points About Living With Neuropathy

If you have . . .	You should . . .
Cardiac Denervation Syndrome ***What it is:*** Neuropathy of the nerves that control the heart and blood vessels. ***Symptoms:*** Resting heart rate >100 beats per minute that does not respond to stress or exercise; blood pressure drops more than 20 points when standing up; changes in breathing or sleep; if heart attack occurs, there may be no warning symptoms of chest pain (silent heart attack).	• Avoid heavy exercise, aerobic exercise, and straining. • Ask your provider to prescribe a stress test before you start any exercise program. • Get physical therapy to help improve strength and balance. • Take prescribed medications that can help normalize your heart rate.

(continued)

TABLE 8.9 Important Points About Living With Neuropathy *(continued)*

If you have . . .	You should . . .
Postural Hypotension ***What it is:*** Neuropathy of the nerves that control blood pressure. ***Symptoms:*** Sudden drop in blood pressure upon standing, causing dizziness, light-headedness, weakness, or fainting.	• Be aware of your risk for falling. • Always get up slowly from a lying position. • Keep the head of the bed elevated 30 degrees. • Wear waist-high elastic support stockings to keep blood from pooling. • Take prescribed medications that can help normalize your blood pressure.
Gastroparesis ***What it is:*** Neuropathy of the nerves that control the upper intestinal tract. Stomach emptying is delayed. ***Symptoms:*** Heartburn, nausea, bloating, gastric reflux, lack of appetite, feeling full after eating only a small amount, vomiting of undigested food (eaten hours or days prior). Glucose levels may be erratic because of the delay in emptying of the stomach after meals.	• Discuss with your provider the option of obtaining a referral to a gastroenterologist (specialist in diseases of the intestine). • Ask for a referral to a dietitian to customize a meal plan. • Follow a low-fat, low-fiber diet. Eat small frequent meals (6 feedings with 30–45 g carbohydrates each). Meals that are mostly liquid may be better tolerated.* • Avoid foods that aggravate reflux: peppermint, chocolate, fat, and caffeine. Avoid chewing gum, which leads to swallowing of air.* • To reduce reflux, sit up for about 1 hour after meals; avoid lying down right away. Avoid late-night snacking. Raise the head of the bed 6 to 8 inches (by placing pillows between mattress and springs or raising the head of the bed with blocks).† • Take prescribed medications (eg, metoclopramide [Reglan®] or erythromycin‡) that can help your intestine move food along. • If you take rapid-acting insulin, discuss with your provider about timing the injection after you eat, once you know the blood glucose has peaked.§ • Discuss the appropriateness of insulin pump and continuous glucose monitoring therapies with your provider.¶
Lower Intestinal Tract Dysfunction ***What it is:*** Neuropathy of the nerves that allow for proper movement of waste through the lower intestinal tract. ***Symptoms:*** Constipation and/or diarrhea (sometimes alternating), bowel incontinence.	• For constipation: increase fiber, drink enough water, be more active, use stool softeners. Use bulk laxatives like psyllium (Metamucil®) as prescribed. • For diarrhea, include fiber in the diet to increase bulk. Take prescribed medications to control bowels.
Male Sexual Dysfunction ***What it is:*** Neuropathy of the nerves that allow a man to respond to sexual situations. Other processes, such as circulatory problems, low sex hormone levels, and drugs may contribute to the problem. See the Supplement (Sexual Dysfunction) for detailed instruction plan on treatment options for erectile dysfunction. ***Symptoms:*** Erectile dysfunction (ED)—unable to attain and/or maintain an erection.	• Ask your provider if any of your current medications may be causing ED. See Table S.1, Medications That May Cause Sexual Dysfunction, in this book's Supplement. • Ask your provider if you are a candidate for medications that help with ED (eg, alprostadil [Muse®, Caverject®], sildenafil [Viagra®], tadalafil [Cialis®], vardenafil [Levitra®]). • Ask your provider about mechanical devices that can help you achieve an erection (eg, vacuum devices, penile prosthesis). • Ask your provider about obtaining a referral to a urologist, a doctor who specializes in ED treatment. • Avoid alcohol. If you smoke, stop. Alcohol and smoking can make ED worse. • Include your sex partner in any decisions about therapy.

TABLE 8.9 Important Points About Living With Neuropathy *(continued)*

If you have . . .	You should . . .
Female Sexual Dysfunction ***What it is:*** Neuropathy of the nerves that allow a woman to respond to sexual situations. Other things such as depression, illness, or hormonal changes (such as during menopause) may contribute to the problem. See the Supplement (Sexual Dysfunction) for detailed instruction plan on treatment options for sexual dysfunction. ***Symptoms:*** Decreased sexual desire, difficulty in getting sexually aroused, pain during intercourse, vaginal dryness.	• Ask your provider if medications such as estrogen vaginal cream may be prescribed. • Ask your provider if any of your current medications may be causing sexual side effects. See Table S.2, Medications That May Cause Sexual Dysfunction, and Table S.6, Medications That May Cause Vaginal Dryness, in this book's Supplement. • Ask your provider about obtaining a referral to a gynecologist who is knowledgeable about female sexual dysfunction. • Use a water-based lubricant during sex. • Include your sex partner in any decisions about therapy.
Bladder Dysfunction ***What it is:*** Neuropathy of the nerves that control sensation of a full bladder. ***Symptoms:*** Early stages—infrequent urination because of lost urge; later stages—unable to fully empty the bladder, dribbling of urine, incontinence.	• Go to the bathroom frequently and try to urinate completely. • Feel your lower abdomen to find out if the bladder is full. • Report any signs and symptoms of a urinary tract infection to your provider promptly. • If antibiotics are prescribed for a urinary tract infection, take them all.
Sweating Disturbances (Sudomotor Dysfunction) ***What it is:*** Neuropathy of the nerves that control sweating. ***Symptoms:*** Intolerance to heat; profuse sweating of the upper part of the body, especially when eating certain foods (spicy foods, cheese); lack of sweating, especially in the feet, which can cause excessively dry and cracked skin.	• Avoid foods that trigger sweating. • Be aware of the temperature, and limit your exposure to heat. • Practice good foot care, with special attention to using moisturizer.
Hypoglycemia Unawareness ***What it is:*** Neuropathy of the nerves that allow you to recognize and react to hypoglycemia (low blood glucose). ***Symptoms:*** Lack of warning symptoms that the blood glucose level is low; inability of the liver to release stored glucose during hypoglycemia.	• Take steps to avoid hypoglycemia, because repeated episodes of hypoglycemia reduce future symptoms of low blood glucose.[#] • Monitor blood glucose frequently, especially before driving. • Ask your provider whether your glucose target should be raised in order to limit your risk for hypoglycemia. • Always wear medical identification that states you have diabetes. • Teach your family and close associates how to help you if you have hypoglycemia. • Ask your provider for a prescription for a glucagon emergency kit. • Have your close associates train on how to use a glucagon emergency kit. • Talk with your provider about insulin pump and continuous glucose monitoring therapies.

[*]SL Tomar, S Asma, "Smoking attributable periodontitis in the United States: findings from the NHANES III," *J Periodontol* 71 (2000): 743-51.
[†]CR Parrish, JG Pastors, "Nutritional management of gastroparesis in people with diabetes," *Diabetes Spectr* 20, no. 4 (2007): 231-4.
[‡]M Kalyani, K Onyemere, MP Jones, "Oral erythromycin and symptomatic relief of gastroparesis: a systematic review," *Am J Gastroenterol* 98, no. 2 (2003): 259-63.
[§]American Diabetes Association, "Gastroparesis and diabetes" (cited 2015 July 9), on the Internet at: http://www.diabetes.org/living-with-diabetes/complications/gastroparesis.html.
[¶]International Diabetes Federation, *IDF Consensus Statement on Sleep Apnea and Type 2 Diabetes* (Brussels, Belgium: IDF, 2008).
[#]P Mistiaen, E Poot, S Hickox, et al, "Preventing and treating intertrigo in the large skin folds of adults: a literature overview," *Dermatol Nurs* 16 (2004): 43-6, 49-57.
Sources: AJM Boulton, AI Vinik, JC Arezzo, et al, "Diabetic neuropathies: a statement by the American Diabetes Association," *Diabetes Care* 28, no. 4 (2005): 956-62; GM Caputo, PR Cavanagh, JS Ulbrecht, et al, "Assessment and management of foot disease in patients with diabetes," *N Engl J Med* 331, no. 13 (1994): 854-60.

Sleep Health

 The International Diabetes Federation (IDF) issued a consensus statement and "call to action" about obstructive sleep apnea at the 2008 American Diabetes Association Scientific Sessions. Because of the high incidence of undiagnosed sleep apnea, healthcare providers who treat those with type 2 diabetes should routinely screen for sleep apnea. Conversely, all patients with known sleep apnea should be screened for type 2 diabetes.[89]

Consider using the "Berlin Questionnaire"[90] found in the "Resources" section at the end of this module to assess your patients for sleep apnea. The patient completes page 1. Page 2 is the score sheet and is completed by staff. A copy of the score sheet should be forwarded to the referring provider for continuity of care.

Do you wake up tired or feel sleepy during the day? Do you snore loudly? If you said yes, then you have some of the symptoms of sleep apnea. Sleep apnea is a serious condition that affects over half of all people with type 2 diabetes, but most don't know it.[91]

In the overall population of people with type 2 diabetes, up to 23% may have sleep apnea.[92] In 1 study that was done with people who have diabetes, up to 80% of those who were obese also had sleep apnea.[93] In addition, sleep apnea puts you at higher risk for heart disease.

Sleep apnea is defined by periods of no breathing for 10 seconds or more.

When there is not enough intake of air, the oxygen level in the blood drops below normal. After a time of not breathing, the lungs make an automatic effort to take in a big breath, which can sound like choking or coughing to a sleep partner. The repeated periods of low oxygen levels in sleep apnea cause a major stress to the body. In response to this stress, hormones that raise both blood pressure and blood glucose levels are released into the blood. See Table 8.10 for symptoms of sleep apnea.

If you have the symptoms of sleep apnea, discuss it with your provider. If you are at high risk for sleep apnea, your provider may prescribe a sleep study. A sleep study requires an overnight stay at a sleep lab. Before going to sleep, several wires are attached to your body to measure your breathing, muscle movements, and oxygen level. A specialist reviews the results to find out if you stop breathing during the night, and if so, for how long.

If you are found to have sleep apnea, be encouraged that there are effective treatments.

- If you are overweight, weight loss is often effective in treating mild sleep apnea.
- If you are a smoker, stop smoking.
- Treat nasal congestion.

TABLE 8.10 Symptoms of Sleep Apnea

When Awake	When Asleep
Sleepiness	Loud snoring
Poor concentration	Restless sleep
Short-term memory loss	Choking or coughing
Morning headache	Frequent urination
Morning sore throat	Heavy sweating
Erectile dysfunction	Sleep partner witnesses signs of high blood pressure, periods of not breathing

Module 8   *Reducing Risks*   321

- Sleep on your side.
- Avoid the use of tranquilizers and sleeping pills.
- Avoid alcohol close to bedtime.
- If sleep apnea is moderate or severe, the recommended treatment is CPAP.

CPAP stands for *continuous positive airway pressure*. A mask is fitted to the face to deliver air with each intake of breath. There is just enough pressure in this airflow to prevent the airway from collapsing. Studies show that people who have both type 2 diabetes and sleep apnea benefit from CPAP in more ways than just better breathing. Effective CPAP therapy helps control high blood pressure.[92] While research is mixed on CPAP use improving blood glucose control, treatment has been shown to improve quality of life and help with blood pressure control.[93]

There are some other treatment options to CPAP that may be helpful for those who cannot tolerate CPAP. One is called expiratory positive airway pressure (EPAP) and consists of small devices that are placed over each nostril before going to bed. There is also a mouthpiece that you can get from your dentist that may help with sleep apnea.

T&L **Invite participants who have successfully used CPAP to share with others in the group how it made a positive difference in their daily life.** Consult preprogram patient assessments to identify who is on CPAP and make an inquiry beforehand. Gain permission to call on them in a group setting. Adults with social/interpersonal intelligence learn by telling their story; hearing and telling stories helps those with verbal/auditory intelligence learn.

Dental Health

Periodontal disease, while not more common in people with diabetes, tends to be more serious among those with diabetes.[94,95]

It can start with a common gum problem, called gingivitis. The bacteria in plaque infect the gums and the bones around the teeth. Some people with gum disease are unaware because they have no symptoms. When symptoms are present, they include red, swollen gums that easily bleed. If the growth of plaque reaches below the gum line, it can eventually infect the bones and tissues that support the teeth. This is called periodontitis. Symptoms can include loose teeth and bad breath. If untreated, periodontitis can lead to tooth loss. Periodontal disease can also make blood glucose control more difficult.[95]

Chronic dry mouth, called *xerostomia*, is another common concern for people with diabetes. Saliva substitutes or fluoride mouth rinses may be helpful, and can be recommended by a dentist. Taking frequent sips of water and restricting intake of caffeine and alcohol may help alleviate dry mouth.[96(p236)]

A yeast infection commonly known as *thrush* is caused by overgrowth of *Candida*, a fungus that naturally resides in the mouth. The symptoms are white patches on the inside of the mouth that may be painful. If rubbed, the patches may bleed. Thrush is more likely to occur when blood glucose levels are elevated for a long time. People who wear dentures are at higher risk for thrush developing on the gums beneath the denture plates.[97(p190)]

Reducing Your Risk for Dental Problems

There are things you can do to lower your risk for dental problems.

- Control your blood glucose as best you can.[94,98]
- Visit your dentist at least twice per year, more often if you have gum disease.[99]
- Don't smoke. Smoking dramatically increases the risk for gum disease.[100,101]
- Brush twice daily and floss daily.[102]

American Association of Diabetes Educators©

- Use a soft toothbrush. Soft bristles bend more easily and can get between teeth better than stiffer bristles. They are also less likely to scratch the gums. However, the American Dental Association emphasizes that any bristle strength (soft, medium, or hard) should be free of sharp or jagged edges and endpoints.[103]
- Maintain a healthy meal plan and limit between-meal snacks.
- Denture wearers: Clean and rinse dentures daily. Remove dentures while sleeping to lessen the risk for thrush.[97(p190)]

Skin Health

Your skin is your body's first line of defense. Any breaks in the skin put you at risk for infection. If your glucose level is elevated, the risk for infection is increased.

Reducing Your Risk for Skin Problems

There are things you can do to lower your risk for skin problems.

- Keep your skin clean.
- Dry well after bathing. Take steps to keep skin free of excess moisture. Areas of skin-on-skin friction, such as between the toes, the armpits, the groin, and beneath the breasts, can become irritated if kept too moist. Too much moisture plus elevated blood glucose levels can lead to a bacterial or fungal skin infection.

  Symptoms of skin infection include redness, itching, and discomfort. The skin may ooze clear fluid, or a red rash may erupt. Using powder (talc or cornstarch) in skin-fold areas has little or no proven benefit. In fact, these substances may further irritate the skin or allow fungus to thrive.[104]

  Wearing lightweight, absorbent clothing that is not too tight is helpful in preventing and treating skin infection. Avoid clothing made of wool or synthetic fibers (eg, nylon, spandex).[105,106] If you have frequent skin problems, ask your provider if an antibacterial or antifungal medication is in order.

- Always use sunscreen when spending time outdoors.[4,107(p469)] Vigorously scratching skin when it feels dry and itchy from sunburn can break the skin. Any blisters that form after a severe sunburn are a possible source of infection if they are broken open. If you get sunburned, use skin moisturizer to reduce dryness and itching. The physical stress of severe sunburn can cause your blood glucose level to rise.

Advanced Detail

Regarding Body Art and Diabetes

Is it safe for a person with diabetes to get a tattoo?

Getting body art—tattoos and piercings—carries an element of risk for anyone, whether or not they have diabetes. Risks include:

- **Allergy**—Allergy to the pigments in tattoo ink (especially red ink) can cause swelling, itching, and redness at the site. Scar tissue and small nodules under the skin can result from an ink allergy.[108]

  Even the ink used for some temporary tattoos can cause an allergic reaction. Natural henna tattoos use a vegetable coloring to paint the skin. Some artists, however, add the chemical from black hair dye—PPD (para-phenylenediamine)—to the henna to make the temporary tattoos last for weeks instead of days. This results in a black henna tattoo, which has been associated with skin reactions and even major allergic reactions.

If a person is exposed to PPD and then takes certain medications, an allergic reaction can occur. Medications that can spark the reaction after exposure to PPD include certain heart, blood pressure, and diabetes medications.[109]

❖ **Infection**—Each of the skin punctures in a piercing or tattoo is an entry point for germs. If the germ enters the bloodstream, a full-body infection (sepsis) can occur. People at high risk for infection include those with conditions that affect their immune system—people with HIV/AIDS, people who have received an organ transplant and take immunosuppressant drugs, and people with diabetes.[108] How does diabetes affect healing? When the glucose level is elevated, the immune system doesn't work as it should. This means that white blood cells are slower to attack invading organisms, and infection is more likely.[110,111]

Most people have heard about the risks for contracting hepatitis C and HIV from unsanitary practices in body art. These diseases can be spread if the body artist uses improper sanitation practices.

There is no federal regulation of body art salons. Some states may require licensing to perform tattoos. The FDA regulates the color pigments that are used for making cosmetics. But no pigments are FDA-approved for injection into the skin.

❖ Research has found that some pigments used in tattoos contain lead. Some salons use pigments that come from industrial-grade auto body paint because the color lasts longer in the skin. These paints can contain lead or other potentially dangerous chemicals.[112]

If you choose to get body art despite the risks, these guidelines may help lessen your risk:

❖ Make sure your diabetes has been in control (A1C <7%) so that you are more likely to heal properly.

❖ Make sure the salon uses a steam *autoclave* machine to disinfect instruments between clients. Bleach and other liquid disinfectants won't kill hepatitis C.

❖ Make sure the artist practices hand-washing and wears new gloves with each customer.

❖ Make sure the tattoo artist does not reuse ink from a previous customer.

❖ Avoid getting body art on the lower extremities or places where circulation may be poor (eg, feet, ankles, calves, buttocks, genitals).

After a tattoo:

❖ Don't pick or scratch the skin.

❖ When bathing, use antibacterial soap on the tattoo.

❖ Use antibacterial ointment on the tattoo until it is healed.

❖ Avoid soaking in a bathtub, pool, or hot tub until the tattoo is healed.

❖ Always wash your hands with an antibacterial soap before touching an unhealed tattoo.

Standard of Medical Care in Diabetes[113]

❖ All people with diabetes should have routine vaccinations that are recommended for the general public.

❖ All people with diabetes aged 6 months or older should have an annual influenza vaccine.

❖ All people with diabetes aged 19 to 59 should have a Hepatitis B vaccination, if never vaccinated for it in the past. Consider it for those over age 60.

American Association of Diabetes Educators©

Standard of Medical Care in Diabetes[114]

❖ A pneumonia vaccine should be given to all people with diabetes who are aged 2 years or older (PPSV23). If the PPSV23 vaccine was given prior to age 65, a onetime vaccination of PCV13 is recommended if the person is now 65 years or older AND it's been more than 1 year since the initial vaccine was given. If the person is 65 years or older and has never been vaccinated, 2 different pneumonia vaccines are recommended—PCV13 followed by PPSV23 6 to 12 months later.

❖ Other people who should have repeated pneumonia vaccination include those with kidney disease or conditions of lowered immunity (eg, after receiving an organ transplant).

Immunizations

In general, people with chronic conditions (including diabetes) have a harder time recovering from influenza (flu) and pneumonia than people who don't have chronic conditions. The death rate from those infections is also much higher for people with chronic conditions.[113,115-118] For these reasons, immunizations are recommended.[114,115,119,120]

Vaccines are safe. They also help you avoid serious complications if you do get the flu or pneumonia.[120,121] Across several studies, the most common reaction to vaccines was mild soreness where the shot was given.[113] The flu vaccine and the pneumonia vaccine can be given at the same visit but in different injection sites.[122]

> **Help skeptical patients build a realistic attitude about vaccinations by:**
>
> • Examining erroneous beliefs, expectations, and assumptions about their vulnerability to poor outcomes after an immunization
> • Presenting evidence that the risk for poor outcomes from pneumonia or influenza is significantly greater than the risk for an adverse vaccine reaction

A flu vaccine is needed each year because the flu vaccine only protects you for 1 year. Different types of the flu are common each year. The vaccine that is considered most effective for the current flu strain is the one you should receive.[123] If you have concerns about taking vaccines, talk to your provider for more information. Pregnant women should have the flu vaccine because their immune systems are weaker. (See the "Resources" section at the end of this module for a patient handout on high-risk populations and influenza.)

People with diabetes who are 6 months and older should also receive a pneumococcal vaccination. Once they are over age 65, a slightly different pneumococcal vaccination should be given. If someone with diabetes is over the age of 65 and has never had a pneumonia shot, the 2 different vaccines should be given 6 to 12 months apart. (See the "Resources" section at the end of this module for a patient handout on pneumonia.)

Adults aged 19 to 59 who have diabetes also benefit from getting the Hepatitis B vaccination. In addition, all people with diabetes should stay current on all of the vaccinations that are recommended for the general population, such as a shingles (Zoster) vaccination after the age of 60 and regular tetanus booster shots. (See the "Resources" section at the end of this module for a patient handout on Hepatitis B vaccination.)

See the "Resources" section at the end of this module for "CDC 2015 Recommended Immunizations for Adults by Age and by Health Condition."

Psychosocial Assessment and Care

> **Standard of Medical Care in Diabetes**
>
> - Regularly assess psychosocial status of people with diabetes.
> - Include routine screening for depression, diabetes-related distress, eating disorders, cognitive impairment anxiety, and other psychosocial problems.
> - It is especially important to screen for and treat depression in those over the age of 65.

People with diabetes have a higher rate of depression than those who do not have diabetes. In addition, the DAWN 2 study indicated that almost half of people with diabetes have a high level of distress linked to having diabetes. Getting more help dealing with the emotional impact of diabetes will help you do the things you need to do to care for yourself and control your diabetes. Talk with your healthcare team if you are feeling overwhelmed about your diabetes or if you just don't feel like you can take care of your diabetes.[124,125]

Reducing Risks Before and During Pregnancy

Preconception Care

Preconception care is a set of preventive and management interventions that identify and modify risk factors that can affect pregnancy outcome. The CDC recommends incorporating preconception care into the routine health care of all women of childbearing age.[126]

> **Standard of Medical Care in Diabetes**
>
> Starting at puberty, preconception counseling should be part of the routine diabetes visit for females of childbearing potential who have diabetes (type 1 or type 2).[127]

Since more than half of all pregnancies in the United States are unplanned or unintended, most women do not receive preconception care, including those with preexisting diabetes or prediabetes, or women with previous GDM.[126]

The following recommendations are from the ACOG and the ADA. Ideally, preconception planning should allow for at least 3 to 4 months' time to achieve glycemic control, as evidenced by the A1C.[128] Every effort should be made to involve significant others in preconception and pregnancy education and care.

For Women With Diabetes WHO ARE NOT PLANNING to Become Pregnant

An effective method of contraception should be used consistently to prevent unplanned or unintended pregnancies.

What have you heard about women with diabetes and childbirth? What concerns you most about your pregnancy?

If participant has had a previous pregnancy with diabetes, ask: *Can you tell me about your last pregnancy? How was your diabetes managed?*

Standard of Medical Care in Diabetes

- Women with diabetes who are not planning a pregnancy should practice birth control.[128]
- Women who may become pregnant and are sexually active and not using birth control should avoid the use of medications that could potentially harm the fetus, such as ACE inhibitors and statins.[128]
- Women with diabetes may use any form of contraception that women without diabetes can use. Birth control options with a high rate of success should be used to prevent pregnancy.[129] See Table 8.11 for contraception options for women with preexisting diabetes or prior history of gestational diabetes.

An unplanned pregnancy puts your unborn baby at risk. During the first 6 to 8 weeks of pregnancy, the baby's organs are being formed. If your blood glucose is elevated during this time, there is a higher risk for birth defects.[130-132]

It's advisable to address participants' feelings and concerns *before* launching into details of preconception/pregnancy care.

TABLE 8.11 Contraceptive Use in Women With Preexisting Diabetes or Prior History of GDM

Contraceptive Type	Efficacy	Safety
Barrier methods: diaphragm, condoms, spermicides, cervical caps*	70%–97% depending on method and if used alone or in combination with another method	No contraindications
Intrauterine devices (IUDs)*	98%–99%	Not recommended if high-risk exposure to sexually transmitted diseases
Oral contraceptives (OCs)*	97%–99.5%	Low-dose progestin or combination of lowest progestin/estrogen dose preferred for women without vascular complications or strong family history of myocardial disease. Women with prior history of GDM should not use progestin-only OCs while breastfeeding
Non-oral hormonal[†] contraceptives (eg, implants, injections, transdermal patches)	99%	May affect glucose and lipid levels

*JL Kitzmiller, L Jovanovic, F Brown, et al, eds, *Managing Preexisting Diabetes and Pregnancy* (Alexandria, Va: American Diabetes Association, 2008); C Kim, KW Seidel, EA Begier, et al, "Diabetes and depot medroyprogesterone contraception in Navajo women," *Arch Inter Med* 161 (2001); SL Kjos, TA Buchanan, "Postpartum management, lactation, and contraception," in EA Reece, DR Coustan, SG Gabbe, eds, *Diabetes in Women: Adolescence, Pregnancy, and Menopause* (Philadelphia: Lippincott Williams & Wilkins, 2004), 441-9.

[†]JL Kitzmiller, L Jovanovic, F Brown, et al, eds, *Managing Preexisting Diabetes and Pregnancy* (Alexandria, Va: American Diabetes Association, 2008); C Kim, KW Seidel, EA Begier, et al, "Diabetes and depot medroyprogesterone contraception in Navajo women," *Arch Inter Med* 161 (2001); CH Chuang, GA Chase, DM Bensyl, CS Weisman, "Contraceptive use by diabetic and obese women," *Women's Health Issues* 15, no. 4 (2005): 167-73; SL Kjos, TA Buchanan, "Postpartum management, lactation, and contraception," in EA Reece, DR Coustan, SG Gabbe, eds, *Diabetes in Women: Adolescence, Pregnancy, and Menopause* (Philadelphia: Lippincott Williams & Wilkins, 2004), 441-9.

Help patients build a positive attitude about diabetes and pregnancy self-care by:

- Examining beliefs, expectations, and assumptions about their vulnerability to pregnancy complications.
- Providing a safe, supportive environment for them to express any fear and anxiety they may be experiencing about the pregnancy.
- Dealing with emotions up front allows for catharsis, which serves to reduce anxiety. Reducing undue anxiety is conducive to the learning process.

Identifying Participant Feelings and Concerns About Pregnancy and Diabetes

Ask participants questions that will stimulate active discussion about the pregnancy complicated by diabetes.

Years ago, it was a common belief, even among doctors, that women with diabetes could not have a normal pregnancy. Many women with diabetes were advised not to get pregnant.

Now, it's well known that controlling your blood glucose before and during pregnancy is one of the keys to help prevent miscarriage, birth defects, and other health problems with your baby.

For Women With Diabetes WHO ARE PLANNING to Become Pregnant

Even with a planned pregnancy, you may not realize you are pregnant for a number of weeks. During the first 6 to 8 weeks of pregnancy, your baby's organs are forming. If your blood glucose is elevated during this time, there is a higher risk for birth defects.[133,134,135(p1386)] If you currently take oral diabetes medication, your doctor will likely switch you to insulin therapy.[127]

Work with your entire healthcare team to set up your plan of care *before* becoming pregnant. Once you are pregnant, you will need to work very closely with your team. This means frequent contact with your primary care physician, a diabetes specialist, your obstetrician, and perhaps a maternal-fetal specialist (a doctor specially trained in managing high-risk pregnancies). Other physician specialists should be included, as needed, to monitor your eyes, kidneys, and blood pressure.[129]

YOU are the most important member of the team. You will be responsible for your choices in eating, activity, monitoring, taking medication, and problem solving. A diabetes educator and dietitian should be part of your team to help you make the needed lifestyle changes to self-manage your diabetes. Ideally, a social worker or trained counselor will be available to help you adjust to the demands of self-care during your pregnancy.[129]

Standard of Medical Care in Diabetes[129]

Women with diabetes should get their A1C under 7% before trying to become pregnant, as long as they can do so without hypoglycemia (low blood glucose).

Standard of Medical Care in Diabetes

Women with diabetes who are planning a pregnancy should be evaluated for the presence of any diabetes complications involving the eyes, kidneys, nerves, and cardiovascular system.[129]

328   Diabetes Education Curriculum

The prepregnancy evaluation should include the following:

- **Eyes**—Have a dilated eye examination by an ophthalmologist or other trained eye specialist.[129]

- **Blood pressure**—You should have your blood pressure checked sitting, lying, and standing.[129]

  If your blood pressure is too high, you should receive the necessary treatment. Some blood pressure medications are not safe to use during pregnancy, however, and your doctor may need to switch you to another type of treatment. Angiotensin-converting enzyme inhibitors and ARBs should not be taken during pregnancy.[2,129,136] (See Table 8.12—Blood Pressure Medications *Not Safe* During Pregnancy.) The following blood pressure medications have been proven safe and effective for use during pregnancy: methyldopa (Aldomet®), labetalol (Normodyne®), diltiazem (Tiazac®), clonidine (Catapres®), and prazosin (Minipress®).[23]

- **Cardiovascular system**—Pregnancy puts a big demand on your heart and circulatory system. You should have a full examination to check for the presence of any heart or circulation problems.[129] **If you take a statin** medication for abnormal lipid levels, your doctor will have to change your treatment. Statin medications are not safe to use during pregnancy.[2,129] (See Table 8.13—Statin Lipid Medications *Not Safe* During Pregnancy.)

TABLE 8.12   Blood Pressure Medications *Not Safe* During Pregnancy

Generic Name	Trade Name	Generic Name	Trade Name
ACE inhibitors		*ARBs*	
Benazepril	Lotensin®	Candesartan	Atacand®
Captopril	Capoten®	Irbesartan	Avapro®
Enalapril	Vasotec®	Losartan	Cozaar®
Fosinopril	Monopril®	Lmesartan	Benicar®
Lisinopril	Prinivil®, Zestril®	Prosartan	Teveten®
Moexipril	Univasc®	Telmisartan	Micardis®
Perindopril	Aceon®	Valsartan	Diovan®
Quinipril	Accupril®		
Ramipril	Altace®		
Trandolapril	Mavik®		

Sources: A Thomas, "Pregnancy with diabetes," in C Mensing, ed, *The Art and Science of Diabetes Self-Management Education: A Desk Reference for Healthcare Professionals*, 3rd ed (Chicago: American Association of Diabetes Educators, 2014), 693; WO Cooper, S Hernandez-Diaz, PG Arbogast, et al, "Major congenital malformations after first-trimester exposure to ACE inhibitors," *N Engl J Med* 354 (2006): 2443-51.

TABLE 8.13   Statin Lipid Medications *Not Safe* During Pregnancy

Generic Name	Trade Name
Atorvastatin	Lipitor®
Fluvastatin	Lescol®
Lovastatin	Mevacor®
Pravastatin	Pravachol®
Rosuvastatin	Crestor®
Simvastatin	Zocor®

American Association of Diabetes Educators©

- **Neurologic system**—You should have a neurologic examination to make sure there are no problems with the nerves that control your body's automatic functions.[129]
- **Laboratory testing**—Preconception laboratory work should at least include blood testing for A1C and thyroid function, as well as blood and urine tests to check your kidney function.[129]

For Women With Diabetes WHO ARE PREGNANT
What Happens With Glucose and Insulin During Pregnancy

Glucose from the mother's blood freely passes through the placenta to the baby. Insulin in the mother's system, however, DOES NOT cross the placenta to the baby.

In the first few weeks of pregnancy, when the baby's organs are being formed, an excess of glucose from the mother can lead to miscarriage or birth defects. In the last trimester of pregnancy, when the baby is growing the fastest, an excess of glucose from the mother will result in an excessive production of insulin in the baby. At this stage, the baby's pancreas is making its own insulin, and it will produce as much insulin as needed to match the amount of glucose coming in from the mother.

Excess insulin in the baby's system works like a growth hormone. It causes the baby to gain too much weight, especially around the head and shoulders. A baby that is larger than its gestational age may be born too soon, before the lungs are fully developed. A large baby can be very difficult to deliver, leading to birth injuries and/or the need for an emergency caesarean delivery.[137-141]

Use anatomical graphics to illustrate the relationship between maternal and fetal blood flow via the placenta. Use of graphics resonates with learners, especially those with strong visual/spatial intelligence.

How Pregnancy Affects Diabetes Care
For Pregnant Women With Type 1 Diabetes

Your glucose levels may drop lower than usual during the first 3 months of pregnancy. Therefore, your insulin dose may need to be adjusted at this time so that you do not experience hypoglycemia (low blood glucose).[133,142] In the second and third trimesters, there is an increase in the levels of hormones (eg, estrogen, progesterone, human placental lactogen) that help sustain your pregnancy. This causes you to be more resistant to insulin, and your glucose levels will be higher, especially fasting and after eating (postprandial).

For this reason, your dose of insulin will need to be increased in order to get your glucose to the goal level. It is not unusual for a woman with type 1 diabetes to require *2 or 3 times the amount of insulin* she needed before becoming pregnant.

For Pregnant Women With Type 2 Diabetes

As the pregnancy progresses, you will need more and more insulin in order to get your glucose to the goal level. Remember, type 2 diabetes causes you to become resistant to insulin. If you are overweight, this resistance to insulin is magnified. When the hormones that help sustain your pregnancy (eg, estrogen, progesterone, human placental lactogen) increase during the second and third trimesters, you become even more insulin resistant.

For Pregnant Women With Gestational Diabetes

In the second or third trimester of pregnancy, when the hormones that help sustain your pregnancy (eg, estrogen, progesterone, human placental lactogen) increase, you become resistant to insulin. If you are overweight, this resistance is magnified. If your pancreas cannot make enough insulin to overcome this resistance, your blood glucose

330 Diabetes Education Curriculum

level rises above normal. Depending on your blood glucose level, your diabetes care may just involve adjusting your eating habits and activity. Medication may be necessary to get your glucose levels to the target.

Blood Glucose Goals

Once you are pregnant, the main task is to try to keep your blood glucose level at the recommended target. Different organizations publish differing glucose targets for pregnancy. Your provider may recommend slightly different glucose goals for your individual situation. See Table 8.14, Recommended Target Blood Glucose During Pregnancy, and Table 8.15, ACOG Target Plasma in GDM.

Managing Diabetes During Pregnancy

Managing diabetes during your pregnancy involves choices about coping, eating, being active, monitoring, taking medication, problem solving, and reducing risks. Let's look at each of those areas.

TABLE 8.14   Recommended Target Blood Glucose During Pregnancy*

	Women With Preexisting Type 1 or Type 2 Diabetes[‡]	Women With Gestational Diabetes[§]
Premeal	60–99 mg/dL (3.3–5.4 mmol/L)	<95 mg/dL (<5.3 mmol/L)
1-hour postmeal (peak postprandial)	100–129 mg/dL (5.5–7.1 mmol/L)	<140 mg/dL (<7.8 mmol/L)
2-hour postmeal (peak postprandial)	100–129 mg/dL (5.5–7.2 mmol/L)	<120 mg/dL (<6.7 mmol/L)
Bedtime/overnight	60–99 mg/dL (3.3–5.4 mmol/L)	
A1C[†]	<6%	

*Plasma values.

[†]Due to the increase in red blood cells during pregnancy, A1C levels fall during pregnancy. A1C should be used as a secondary measure after self-blood glucose monitoring. A1C levels may need to be monitored more frequently in pregnancy (eg, monthly).

[‡]American Diabetes Association, "Standards of medical care in diabetes—2015," *Diabetes Care* 38, Suppl 1 (2015): S1-94; American Association of Clinical Endocrinologists Diabetes Mellitus Clinical Practice Guidelines Task Force, "Medical guidelines for clinical practice for the management of diabetes mellitus," *Endocr Pract* 13, Suppl 1 (2007): 1-68; JL Kitzmiller, JM Block, FM Brown, et al, "Managing preexisting diabetes for pregnancy: summary of evidence and consensus recommendations for care," *Diabetes Care* 31 (2008): 1060-79.

[§]JL Kitzmiller, JM Block, FM Brown, et al, "Managing preexisting diabetes for pregnancy: summary of evidence and consensus recommendations for care," *Diabetes Care* 31 (2008): 1060-79; BE Metzger, TA Buchanan, DR Coustan, et al, "Summary and recommendations of the Fifth International Workshop—Conference own Gestational Diabetes Mellitus," *Diabetes Care* 30, Suppl 2 (2007): S251-60.

TABLE 8.15   ACOG Target Plasma in GDM

Fasting	<90 mg/dL (5.0 mmol/L)
Preprandial	<105 mg/dL (5.8 mmol/L)
1-hour postprandial	<130–140 mg/dL (7.2–7.8 mmol/L)
2-hour postprandial	<120 mg/dL (<6.7 mmol/L)

Source: MB Landon, SG Gabbe, "Gestational diabetes mellitus," *Obstet Gynecol* 118 (2011): 1386.

American Association of Diabetes Educators©

Healthy Coping

Dealing with a pregnancy can feel overwhelming. Dealing with diabetes AND pregnancy can be even more so. You are likely to experience a wide range of feelings during this time of very rapid change in your life. That's normal. The more you arm yourself with good information, the more prepared you'll be, and the better choices you will make. Ask for the support you need. Your healthcare team is there to support you, and you can include your family and friends by letting them know what you need from them during this time.

Healthy Eating

Weight Gain

How much weight you should gain during pregnancy partly depends on your prepregnant weight and whether you are carrying 1 or more babies. You need to take in enough calories each day to allow for your body's needs and the proper growth of your baby. Research shows that your baby won't develop properly if you don't gain enough weight during your second and third trimesters.[143] Weight loss during pregnancy is not recommended.[144] When you lose weight from taking in too few calories, fat is burned, and ketones are produced in response. An excessive amount of ketones during pregnancy has been linked to lower IQ scores in the child.[145(p300),146]

Meal Planning

Your individual situation—age, height, weight, activity level, and stage of pregnancy—is taken into account when a meal plan is developed. Eating at regular times will help you avoid hypoglycemia. Work closely with your dietitian to customize a meal plan that suits your food preferences, schedule, and culture. One of the most important aspects of your meal plan will be spreading the carbohydrates throughout the day into 3 small meals and 2 to 4 snacks.[147] Your meal plan will need to be adjusted as your needs and blood glucose levels change throughout the pregnancy.

Vitamins and Minerals

Getting enough of certain vitamins and minerals is very important during pregnancy. This includes calcium, iron, folate, vitamin D, and magnesium. Your meal plan should contain foods with these vitamins and minerals. Getting enough folate is especially important during early pregnancy to help prevent spinal cord defects (eg, spina bifida) in the baby. Your provider will probably also prescribe a prenatal supplement to ensure you get adequate amounts of these elements. See Module 2: Healthy Eating and Module 4: Taking Medication for more details on vitamins and minerals.

Morning Sickness

If severe vomiting occurs after taking rapid-acting or short-acting insulin, you are at risk for hypoglycemia (low blood glucose). In this case, taking an injection of glucagon can help you prevent hypoglycemia until vomiting subsides. Glucagon is a hormone that forces the liver to quickly release glucose into the bloodstream. If you have severe vomiting, contact your provider for options.[148(p7)]

High-Intensity Sweeteners

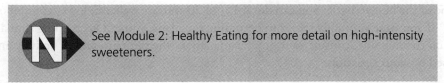
See Module 2: Healthy Eating for more detail on high-intensity sweeteners.

The following high-intensity sweeteners have been proven safe and are approved by the FDA for use during pregnancy.[149,150]

Chemical Name	Brand Name(s)
Acesulfame potassium	Sweet One®, Sunett®
Advantame	FDA approved May 2014—no brand name available at press time
Aspartame	NutraSweet®, Equal®
Neotame	FDA approved 2002—no brand name available at press time
Saccharin	Sweet'N Low®, Sugar Twin®, Sweet Twin®, NectaSweet®
Sucralose (yellow packet)	Splenda®

Alcohol

You should avoid drinking alcohol while pregnant, as this poses risks to your baby.[151]

Mercury

Certain types of fish often contain high levels of mercury. Mercury crosses the placenta and can cause damage to your baby's nervous system.[152] According to the FDA, you should avoid eating the following types of fish while pregnant: shark, swordfish, jack mackerel, and tilefish. Limit your intake of all other types of fish to 8 to 12 ounces per week.[152] When choosing tuna, be aware that albacore tuna contains more mercury than chunk light tuna.[153]

Listeriosis

Listeriosis is a bacterial infection that can be transmitted from you to your unborn baby. It can cause you to miscarry, have a preterm delivery, or have other complications. The *Listeria* bacteria are more likely to be found in certain types of food. To reduce the risk for *Listeria* infection, you should avoid the following foods while pregnant[128(p686-7)]:

- Deli meats, hot dogs, and lunch meats (unless reheated until steaming hot)
- Soft cheeses (eg, feta, Brie, Camembert, blue-veined, queso blanco, and queso fresco; hard cheese and pasteurized cheese are recommended)
- Refrigerated paté and refrigerated meat spreads (canned and shelf-stable paté and meat spreads can be consumed)
- Refrigerated smoked seafood (unless it is cooked)
- Raw or unpasteurized milk

Being Active

Unless you have complications, you should get at least 150 minutes (2 hours and 30 minutes) a week of moderate-intensity or 75 minutes (1 hour and 15 minutes) a week of vigorous-intensity aerobic physical activity, or an equivalent combination of moderate- and vigorous-intensity aerobic activity.[154(pvii)] Breaking your activity into 3 sessions of 10 minutes is effective.[154(pvii)] If you were sedentary prior to becoming pregnant, don't attempt to start a vigorous exercise program during pregnancy.

Walking is one of the best activities you can do. A 15- to 20-minute walk can lower your blood glucose level by 20 to 40 points.[155] If you were very active prior to becoming pregnant, you can keep doing similar activities during pregnancy. To be on the safe side, consult your physician(s) about the right amount of activity and any limitations you may have based on your situation.

Tips for Safety During Physical Activity[155]

- If you take insulin, be sure to monitor your blood glucose level before and after activity sessions. Be aware that insulin increases your risk for hypoglycemia (low blood glucose).

American Association of Diabetes Educators©

Module 8   *Reducing Risks*   333

- Avoid activity during the times that insulin is peaking. Don't inject insulin into your arm or leg if your exercise is going to work the muscles in those extremities.

- Always have some quick-acting carbohydrate handy during your activity sessions, in case of an episode of hypoglycemia.

- Avoid becoming overheated during activity. Avoid outside activity during the hottest time of the day. Wear clothes that breathe.

- Drink enough fluids (water is best) so that you don't become dehydrated during activity.

- If your heart rate exceeds 140 beats per minute and/or you become short of breath, you are exercising too intensely. Slow down your pace.

- Using your hands, feel your belly for any contractions during activity. If you have any contractions, stop the activity.

- If you have any of the following conditions, you should not exercise: preterm labor, premature rupture of membranes, or extremely high or low blood glucose levels.

Monitoring

Glucose Monitoring

Checking your blood glucose levels before and after meals will help show how well your body is processing the carbohydrates in your food. Your provider will advise you on the frequency of checking your glucose. If you take insulin, it will be adjusted based on your glucose results. Research shows that after-meal glucose monitoring is valuable because it's closely related to a lower chance of complications with both mother and baby.[156]

Ketone Monitoring

Your provider may advise you to check your urine for ketones. Ketone testing is always recommended for those with type 1 diabetes during times of illness, weight loss, or reduced food intake. In early pregnancy, morning sickness often causes nausea and vomiting. This is a time to check your urine for ketones. The presence of ketones (especially when your glucose is normal or low) is a sign that your body is in a state of starvation. If this is the case, you need to consult your healthcare team to treat the nausea and vomiting so that you can keep food down.

Ketone testing can be done by dipping a dipstick in urine, watching for the color change, and comparing it with a results chart. There is also a glucose meter on the market that can test for blood ketones, using a special strip.

A1C Monitoring

A1C monitoring is recommended every 4 to 6 weeks for pregnant women with type 1 or type 2 diabetes. The A1C measures your average glucose level over the past 2 to 3 months. The goal is to get your A1C within 1% of the normal range. This tight control is necessary to help prevent problems with the baby's development.[155] In pregnancy, A1C levels may need to be monitored more frequently (eg, monthly) because of the alteration in red blood cell kinetics.

Tests to Monitor Your Baby

During your pregnancy, you will have lots of tests to monitor the health of your baby. Understanding what these tests are for may help allay any anxiety you have. Some of the tests may include[157]:

- fetal movement counts
- the nonstress test
- biophysical profile
- modified biophysical profile
- contraction stress test
- Doppler ultrasound of the umbilical artery

American Association of Diabetes Educators©

For details about each test, see "Tests to Monitor Your Baby" in the "Resources" section at the end of this module. Consider using it as a patient handout.

Taking Medication

Oral Diabetes Medications

If you take oral diabetes medication to manage your diabetes, your doctor may switch you to insulin therapy once you become pregnant.[142]

Insulin Injections

Research shows that an insulin regimen that involves 4 injections per day improves both glucose control and birth outcomes.[128(p700)] The purpose of multiple injections is to try to closely mimic what a normal pancreas does when there is no diabetes. A common regimen is:

- *Before breakfast*—a combination injection of intermediate-acting insulin AND rapid-acting insulin. The rapid-acting insulin is meant to control the glucose rise after breakfast; the intermediate-acting insulin is meant to control the glucose rise in the late afternoon.
- *Before lunch*—an injection of rapid-acting insulin. This injection is meant to control the glucose rise after lunch.
- *Before dinner*—an injection of rapid-acting insulin. This injection is meant to control the glucose rise after dinner.
- *At bedtime*—an injection of intermediate-acting insulin. This injection is meant to control the glucose rise during the night until breakfast.

It is safe to take insulin injections in the abdomen during pregnancy.[158] In later pregnancy, when the skin of the stomach can become very stretched, with little fat beneath the skin, if you can pinch up an inch of the skin, you can continue to inject into the pinched-up area. If you can't pinch up an inch, choose an area at the side of your stomach that has more fat.

Insulin Pump Therapy

Insulin pump therapy (continuous subcutaneous insulin infusion) is becoming the recommended treatment for pregnant women who had diabetes before becoming pregnant. The greatest concerns are cost of pump therapy and the potential for frequent and severe hyperglycemia if there is an interruption in the delivery of insulin, eg, a kinked tube or an infection at the infusion site.[128(p701)]

Using a pump allows a person to be more spontaneous and flexible in terms of meal times.[159] Pump therapy requires a very motivated person who is willing to take on extra responsibility. Advanced carbohydrate counting is usually the type of meal planning that is most helpful when using a pump.

Engage learners in critical thinking activities pertaining to any episodes of hypoglycemia experienced. Those with logical/mathematical intelligence will especially benefit from this approach to learning.

Problem Solving

Hypoglycemia

Treat any blood glucose level below 60 mg/dL (3.33 mmol/L) with a quick-acting carbohydrate. After hypoglycemia is resolved, always question why your blood glucose dropped too low:

- "Did I take too much insulin?"
- "Did I delay or skip a meal, or fail to eat enough?"
- "Did I get more physical activity than normal (could be from shopping or yard or house work)?

Once you pinpoint the cause, you can take steps to prevent it from happening again.

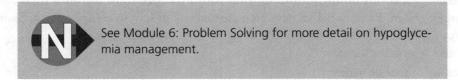

See Module 6: Problem Solving for more detail on hypoglycemia management.

Always have some quick-acting carbohydrate handy, in case of an episode of hypoglycemia. Glucose tablets are easy to carry, and they are the most predictable treatment for hypoglycemia. Each 5-g glucose tablet should raise your glucose level by about 10 points. Standard treatment is to take 3 or 4 glucose tablets, which should raise your glucose level by 30 points.[48(p534)]

Reducing Risks for Complications[128(p702)]

If you experience the following events during your pregnancy, call your provider right away to reduce your risk for serious complications:

- **Hyperglycemia** (high blood glucose) that you can't manage at home with insulin therapy.
- **Persistent presence of ketones.**
- **Uncontrolled vomiting** (also known as hyperemesis gravidarum).
- **Decreased movement of the fetus.** After 28 weeks or so, you should begin to monitor your baby's movements. This monitoring is sometimes called fetal movement counts or kick counts. There are different ways that kick counts can be done. Your healthcare provider will tell you how often to do it and when to notify him or her.[158]

Advanced Detail

Family members should be trained to inject you with glucagon in an emergency involving hypoglycemia. If you lost consciousness because of a severely low blood glucose level, you would be unable to take any oral treatment such as glucose tablets or milk. Ask your provider whether your situation calls for glucagon. Glucagon requires a prescription.

See Module 6: Problem Solving for detailed information on glucagon administration.

336   Diabetes Education Curriculum

◆ **Signs and symptoms of preeclampsia.**[160] This is a serious condition that can occur after 20 weeks of pregnancy, typically in the third trimester. When it occurs before 32 weeks of pregnancy, it is called early-onset preeclampsia. It also may occur postpartum.

Preeclampsia is a serious blood pressure disorder that can affect all of the organs in a woman's body. A woman has preeclampsia when she has high blood pressure and other signs that her organ systems are not working normally. One of these signs is *proteinuria* (an abnormal amount of protein in the urine). A woman with preeclampsia whose condition is worsening will develop other signs and symptoms known as "severe features." These include a low number of *platelets* in the blood, abnormal kidney or liver function, pain over the upper abdomen, changes in vision, fluid in the lungs, or a severe headache. A very high blood pressure reading also is considered a severe feature.[160]

If preeclampsia occurs during pregnancy, your baby may need to be delivered right away, even if he or she is not fully grown. Preterm babies have an increased risk of serious complications. Some preterm complications can last the lifetime of the child and require ongoing medical care.[160]

Signs and symptoms include:[160]

—Swelling of face or hands

—A headache that will not go away

—Seeing spots or changes in eyesight

—Pain in the upper abdomen or shoulder

—Nausea and vomiting (in the second half of pregnancy)

—Sudden weight gain

—Difficulty breathing

◆ **Vaginal bleeding or discharge.**

◆ **Preterm labor (uterine contractions).**

Postpartum Concerns

Continued diabetes self-management is important. After your baby is born, continue the healthy habits that you learned while pregnant to help YOU be healthier in the future.

Healthy Eating

Work with your dietitian to adjust your meal plan to your needs after the baby is born. If you will be breastfeeding, your calorie needs will be higher than during the pregnancy.

Being Active

Once your provider approves, you should resume activity. Being active is an important part of getting back to your prepregnancy weight and helping with glucose control.

Monitoring

Keep checking your glucose regularly. Share results with your provider at follow-up. The ADA recommends the following glucose targets for most nonpregnant adults: before meals, 80 to 130 mg/dL (3.9–7.2 mmol/L); 1 to 2 hours after meals, <180 mg/dL (<10 mmol/L).[2]

Some providers recommend even tighter glucose targets (from AACE): before meals, <110 mg/dL (6.10 mmol/L); 2 hours after meals, <140 mg/dL (7.77 mmol/L).[6] Discuss target blood glucose levels with your provider.

Taking Medication

The hormones that helped sustain the pregnancy return to normal levels after delivery. This will change your glucose patterns, so your medication regimen will need to change in response. Your plans to breastfeed will affect your medication plan.

American Association of Diabetes Educators©

If you will be taking insulin, you will find that breastfeeding may lower the amount of insulin you require. Oral diabetes medications are not recommended when breastfeeding.[128(p701)]

Reducing Risks

Breastfeeding is recommended for women with preexisting diabetes, as well as those with recent gestational diabetes.[161] Studies show that breastfeeding improves glucose tolerance and lowers glucose levels.[162,163]

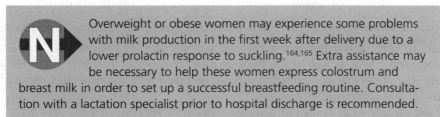

Overweight or obese women may experience some problems with milk production in the first week after delivery due to a lower prolactin response to suckling.[164,165] Extra assistance may be necessary to help these women express colostrum and breast milk in order to set up a successful breastfeeding routine. Consultation with a lactation specialist prior to hospital discharge is recommended.

- Women who have gestational diabetes are at high risk for developing type 2 diabetes later in life.[161,164-166] A healthy lifestyle is one key to lowering your chances of getting type 2 diabetes later on. The principles of healthy eating that you learned during your pregnancy should be continued, with the right calorie level, of course. And being active will help if you need to lose weight. These lifestyle choices are good for the whole family, and can help reduce the future risk for obesity and type 2 diabetes in your children.

- If you had gestational diabetes, it is important that you are screened for diabetes or prediabetes 6 to 12 weeks after delivery and every 1 to 3 years after depending on your risk factors.

Coping

Naturally, taking care of your baby will require a lot of energy. Be sure to ask your family and friends to help you during this time. If you breastfeed, you may find that the hormone released when your baby nurses (oxytocin) helps relax you. Oxytocin has been found to reduce stress and alter a person's response to stressful events.

Advanced Detail

Reducing Risks While Traveling

See the "Resources" section for "Tips for Managing Diabetes While Traveling." Consider using as a patient handout as needed.

Traveling might be on your agenda for work or for pleasure. Here are some tips that can help you manage diabetes while away from home.

Healthy Eating

- Always keep some extra food with you in case of delays. Crackers and cheese, peanut butter, hard candy, and glucose tablets will get you through until a meal is possible.
- In foreign countries, avoid tap water. Drink bottled water or bottled drinks instead. Remember to ask for drinks without ice cubes. Use bottled water for brushing your teeth.
- Avoid food from street vendors.

338   Diabetes Education Curriculum

Being Active

- ◆ On long trips in the car or on an airplane, make it a point to move your legs every 1 to 2 hours. This can help lower your risk for blood clots, which can form after prolonged inactivity.

- ◆ When on business travel, use the hotel fitness center. If no fitness center is available, check the hotel television station for exercise programming. Take short walks during lunch or breaks in meetings.

Monitoring

- ◆ Check your glucose level frequently during long travel, and as soon as you arrive at your destination.

- ◆ Take extra care to keep your meter and monitoring supplies safe from harm. The cargo compartments of buses, airplanes, and trains, as well as the trunk of a car, may be too hot or too cold for your meter and supplies. Carry your meter and all monitoring supplies on board with you when traveling by these modes of transportation.

- ◆ Be aware of the current Transportation Safety Administration (TSA) regulations that apply to most modes of public transportation. Notify the TSA officer that you have diabetes and are carrying monitoring supplies with you. Blood glucose meters, test strips, lancets, alcohol swabs, and control solutions are allowed past the security checkpoint after screening. Sharps disposal containers or similar hard shatterproof disposal containers for storing used lancets and test strips are also allowed.

Taking Medication

- ◆ Before you travel to a foreign country, get a letter from your doctor that describes your diabetes management, including the need for monitoring and medications. List any allergies (medication, food, substances) that you may have. Carry signed prescriptions for all your medications in case you run out or your supplies are lost during your travel. (Check on prescription requirements in the area you will be traveling to.)

- ◆ Pack twice as much medication as you think you will need on your trip. If you take insulin, be sure to pack twice the number of syringes or pen needles you think you'll need. If you use a pump, bring extra supplies and batteries.

- ◆ While traveling, keep your medication in your carry-on baggage. Don't risk losing your medication by packing it in checked luggage. The cargo compartments of buses, airplanes, and trains, as well as the trunk of a car, may be too hot or too cold for insulin.

- ◆ Insulin does not need to be refrigerated, but if you are planning extended time outdoors in very warm or cold weather, insulated travel packs, minicoolers, and refrigerated gel packs are good options for storing insulin.

- ◆ If you take insulin, be aware that it may be available in U-40 or U-80 strength in countries outside the United States. U-40 or U-80 means that there are 40 or 80 units of insulin in each milliliter of liquid (as opposed to the vials in the United States, which contain 100 units of insulin per milliliter of liquid). U-40 and U-80 insulin require a special syringe. If you take your usual number of units using U-40 or U-80 insulin, you will get less insulin than what you need.

- ◆ When drawing up insulin on board an airplane, remember that the cabin is pressurized. Therefore, you do not need to inject air into the vial prior to drawing up your dose.

- ◆ Always discuss international travel with your provider so that you can safely plan for your insulin needs. Many insulin users find that a daily injection of long-acting insulin plus premeal rapid-acting insulin injections provides flexibility during international travel. If you travel east, your day is shortened, so you may need less insulin than usual. If you travel west, your day is lengthened, and you may need more insulin than usual.

American Association of Diabetes Educators©

Reducing Risks

◈ Always carry or wear medical identification.

◈ If you are traveling to a foreign country, be able to ask for assistance in that language. Write these phrases on a card you can pull out when needed. Better yet, learn how to say "I have diabetes," "I need a doctor," and "I need orange juice." There are also phone apps that can help translate English into other languages.

◈ For a list of doctors in other countries who speak English, you can call the International Association for Medical Assistance to Travelers at 1-716-754-4883 or http://www.iamat.org. If you don't have this list but have a medical emergency in a foreign country, contact the American Consulate, American Express, or local medical schools to get a list of doctors.

◈ Travel time is not a good time to break in a new pair of shoes. When traveling, carry an alternate pair of good-fitting shoes, especially if you will be doing lots of walking. Carry antibacterial ointment and some bandages in case you develop a blister on your feet. If you plan to swim in lakes, rivers, or the ocean, wear water shoes to protect your feet from injury.

◈ In case of diarrhea or upset stomach during travel, carry over-the-counter medications such as loperamide (Imodium-AD®), Pepto-Bismol®, or Kaopectate®.

◈ Use sunblock to protect your skin if you'll be outside for an extended time.

Advanced Detail

Reducing Risks During Disaster Conditions

Standard of Medical Care in Diabetes[167]

People with diabetes should keep a disaster kit ready in case of a disaster. The kit should include necessary items required to manage diabetes. It should be reviewed at least twice a year.

Everyone needs to be prepared for emergencies, whether they are natural disasters or otherwise. For people with diabetes, emergency preparedness takes on extra importance. Being prepared will help lessen the impact of the situation on your diabetes.[168,169]

People with diabetes should keep a waterproof and insulated disaster kit ready. Be sure everyone in your household knows where the kit is located. Store the kit where it will not be exposed to extreme temperatures. Items to include in the kit are as follows[2]:

◈ Glucose meter

◈ Glucose testing strips

◈ Lancets

◈ Medication

◈ Syringes (if using insulin)

◈ Glucose tablets or gel

◈ Glucagon emergency kit

◈ Antibiotic ointment

◈ If you wear glasses or contacts, add an extra pair to your kit

◈ Waterless antibacterial hand rinse

American Association of Diabetes Educators©

- List of all medications and pharmacy prescription numbers (if you get relocated during a disaster, pharmacies will often refill prescriptions based on this number)
- If possible, include a copy of your latest laboratory tests and procedures

You should look through your disaster kit twice a year to make sure nothing is missing. Replace any expired medications or glucose test strips. It is also desirable to have additional supplies at your place of work.

Identifying Barriers to Reducing Risks

Even though you know that keeping up with regular doctor visits and preventive care is good for you, there may be barriers that prevent you from making healthy choices about reducing your risk for diabetes complications. For every barrier there may be many possible solutions.

What might work to overcome this barrier? Let's brainstorm together and learn from one another's experiences.

Reality Scenario	Problem Solving — Possible Solutions/What Would *You* Do?
Interpersonal *I want to get the needed tests done each year, but I don't feel comfortable making suggestions to my doctor about my care. It's intimidating. It's as if I'm challenging the treatment my doctor has prescribed. After all, I didn't go to medical school, my doctor did.*	• Every patient has the right to question what his or her provider recommends. Doctors are very busy and may not be up to date on every aspect of diabetes care. You have the right to offer your own ideas for alternate treatment. • Show your doctor your personal care record, with needed tests and how often they should be done. Tell him or her you want to keep up with the tests that the American Diabetes Association recommends. • Write down your questions and concerns in advance. Ask the doctor to read the list of questions/concerns. • Bring a person to the appointment with you for moral support. Make sure he or she understands your position about your care. Ask that person to speak up if you can't voice your concerns.
Transportation problems *I don't have reliable transportation. It's hard to get to all the necessary medical appointments.*	• Check your insurance benefits. Many major plans include coverage for transportation to medical appointments. Some imaging centers provide free transportation services. If you need to make an appointment for X-rays, MRIs, CT scans, etc, call your local imaging centers to find out if they offer transportation. • If you have Medicaid, you may qualify for medical appointment transportation through local medical transportation companies. Check your benefits. • Veterans may also be eligible for transportation to VA treatment centers. Check with your VA center. • If you are a senior, the National Council on Aging (NCOA) has a Web site that can help you find services in your local area. Transportation for medical appointments may be available. • Visit the NCOA's BenefitsCheckUp Web site: http://www.benefitscheckup.org/moreprograms.cfm?partner_id=0. • Consider public transportation. Some public transportation companies offer seniors a discount. • Ask a friend or family member to drive you. If you have lots of appointments, try to schedule more than one on a given day, so the number of trips is minimized.

American Association of Diabetes Educators©

Reality Scenario	Problem Solving Possible Solutions/What Would *You* Do?
Physical limitations *I can't do a proper foot exam because I have trouble reaching/seeing/feeling my feet.*	• Use a mirror to help visualize your feet. Try a mirror with an attachment that allows you to prop it up on a hard surface (the floor or a chair) and angle it upward so you can see your foot. A mirror with a telescoping handle is also very helpful if you can't bend your legs or back to examine your feet. • Ask someone else in your home to take a look at your feet every day. • If you live alone, a friend, neighbor or family member may be willing to help you.
Psychobiologic *I want to quit smoking but it's too hard.*	See the "Resources" section at end of this chapter for "Tips to Quit Smoking."
Financial *I can't afford special diabetic shoes.*	• Check your insurance benefits. You may have coverage for special shoes and/or inserts. If you have Medicare Part B and you meet certain criteria, you can get special shoes and/or inserts. See the "Resources" section at the end of this module for "Medicare Part B Coverage of Therapeutic Shoes and Inserts," which may be used as a patient handout. • If you have no insurance coverage for special shoes, look for shoes that are supportive, are wide and deep enough in the toe area so that your toes don't rub, and have shock-absorbing soles. Many reasonably priced athletic or walking shoes meet these requirements.
How can I see a dentist twice a year? I don't have dental insurance, and I can't afford to.	• You may also be eligible for free or reduced care through a federally qualified health center. • Check for dental schools in your area, where costs for dental care are usually reduced. Sometimes fees for professional services are reduced or patients are only charged for equipment and supplies. Dental schools: http://www.ada.org/en/education-careers/dental-schools-and-programs. State dental societies may be able to direct you to dental patient assistance programs. State and local dental societies: http://www.ada.org/en/about-the-ada/national-state-local-dental-societies.

Identifying Facilitators for Reducing Risks

As important as it is to identify barriers to reducing risks, it's just as important to consider the positives, or facilitators, in our situation. Looking deeper, you may find that there are more positives than you thought.

 What are some things that can help you reduce your risk for diabetes complications?

Common Facilitators

- Social support—family members, coworkers, etc
- Resources—free resources for smoking cessation, transportation services to medical office visits, dental schools for low-cost dental care, full use of insurance plan benefits
- Reminders and cues—personal diabetes care wallet card, notes of encouragement (positive affirmations)
- Rewards—incentives to maintain motivation

Setting a SMART Goal to Reduce Risks

S—Specific: exactly what you want to do
M—Measurable: you can measure it (how much, how often, etc)
A—Attainable: challenging but not out of reach
R—Realistic: given person's situation, can it be done?
T—Timeline: short term, for next 2 to 4 weeks

The participant sets individual goals for reducing risks. The educator and the participant schedule a date to evaluate progress with behavior change.

Using a mnemonic like SMART to help remember an idea can be a useful teaching tool, especially for those with verbal/auditory intelligence.

Follow-up/Outcomes Measurement

Per the Standards for Outcomes Measurement of Diabetes Self-Management Education, the **first follow-up should be conducted within 2 to 4 weeks** after the initial teaching session on reducing risks. At this follow-up, success in implementing risk-reduction behavior can be assessed. **Subsequent follow-up is recommended at 3- to 6-month intervals thereafter.** Use the following table as a guide for identifying outcomes measures and how to measure them. Measurement of these outcomes may be objective or subjective.[170]

The exception to this schedule would be during pregnancy. The first follow-up should be conducted within 1 week and subsequent visits at 2 to 4 weeks.

Self-Care Behavior: Reducing Risks Outcomes Measures	Self-Care Behavior: Reducing Risks Methods of Measurement
Immediate outcome: Learning Immediate outcomes of learning can be assessed right away after the educational encounter. Immediate outcomes include: K: Acquiring *knowledge* (*what to do*) S: Acquiring *skills* (*how to do it*) CM: Developing *confidence and motivation* (*want to do it*) PS: Developing *problem-solving/coping skills* to overcome barrier (*can do it*)	Immediate outcomes of learning can be measured by patient knowledge testing (paper-and-pen testing, or questioning to determine that patient understands information taught). Immediate outcomes for acquiring a skill can be measured by patient's demonstration of that skill. Following are various methods of measuring immediate outcomes for the self-care behavior of *reducing risks*.
Standards of care (K)	<u>Subjective:</u> Patient describes the standards of care—necessary tests and their frequency (eg, dilated eye examination annually).
Therapeutic goals (K)	<u>Subjective:</u> Patient states recommended therapeutic goals for tests in the standards of care (eg, blood pressure <140/90 mm HG).
Self-examination of foot and foot care (K,S)	<u>Subjective:</u> Patient explains proper foot care, as well as findings that should be reported to provider. <u>Objective:</u> Patient demonstrates proper self-examination of foot.
Self-monitoring of blood pressure (K,S)	<u>Subjective:</u> Patient explains proper operation of home blood pressure monitor. <u>Objective:</u> Patient demonstrates proper technique for taking blood pressure.

Self-Care Behavior: Reducing Risks Outcomes Measures	Self-Care Behavior: Reducing Risks Methods of Measurement
Maintaining personal care record (K,S)	Subjective: Patient explains how to effectively use personal care record. Objective: Patient documents his or her personal care record (dates that tests were done/are due, results of tests, etc).
Potential barriers (financial, physical limitations, time constraints, communication problems with provider) and facilitators to risk reduction (PS)	Subjective: Considering his or her individual situation, patient describes anticipated obstacle(s) that may limit the ability to reduce risks (access preventive care services or perform risk-reduction behaviors). Patient describes facilitators that may help him or her reduce risk (access preventive care services or perform risk-reduction behaviors).
Strategy to overcome potential barriers to risk reduction (PS)	Subjective: Patient develops a plan to deal with anticipated obstacle(s) to risk reduction.
Intermediate outcome: Behavior change	Intermediate outcomes measures can be assessed over time: after the educational encounter and once the patient has had adequate time to implement new behavior(s) in a real-life setting. *Behavior change* is an intermediate outcomes measure. It is the ultimate outcome of DSME/T. At follow-up intervals, knowledge and skills (discussed above) should be reassessed, as well as behavior change.
Risk-reduction behavior: accessing preventive care services	Subjective: Patient self-report of accessing preventive care services (eg, getting eye examination) Objective: Documentation (eg, medical records audit, examination code audit, patient's personal care record) of preventive care services obtained: • Office visits—primary care, specialists, educator, dietitian, etc • Blood pressure at each visit to primary care provider • Aspirin therapy (if clinically indicated) • Foot examinations—inspection, comprehensive • Dilated eye exams • Laboratory tests—A1C, lipids, urine for protein • Immunizations—influenza, pneumonia, Hepatitis B • Counseling to stop smoking (if applicable) • Prepregnancy counseling (if applicable) • Dental visits
Risk-reduction behavior: foot care and self-examination of foot	Subjective: Patient self-report of frequency of self-examination of foot and relevant findings. Objective: Patient demonstration of proper self-examination of foot; observation of patient's footwear.
Risk-reduction behavior: self-monitoring of blood pressure	Subjective: Patient self-report of frequency of self-monitoring of blood pressure. Objective: Patient demonstration of proper technique for taking his or her blood pressure; patient's documentation of blood pressure results.
Risk-reduction behavior: smoking cessation (if applicable)	Subjective: Patient self-report of smoking status (eg, quit smoking, number of cigarettes smoked per day, efforts to quit).
Risk-reduction behavior: aspirin therapy (if applicable)	Subjective: Patient self-report of taking aspirin per provider's order
Barrier identification and resolution (PS)	Subjective: Patient self-report of barriers faced and facilitators and strategies used during efforts to implement risk-reduction behaviors
Plan for future behavior change (PS)	Subjective: Patient self-report of plans to reduce risk and behavior strategies going forward.

American Association of Diabetes Educators©

REFERENCES

1. Boren SA, Gunlock TL, Schaefer J, Albright A. Reducing risks in diabetes self-management: a systematic review of the literature. Diabetes Educ. 2007;33(6):1053-77.

2. American Diabetes Association. Standards of medical care in diabetes—2015. Diabetes Care. 2015;38 Suppl 1: S1-94.

3. D'Eramo Melkus G. Reducing risks in diabetes self-management: a commentary. Diabetes Educ. 2007;33(6):1078-9.

4. Constance A. Reducing risks. In: Mensing C, ed. The Art and Science of Diabetes Self-Management Education Desk Reference. 3rd ed. Chicago: American Association of Diabetes Educators; 2014:287-307.

5. Sacks DB, Bruns DE, Goldstein DE, et al. Guidelines and recommendations for laboratory analysis in the diagnosis and management of diabetes mellitus. Clin Chem. 2002;48:431-72.

6. American Association of Clinical Endocrinologists. AACE Diabetes Mellitus Clinical Practice Guidelines Task Force. Medical guidelines for the clinical practice for developing a diabetes mellitus comprehensive care plan. Endocr Pract. 2011;17 Suppl 2:1-53.

7. Skyler JS, Bergenstal R, Bonow RO, et al. Intensive glycemic control and the prevention of cardiovascular events: implications of the ACCORD, ADVANCE, and VA Diabetes Trials: a position statement of the American Diabetes Association and a scientific statement of the American College of Cardiology Foundation and the American Heart Association. Diabetes Care. 2009;32:187-92.

8. Diabetes Control and Complications Trial Group. The effect of intensive treatment of diabetes on the development and progression of long-term complications in insulin-dependent diabetes mellitus. N Engl J Med. 1993;329:977-86.

9. UK Prospective Diabetes Study Group. Intensive blood glucose control with sulphonylurea or insulin compared with conventional treatment and risk for complications in patients with type 2 diabetes (UKPDS 33). Lancet. 1998;352:837-53.

10. UK Prospective Diabetes Study Group. Effect of intensive blood glucose control with metformin on complications in overweight patients with type 2 diabetes (UKPDS 34). Lancet. 1998:352:854-62.

11. Ohkubo Y, Kishikawa H, Araki E, et al. Intensive insulin therapy prevents the progression of diabetic microvascular complications in Japanese patients with non-insulin-dependent diabetes mellitus: a randomized prospective 6-year study. Diabetes Res Clin Pract. 1995;28:103-17.

12. Stratton IM, Adler AI, Neil HA, et al. Association of glycaemia with macrovascular and microvascular complications of type 2 diabetes (UKPDS 35): prospective observational study. BMJ. 2000;321:405-12.

13. The DCCT Trial/Epidemiology of Diabetes and Complications (EDIC) Research Group. Retinopathy and nephropathy in patients with type 1 diabetes 4 years after a trial of intensive therapy. N Engl J Med. 2000;342:381-9.

14. Martin CL, Albers J, Herman WH, et al. Neuropathy among the diabetes control and complications trial cohort 8 years after trial completion. Diabetes Care. 2006;29:340-4.

15. Holman RR, Paul SK, Bethel MA, et al. 10-year follow-up of intensive glucose control in type 2 diabetes. N Engl J Med. 2008;359:1577-89.

16. UK Prospective Diabetes Study Group. Intensive blood glucose control with sulphonylureas or insulin compared with conventional treatment and risk of complications in patients with type 2 diabetes (UKPDS 38). Lancet. 1998; 352(9131):837-53.

17. Arguedas JA, Leiva V, Wright JM. Blood pressure targets for hypertension in people with diabetes mellitus. Cochrane Database Syst Rev. 2013 Oct 30;10:CD008277.

18. James PA, Oparil S, Carter BL, et al. 2014 evidence-based guideline for the management of high blood pressure in adults: report from the panel members appointed to the Eighth Joint National Committee (JNC 8). JAMA. 2014;311:507-20.

19. Zoungas S, Chalmers J, Neal B, et al, ADVANCE-ON Collaborative Group. Follow-up of blood-pressure lowering and glucose control in type 2 diabetes. N Engl J Med. 2014;371:1392-406.

20. ACCORD Study Group, Cushman WC, Evans GW, et al. Effects of intensive blood-pressure control in type 2 diabetes mellitus. N Engl J Med. 2010;362:1575-85.

21. Adler AI, Stratton IM, Neil HA, et al. Association of systolic blood pressure with macrovascular and microvascular complications of type 2 diabetes (UKPDS 36): prospective observational study. BMJ. 2000;321:412-9.

22. American Diabetes Association. Cardiovascular disease and risk management—2015. Diabetes Care. 2015;38 Suppl 1:S49-57.

23. Sibai BM. Treatment of hypertension in pregnant women. New Engl J Med. 1996;335:257-65.

24. American Diabetes Association. Children and adolescents—2015. Diabetes Care. 2015;38 Suppl 1:S70-6.

25. American Diabetes Association. Type 2 diabetes in children and adolescents: consensus statement. Diabetes Care. 2000;23:381-9.

26. Copeland KC, Silverstein J, Moore KR, et al. Management of newly diagnosed type 2 diabetes mellitus (T2DM) in children and adolescents. Pediatrics. 2013;131:364-82.

27. Bernstein EF, Fronek A. Current status of non-invasive tests in the diagnosis of peripheral arterial disease. Surg Clin North Am. 1982;62:473-87.

28. Criqui MH. Peripheral arterial disease: epidemiological aspects. Vasc Med. 2001;6 Suppl 1:3-7.

29. American Diabetes Association. Microvascular complications and foot care—2015. Diabetes Care. 2015;38 Suppl 1: S58-66.

30. American Diabetes Association. Peripheral arterial disease in people with diabetes: consensus statement. Diabetes Care. 2003;26:3333-41.

31. Sega R, Facchetti R, Bombelli M, et al. Prognostic value of ambulatory and home blood pressures compared with office blood pressure in the general population: follow-up results from the Pressioni Arteriose Monitorate e Loro Associazioni (PAMELA) study. Circulation. 2005;111:1777-83.

32. O'Brien E, Asmar R, Beilin L, et al, for the European Society of Hypertension Working Group on Blood Pressure Monitoring. European Society of Hypertension recommendations for conventional, ambulatory and home blood pressure measurement. J Hypertens. 2003;21:821-48.

33. Pickering TG, Miller NH, Ogedegbe G, et al. Call to action on use and reimbursement for home blood pressure monitoring: executive summary: a joint scientific statement from the American Heart Association, American Society of Hypertension, and Preventive Cardiovascular Nurses Association. Hypertension. 2008;52:1-9.

34. US Food and Drug Administration. Non-invasive blood pressure (NIBP) monitor guidance (cited 2015 Jul 9). On the Internet at: http://www.fda.gov/RegulatoryInformation/Guidances/ucm080219.htm.

35. dabl® Educational Trust. Blood pressure monitors—validations, papers and reviews (cited 2015 Jul 9). On the Internet at: http://www.dableducational.org/sphygmomanometers.html.

36. Scrier RW, Estacio RO, Esler A, Mehler P. Effects of aggressive blood pressure control in normotensive type 2 diabetic patients on albuminuria, retinopathy and strokes. Kidney Int. 2002;61(3):1086-97.

37. Sacks FM, Sventkey LP, Vollme WM, et al. Effects on blood pressure of reduced sodium and the dietary approached to stop hypertension (DASH) diet. N Engl J Med. 2001;344:3-10.

38. Chobanian AV, Bakris GL, Black HR, et al. The Seventh Report of the Joint National Committee on Prevention, Detection, Evaluation and Treatment of High Blood Pressure: the JNC 7 report. JAMA. 2004;289:2560-72.

39. Vollner WM, Sacks FM, Ard J, et al. Effects of diet and sodium intake on blood pressure. Ann Intern Med. 2001; 135:1019-28.

40. Hermida RC, Ayala DE, Mojon A, Fernandez JR. Influence of time of day of blood pressure-lowering treatment on cardiovascular risk in hypertensive patients with type 2 diabetes. Diabetes Care. 2011;34:1270-6.

41. Zhao P, Xu P, Wan C, Wang Z. Evening versus morning dosing regimen drug therapy for hypertension. Cochrane Database Sys Rev. 2011;10:CD004184.

42. Writing Group of the PREMIER Collaborative Research Group. Effects of comprehensive lifestyle modification on blood pressure control: main results of the PREMIER clinical trial. JAMA. 2003:289(16):2083-93.

43. Whelton SP, Chin A, Xin X, He J. Effect of aerobic exercise on blood pressure. Ann Intern Med. 2002;136:493-503.

American Association of Diabetes Educators©

346 Diabetes Education Curriculum

44. Xin X, He J, Prontini MG, et al. Effects of alcohol reduction on blood pressure: a meta-analysis of randomized controlled trials. Hypertension. 2001;38:1112-7.

45. Primatesta P, Falaschetti E, Gupta S, et al. Association between smoking and blood pressure: evidence from the health survey of England. Hypertension. 2001;37:187-93.

46. Sowers JR, Haffner SM. Treatment of cardiovascular and renal risk factors in the diabetic hypertensive. Hypertension. 2002;40:781-8.

47. Heart Outcomes Prevention Evaluation Study Investigators. HOPE: Effects of ramipril on cardiovascular and microvascular outcomes in people with diabetes mellitus: results of the HOPE study and MICRO-HOPE substudy. Lancet. 2000;355:253-9.

48. Dixon DL, Sisson, EM. Pharmacotherapy: dyslipidemia and hypertension in persons with diabetes. In: Mensing C, ed. The Art and Science of Diabetes Self-Management Education Desk Reference. 3rd ed. Chicago: American Association of Diabetes Educators; 2014:491-540.

49. Green DM, Ropper AH, Kronmal RA, et al. Serum potassium level and dietary potassium intake as risk factors for stroke. Neurology. 2002;59(3):314-20.

50. Khaw KT, Barrett-Connor E. Dietary potassium and stroke-associated mortality: a 12-year prospective population study. N Engl J Med. 1987;316(5):235-40.

51. Lown KS, Bailey DG, Fontana RJ, et al. Grapefruit juice increases felodipine oral availability in humans by decreasing intestinal CYP3A protein expression. J Clin Invest. 1997;99(10):2545-53.

52. Strippoli GF, Craig MC, Schena FP, et al. Role of blood pressure targets and specific antihypertensive agents used to prevent diabetic nephropathy and delay its progression. J Am Soc Nephrol. 2006;17:S153-5.

53. Expert Panel on Detection, Evaluation and Treatment of High Blood Cholesterol in Adults. Executive Summary of the third report of the National Cholesterol Education Program (NCEP) Expert Panel on Detection, Evaluation and Treatment of High Blood Cholesterol in Adults (Adult Treatment Panel III). JAMA. 2001;285: 2486-97.

54. Evert AB, Boucher JL, Cypress M, et al. Nutrition management recommendations for the management of adults with diabetes. Diabetes Care. 2013;36:3821-42.

55. Mukherjee SK, Gold E. Of Inuits and Americans: omega-3s in diabetes treatment. Pract Diabetol. 2003;22(3):28-32.

56. Kris-Etherton PM, Harris WH, Appel LJ, et al. Fish consumption, fish oil, omega-3 fatty acids, and cardiovascular disease. Circulation. 2002;106:2747-57.

57. Pietinen P, Rimm EB, Korhonen P, et al. Intake of dietary fiber and risk of coronary heart disease in a cohort of Finnish men: the ATBC Study. Circulation. 1996;94:2720-7.

58. Rimm EB, Ascherio A, Giovanucci E, Spiegelman D, Stampfer MJ, Willett WC. Vegetable, fruit, and cereal fiber intake and risk of coronary heart disease among men. JAMA. 1996;275:447-51.

59. Brown L, Rosner B, Willett WW, Sacks FM. Cholesterol-lowering effects of dietary fiber: a meta-analysis. Am J Clin Nutr. 1999;69(1):30-42.

60. Kodama S, Tanaka S, Saito K, et al. Effect of aerobic exercise training on serum levels of high-density lipoprotein cholesterol. Arch Intern Med. 2007;167:999-1008.

61. Boden WE, Probstfield JL, Anderson T, et al; AIM-HIGH Investigators. Niacin in patients with low HDL cholesterol levels receiving intensive statin therapy. N Engl J Med. 2011;365:2255-67.

62. Oh R. Practical application of fish oil (omega-3 fatty acids) in primary care. J Am Board Fam Pract. 2005;18:28-36.

63. American Diabetes Association. Position statement. Aspirin therapy in diabetes. Diabetes Care. 2004;27 Suppl 1:S72-3.

64. Kirpitch A, Smith-Ossman S. Diabetic kidney disease. In: Mensing C, ed. The Art and Science of Diabetes Self-Management Education Desk Reference. 3rd ed. Chicago: American Association of Diabetes Educators; 2014: 775-98.

65. American Diabetes Association. Consensus statement. Type 2 diabetes in children and adolescents. Diabetes Care. 2000;23(3):381-9.

American Association of Diabetes Educators©

66. Remuzzi G, Macia M, Ruggenenti P. Prevention and treatment of diabetic renal disease in type 2 diabetes: the BENEDICT study. J Am Soc Nephrol. 2006;17:S90-7.

67. Laffel LM, McGill JB, Gans DJ. The beneficial effect of angiotensin-converting enzyme inhibition with captopril on diabetic nephropathy in normotensive IDDM patients with microalbuminuria. North American Microalbuminuria Study Group. Am J Med. 1995;99:497-504.

68. Snow V, Weiss KB, Mottur-Pilson C. The evidence base for tight blood pressure control in the management of type 2 diabetes mellitus. Ann Intern Med. 2003;138:5887-92.

69. American Academy of Ophthalmology Quality of Care Committee Retina Panel. Preferred Practice Pattern for Diabetic Retinopathy. San Francisco: American Academy of Ophthalmology; 2003.

70. Agardh E, Tababat-Khani P. Adopting 3 year screening intervals for sight-threatening retinal vascular lesions in type 2 diabetic subjects without retinopathy. Diabetes Care. 2011;34:1318-9.

71. Hooper P, Boucher MC, Cruess A, et al. Canadian Ophthalmological Society evidence-based clinical practice guidelines for the management of diabetic retinopathy. Can J Ophthalmol. 2012;47 Suppl 2:S1-30.

72. Kiss S. Eye disease related to diabetes. In: Mensing C, ed. The Art and Science of Diabetes Self-Management Education Desk Reference. 3rd ed. Chicago: American Association of Diabetes Educators; 2014:755-74.

73. American Diabetes Association. Position statement. Retinopathy in diabetes. Diabetes Care. 2004;27:S84-7.

74. Gonzalez VH, Banda RM. Diabetic eye disease. In: Mensing C, ed. The Art and Science of Diabetes Self-Management Education: A Desk Reference for Healthcare Professionals. Chicago: American Association of Diabetes Educators; 2006:511-28.

75. Ahmed J, Ward TP, Bursell SE, Aiello LM. The sensitivity and specificity of nonmydriatic digital stereoscopic retinal imaging in detecting diabetic retinopathy. Diabetes Care. 2006;29:2205-9.

76. The Diabetic Retinopathy Study (DRS) Research Group. Preliminary report of the effects of photocoagulation therapy: DRS Report #1. Am J Ophthalmol. 1976;81:383-96.

77. Early Treatment Diabetic Retinopathy Study (ETDRS) Research Group. Photocoagulation for diabetic macular edema: ETDRS Report #1. Arch Ophthalmol. 1985;103:1796-806.

78. Boulton AJM, Vinik AI, Arezzo JC, et al. Diabetic neuropathies: a statement by the American Diabetes Association. Diabetes Care. 2005;28(4):956-62.

79. Boulton AJ, Armstrong DG, Albert SF, et al. Comprehensive foot examination and risk assessment: a report of the task force of the foot care interest group of the American Diabetes Association, with endorsement by the American Association of Clinical Endocrinologists. Diabetes Care. 2008;31:1679-85.

80. Caputo GM, Cavanagh PR, Ulbrecht JS, et al. Assessment and management of foot disease in patients with diabetes. N Engl J Med. 1994;331(13):854-60.

81. Vinik AI, Vinik EJ. Diabetic neuropathies. In: Mensing C, ed. The Art and Science of Diabetes Self-Management Education Desk Reference. 3rd ed. Chicago: American Association of Diabetes Educators; 2014:799-838.

82. Resnick HE, Valsania P, Phillips CL. Diabetes mellitus and nontraumatic lower extremity amputation in black and white Americans: the National Health and Nutrition Examination Survey Epidemiologic follow-up study, 1971–1992. Arch Intern Med. 1999;159:2470-5.

83. Centers for Disease Control and Prevention. The Surgeon General's 1990 report on the health benefits of smoking cessation. Executive summary. Morbidity and Mortality Weekly Report. 1990 Oct 5 (cited 2015 Jul 9); 39(RR-12): viii-xv. On the Internet at: http://www.cdc.gov/mmwr/preview/mmwrhtml/00001800.htm.

84. McCulloch DK, Campbell IW, Prescott RJ, Clark BF. Effect of alcohol intake on symptomatic peripheral neuropathy in diabetic men. Diabetes Care. 1980;3(2):245-7.

85. American College of Foot and Ankle Surgeons. Diabetic complications and amputation prevention: your proactive measures (cited 2015 Jul 9). On the Internet at: http://www.footphysicians.com/footankleinfo/diabetic-amputations. htm.

86. National Diabetes Education Program. Take care of your feet for a lifetime (cited 2015 Jul 9). On the Internet at: http://ndep.nih.gov/publications/PublicationDetail.aspx?PubId=67.

348 Diabetes Education Curriculum

87. Feldman CB, Davis ED. Sockwear recommendations for people with diabetes. Diabetes Spectr. 2001;14:59-61.

88. Spallone V, Bellavere F, Scionti L, et al. Diabetic Neuropathy Study Group of the Italian Society for Diabetology. Recommendations for the use of cardiovascular tests in diagnosing diabetic autonomic neuropathy. Nutr Metab Cardiovasc Dis. 2011;21:69-78.

89. International Diabetes Federation. IDF Consensus Statement on Sleep Apnea and Type 2 Diabetes. Brussels, Belgium: IDF; 2008.

90. Netzer NC, Stoohs RA, Netza CM, et al. Using the Berlin Questionnaire to identify patients at risk for the sleep apnea syndrome. Ann Intern Med. 1999;131(7):485-91.

91. Einhorn D, Stewart DA, Erman MK, Gordon N. Effect of nasal continuous positive airway pressure treatment on blood pressure in patients with obstructive sleep apnea. Circulation. 2003;107(1):68-73.

92. West SD, Nicoll DJ, Stradling JR. Prevalence of obstructive sleep apnea in men with type 2 diabetes. Thorax. 2006;61:945-50.

93. Foster GD, Sanders MH, Millman R, et al. Sleep AHEAD Research Group. Obstructive sleep apnea among obese patients with type 2 diabetes. Diabetes Care. 2009;32:1017-9.

94. Khader YS, Dauod AS, El-Qaderi SS, Alkafajei A, Batayha WQ. Periodontal status of diabetics compared with nondiabetics: a meta-analysis. J Diabetes Complications. 2006;20: 59-68.

95. Borgnakke WS, Ylöstalo PV, Taylor GW, Genco RJ. Effect of periodontal disease on diabetes: systematic review of epidemiologic observational evidence. J Periodontol. 2013;84 Suppl:S135-52.

96. Austin MM, D'Hondt N. Monitoring. In: Mensing C, ed. The Art and Science of Diabetes Self-Management Education Desk Reference. 3rd ed. Chicago: American Association of Diabetes Educators; 2014:197-245.

97. Dang DK. Taking medication. In: Mensing C, ed. The Art and Science of Diabetes Self-Management Education Desk Reference. 3rd ed. Chicago: American Association of Diabetes Educators; 2014:175-96.

98. Stewart JE, Wager KA, Friedlander AH, Zadeh HH. The effect of periodontal treatment on glycemic control in patients with type 2 diabetes mellitus. J Clin Periodontol. 2001;28(4):306-10.

99. Centers for Disease Control and Prevention. Take charge of your diabetes (cited 2015 Jul 9). On the Internet at: http://www.cdc.gov/diabetes/pubs/pdf/tctd.pdf.

100. Albandar JM, Streckfus CF, Adesanya MR, Winn DM. Cigar, pipe, and cigarette smoking as risk factors for periodontal disease and tooth loss. J Periodontol. 2000;71:1874-81.

101. Tomar SL, Asma S. Smoking attributable periodontitis in the United States: findings from the NHANES III. J Periodontol. 2000;71:743-51.

102. Martin L. Diabetes and your smile (cited 2015 Jul 9). On the Internet at: http://www.mouthhealthy.org/en/az-topics/d/diabetes.

103. American Dental Association. Learn more about toothbrushes (cited 2015 Jul 9). On the Internet at: http://www.ada.org/en/science-research/ada-seal-of-acceptance/product-category-information/toothbrushes.

104. Guitart J, Woodley DT. Intertrigo: a practical approach. Compr Ther. 1994;20:402-9.

105. Mistiaen P, Poot E, Hickox S, Jochems C, Wagner C. Preventing and treating intertrigo in the large skin folds of adults: a literature overview. Dermatol Nurs. 2004;16:43-6, 49-57.

106. Janniger CK, Schwartz RA, Szepietowski JC, Reich A. Intertrigo and common secondary skin infections. Am Fam Physician. 2005;72:833-40.

107. Johnson-Gutierrez EG. Chronic complications. In: Mensing C, ed. The Art and Science of Diabetes Self-Management Education: A Desk Reference for Healthcare Professionals. Chicago: American Association of Diabetes Educators; 2006:461-74.

108. Zanni GR. Tattoo safety: what to know before getting inked. US News & World Report. 2013 Aug 17. On the Internet at: http://health.usnews.com/health-news/health-wellness/articles/2013/08/17/tattoo-safety-what-to-know-before-getting-inked.

American Association of Diabetes Educators©

Module 8 *Reducing Risks*   349

109. American Academy of Dermatologists. Consumer alert: black henna tattoos can cause serious skin reactions (cited 2015 Jul 9). On the Internet at: http://www.newswise.com/articles/consumer-alert-black-henna-tattoos-can-cause-serious-skin-reactions.

110. McMahon MM, Bistrian BR. Host defences and susceptibility to infection in patients with diabetes mellitus. Infect Dis Clin North Am. 1995;9:1-9.

111. MacRury SM, Gemmell CG, Paterson KR, MacCuish AC. Changes in phagocytic function with glycaemic control in diabetic patients. J Clin Pathol. 1989;42:1143-7.

112. US Food and Drug Administration. Consumer Health Information. Think before you ink: are tattoos safe? (cited 2015 Jul 9). On the Internet at: http://www.fda.gov/downloads/ForConsumers/ConsumerUpdates/UCM143401.pdf.

113. American Diabetes Association. Foundation of care, education, nutrition, physical activity, smoking cessation, psychosocial care and immunization. Diabetes Care. 2015;38 Suppl 1:S20-30.

114. Centers for Disease Control. Key facts about influenza (flu) & flu vaccine (cited 2015 Jul 9). On the Internet at: http://www.cdc.gov/flu/keyfacts.htm.

115. Smith SA, Poland GA. Use of influenza and pneumococcal vaccines in people with diabetes. Diabetes Care. 2000; 23:95-108.

116. Bouter KP, Diepersloot RJ, van Romunde LK, et al. Effect of epidemic influenza on ketoacidosis, pneumonia and death in diabetes mellitus: a hospital register survey of 1976–1979 in the Netherlands. Diabetes Res Clin Pract. 1991;12:61-8.

117. Cameron AS, Roder DM, Esterman AJ, Moore BW. Mortality from influenza and allied infections in South Australia during 1968–1981. Med J Aust. 1985;142:14-7.

118. Barker WH, Mullooly JP. Pneumonia and influenza deaths during epidemics: implications for prevention. Arch Intern Med. 1982;142:85-9.

119. Tomczyk S, Bennett NM, Stoecker C, et al. Use of 13-valent pneumococcal conjugate vaccine and 23-valent pneumococcal polysaccharide vaccine among adults aged ≥65 years: recommendations of the Advisory Committee on Immunization Practices (ACIP). MMWR Morb Mortal Wkly Rep. 2014;63:822-5.

120. Fiore AE, Uyeki TM, Broder K. Prevention and control of influenza with vaccines: recommendations of the Advisory Committee on Immunization Practices (ACIP), 2010. MMWR Morb Mortal Wkly Rep. 2010;59(RR08):1-62.

121. Colquhoun AJ, Nicholson KG, Botha JL, Raymond NT. Effectiveness of influenza vaccine in reducing hospital admissions in people with diabetes. Epidemiol Infect. 1997;119:335-41.

122. National Foundation for Infectious Diseases. Improving influenza vaccination rates in adults and children with diabetes: identifying and overcoming immunization barriers in this high-risk population—a call to action (cited 2015 Jul 9). On the Internet at: http://www.diabeteshealth.com/national-foundation-for-infectious-diseases-urges-increased-influenza-vaccination-rates-for-persons-with-diabetes/.

123. Schaffner W, Rehm SJ, Elasy TA. Influenza vaccination: an unmet need in patients with diabetes. Clin Diabetes. 2007;25:145-9.

124. Bot M, Pouwer F, Zuidersma M, van Melle JP, de Jonge P. Association of coexisting diabetes and depression with mortality after myocardial infarction. Diabetes Care. 2012;35:503-9.

125. Nicolucci A, Kovacs Burns K, Holt RIG, et al; DAWN2 Study Group. Diabetes Attitudes, Wishes and Needs second study (DAWN2): cross-national benchmarking of diabetes related psychosocial outcomes for people with diabetes. Diabet Med. 2013;30:767-77.

126. Centers for Disease Control and Prevention. Recommendations to improve preconception health and health care—United States. MMWR Morb Mortal Wkly Rep. 2006;55(RR06):1-23.

127. American Diabetes Association. Management of diabetes in pregnancy. Diabetes Care. 2015;38:77-9.

128. Thomas A. Pregnancy with diabetes. In: Mensing C, ed. The Art and Science of Diabetes Self-Management Education Desk Reference. 3rd ed. Chicago: American Association of Diabetes Educators; 2014:683-718.

American Association of Diabetes Educators©

350   Diabetes Education Curriculum

129. American Diabetes Association. Position statement. Preconception care of women with diabetes. Diabetes Care. 2004;27 Suppl 1:S76-8.

130. Mills JL, Baker L, Goldman AS. Malformations in infants of diabetic mothers occur before the seventh gestational week: implications for treatment. Diabetes. 1979;28:292-3.

131. Jensen D, Damm P, Moelsted-Pedersen L, et al. Outcomes in type 1 diabetic pregnancies. Diabetes Care. 2004:27:2819-23.

132. Wren C, Birrell G, Hawthorne G. Cardiovascular malformations in infants of diabetic mothers. Heart. 2003; 89:1217-20.

133. Catalano PM, Buchanan TA. Metabolic changes during normal and diabetic pregnancies. In: Reece EA, Coustan DR, Gabbe SG, eds. Diabetes in Women: Adolescence, Pregnancy and Menopause. Philadelphia: Lippincott Williams & Wilkins; 2004:129-45.

134. American Diabetes Association. Standards of medical care in diabetes—2015. Diabetes Care. 2015;38 Suppl 1: S1-93.

135. Landon MB, Gabbe SG. Gestational diabetes mellitus. Obstet Gynecol. 2011;118(6):1379-93.

136. Cooper WO, Hernandez-Diaz S, Arbogast PG, et al. Major congenital malformations after first-trimester exposure to ACE inhibitors. N Engl J Med. 2006;354:2443-51.

137. Akinbi HT, Gerdes JS. Macrosomic infants of nondiabetic mothers and elevated C-peptide levels in cord blood. J Pediatr. 1995;127:481-4.

138. Schwartz R, Gruppuso PA, Petzold K, et al. Hyperinsulinemia and macrosomia in the fetus of the diabetic mother. Diabetes Care. 1994;17:640-8.

139. Salvesen DR, Brudenell JM, Proudler AJ, et al. Fetal pancreatic beta-cell function in pregnancies complicated by maternal diabetes mellitus: relationship to fetal acidemia and macrosomia. Am J Obstet Gynecol. 1993;168:1363-9.

140. Dornhorst A, Nicholls JS, Ali K, et al. Fetal proinsulin and birth weight. Diabet Med. 1994;11:177-81.

141. Krew MA, Kehl RJ, Thomas A, Catalano PM. Relation of amniotic fluid C-peptide levels to neonatal body composition. Obstet Gynecol. 1994;84:96-100.

142. Landon MB, Gabbe SG. Diabetes mellitus. In: Barron WM, Lindheimer MD, Davison JM, eds. Medical Disorders in Pregnancy. St Louis, Mo: Mosby; 2000:71-100.

143. Strauss RS, Dietz WH. Low maternal weight gain in the second or third trimester increases the risk for intrauterine growth retardation. J Nutr. 1999;19:988-93.

144. National Academy of Sciences. Nutrition During Pregnancy. Washington, DC: National Academy Press; 1990.

145. Churchill JA, Berendes HW. Intelligence of children whose mothers had acetonuria during pregnancy. In: Perinatal Factors Affecting Human Development. Publication No. 185. Washington, DC: Pan American Health Organization; 1969.

146. Rizzo T, Metzger BE, Burns WJ, et al. Correlations between antepartum maternal metabolism and child intelligence. N Engl J Med. 1991;325:911-6.

147. American Dietetic Association. Medical Nutrition Therapy Evidence-Based Guidelines for Practice: Nutrition Practice Guidelines for Gestational Diabetes Mellitus [CD-ROM]. Chicago: American Dietetic Association; 2001.

148. Coustan DR, ed. Medical Management of Pregnancy Complicated by Diabetes. 5th ed. Alexandria, Va: American Diabetes Association; 2013.

149. US Food and Drug Administration. High-intensity sweeteners (cited 2015 Jul 9). On the Internet at: http://www.fda.gov/Food/IngredientsPackagingLabeling/FoodAdditivesIngredients/ucm397716.htm.

150. American Diabetes Association. Position statement. Evidence-based nutrition principles and recommendations for the treatment and prevention of diabetes and related complications. Diabetes Care. 2003;26 Suppl 1:S51-61.

151. Centers for Disease Control and Prevention. Notice to readers: Surgeon General's advisory on alcohol use in pregnancy. MMWR Morb Mortal Wkly Rep. 2005;54(9):229.

152. Evans ED. The FDA recommendations on fish intake during pregnancy. J Obstet Gynecol Neonatal Nurs. 2002; 31:715-20.

American Association of Diabetes Educators©

Module 8 *Reducing Risks* 351

153. US Department of Health and Human Services and US Environmental Protection Agency. What you need to know about mercury in fish and shellfish: 2004 EPA and FDA advice for women who may become pregnant, women who are pregnant, nursing mothers, young children (cited 2015 Jul 9). On the Internet at: http://www.fda.gov/Food/FoodborneIllnessContaminants/Metals/ucm393070.htm.

154. US Department of Health and Human Services. 2008 Physical Activity Guidelines for Americans. Atlanta, Ga: US Department of Health and Human Services, Centers for Disease Control and Prevention, National Center for Chronic Disease Prevention and Health Promotion; 2008.

155. National Guideline Clearinghouse (NGC). Guideline summary: pregestational diabetes mellitus. In: National Guideline Clearinghouse (NGC). Rockville, Md: American College of Obstetricians and Gynecologists; 1984 Apr (revised 2005 Mar 1). On the Internet at: http://www.guideline.gov.

156. Manderson JG, Patterson CC, Hadden DR, et al. Preprandial versus postprandial blood glucose monitoring in type 1 diabetic pregnancy: a randomized controlled clinical trial. Am J Obstet Gynecol. 2003;189:507-12.

157. babyMed.com. Fetal health monitoring (cited 2015 Jul 9). On the Internet at: http://www.babymed.com/pregnancy/fetal-health-monitoring.

158. Jovanovic L. Gestational diabetes FAQ (cited 2015 Jul 9). On the Internet at: http://www.bd.com/us/diabetes/page.aspx?cat=7001&id=7564#15.

159. Rudolf MC, Coustan DR, Sherwin RS, et al. Efficacy of the insulin pump in the home treatment of pregnant diabetics. Diabetes. 1981;30:891-5.

160. American College of Obstetricians and Gynecologists. Education pamphlet FAQ034. Preeclampsia and high blood pressure during pregnancy. 2014 Sept (cited 2015 Jul 9). On the Internet at: http://www.acog.org/Patients/FAQs/Preeclampsia-and-High-Blood-Pressure-During-Pregnancy.

161. Tigas S, Sunehag A, Haymond MW. Metabolic adaptation to feeding and fasting during lactation in humans. J Clin Endocrinol Metab. 2002;87:302-7.

162. Kjos SL, Henry O, Lee RM, Buchanan TA, Mishell DR Jr. The effect of lactation on glucose and lipid metabolism in women with recent gestational diabetes. Obstet Gynecol. 1993;82:451-5.

163. Rasmussen KM, Kjolhede CL. Prepregnant overweight and obesity diminish the prolactin response to suckling in the first week postpartum. Pediatrics. 2004;113:e465-71.

164. Donath SM, Amir LH. Does maternal obesity adversely affect breastfeeding initiation and duration? Breastfeed Rev. 2000;8:29-33.

165. American College of Obstetrics and Gynecology Committee on Practice Bulletins-Obstetrics. ACOG Practice Bulletin: clinical management guidelines for obstetricians-gynecologists. Obstet Gynecol. 2001;98:525-38.

166. Metzger BE, Coustan DR. Proceedings of the Fourth International Workshop-Conference on Gestational Diabetes Mellitus. Diabetes Care. 1998;21 Suppl 2:B1-167.

167. American Diabetes Association. Standards of Medical Care 2009. Diabetes Care. 2009;32 Suppl 1:S13-61.

168. American Diabetes Association. Statement on emergency and disaster preparedness: a report of the Disaster Response Task Force. Diabetes Care. 2007;30:2395-8.

169. Cefalu WT, Smith SR, Blonde L, Fonseca F. The Hurricane Katrina aftermath and its impact on diabetes care: observations from "ground zero": lessons in disaster preparedness of people with diabetes. Diabetes Care. 2006;29:158-60.

170. Mulcahy K, Maryniuk M, Peeples M, et al. Diabetes self-management education core outcomes measures: technical review. Diabetes Educ. 2003;29(5):768-803.

American Association of Diabetes Educators©

352   Diabetes Education Curriculum

REDUCING RISKS: RESOURCES

Diabetes Goal Tracker Mobile App 352

Tips to Quit Smoking 352

Resources for People With Impaired Vision. 353

Resources for People With Hearing Impairments 354

Medicare Part B Coverage for Therapeutic Shoes and Inserts. 354

Berlin Questionnaire (Sleep Apnea). 355

Tests to Monitor Your Baby. 357

Tips for Managing Diabetes While Traveling. 357

Sick-Day Management 359

Immunizations 359

    Diabetes and Adult Vaccines. 360

    CDC 2015 Recommended Immunizations for Adults: By Age 362

    CDC 2015 Recommended Immunizations for Adults: By Health Condition 363

    Treating Influenza. 364

    Diabetes and Hepatitis B Vaccination 366

    Diabetes and Pneumonia: Get the Facts 368

Diabetes Goal Tracker Mobile App

https://www.diabeteseducator.org/patient-resources/diabetes-goal-tracker-app

Available in English and Spanish*, this tool helps you set goals based on the 7 proven diabetes management approaches:

1. Eating healthier
2. Increasing your level of activity
3. Monitoring your medications as prescribed
4. Learning how to problem solve ordinary and unusual situations
5. Coping with emotional issues
6. Reducing your risk for complications

You can find our app by searching for "AADE Diabetes Goal Tracker" on iTunes or the Google Play Store. Download the free app today!

Tips to Quit Smoking

1. Set a quit date.
2. Change your environment: Get rid of all cigarettes, lighters, and ashtrays at work, at home, and in your car. Clean up areas where you regularly smoked (car, home).

* To use the app in Spanish you need to have your language preference listed as Spanish.

American Association of Diabetes Educators©

3. List reasons why you want to quit (be healthier, protect family from smoke, save money) and remind yourself of those reasons every day. It may also be helpful to write them down and post them somewhere that you will see them often.

4. Identify your smoking triggers and make a plan to deal with them.

5. Find ways to cope with the withdrawal from nicotine (meds, nicotine replacement, and behavior modification can help).

6. Get the support you need:

—Tell your family, friends, and coworkers you are trying to quit.

—Tell your doctor. Ask for smoking cessation medication.

—Plug into a smoking cessation program.

• Call a quit line such at 1-800-QUIT NOW (1-800-784-8669).

• Join an online quit program like Freedom from Smoking Online from the American Lung Association (ffsonline.org).

• Sign up for text messaging at smokefree.gov.

• Download a quit-smoking app.

• Attend a smoking cessation program.

Studies show that smokers who use smoking cessation counseling services are twice as likely to quit as those who don't use such services. If you've tried to quit before and failed, don't give up. Most people who eventually quit for good try many times before they are successful.

Resources for People With Impaired Vision

American Council of the Blind (ACB) The nation's leading membership organization of blind and visually impaired people. It was founded in 1961. The ACB has affiliates in all 50 states and the District of Columbia. The ACB "strives to improve the well-being of all blind and visually impaired people by encouraging and assisting all blind persons to develop their abilities." The Braille Forum is a free monthly national publication produced by the ACB. It is produced in braille, large print, cassette, and IBM-compatible computer disc and contains articles of interest to blind and visually impaired people. Web site: http://www.acb.org

American Foundation for the Blind (AFB) A national nonprofit organization that expands possibilities for people with vision loss. Its priorities include broadening access to technology, elevating the quality of information and tools for the professionals who serve people with vision loss, and promoting independent and healthy living for people with vision loss by providing them and their families with relevant and timely resources. Web site: http://www.afb.org, e-mail: afbinfo@afb.net

Guide Dog Foundation for the Blind, Inc. This organization is focused on improving the quality of life for people who are blind, visually impaired, or with other special needs through the support of training guide dogs and providing guide dogs. Web site: http://www.guidedog.org, e-mail: info@guidedog.org

Lighthouse Guild Vision & Health A leading resource on vision impairment. Its goal is to "assist people with vision loss to develop the skills they need, at home and in the workplace, to lead productive independent lives." Newsletters include Lighthouse News, which is free and is published 3 times a year. Web site: http://www.lighthouseguild.org

National Council of State Agencies for the Blind (NCSAB) The mission of the NCSAB is to promote through advocacy, coordination, and education the delivery of specialized services that enable individuals who are blind and visually impaired to achieve personal and vocational independence. The Web site includes a directory of state agencies. The organization offers specialized services for older adults losing their sight, specialized education services for students with vision loss, and specialized services to enhance employment opportunities for people who are visually impaired. Web site: http://www.ncsab.org

American Association of Diabetes Educators©

354   Diabetes Education Curriculum

National Federation of the Blind (NFB) The purpose of the NFB is to foster "the complete integration of the blind into society on the basis of equality." Members of NFB contact people who are newly blind to help them with adjustment. The NFB provides information about available services from governmental and private agencies, as well as facts about laws and regulations concerning the blind. Web site: http://www.nfb.org

Resources for People With Hearing Impairments

National Association of State Agencies of the Deaf and Hard of Hearing There are approximately 38 state agencies of the deaf and hard of hearing. To help you get started, the association provides information and referral. Download the roster of all state agencies of the deaf and hard of hearing (NASADHH Directory Public). The roster includes the agency name, address, telephone and Internet contact information. If there is no state agency in your state, contact your vocational rehabilitation agency and see if there is a program for deaf, hard of hearing, or deaf-blind. Web site: http://nasadhh.org/about-us/

State Vocational Rehabilitation Agencies Each state has a vocational rehabilitation agency designed to assist individuals with disabilities meet their employment goals. Services include career and technical education/ training, on-the-job training, guidance and counseling, and ancillary support services.

The following list includes links to Web sites and other contact information for vocational rehabilitation agencies in US states and territories: http://www.fda.gov/downloads/AboutFDA/WorkingatFDA/UCM277757.pdf

Medicare Part B Coverage for Therapeutic Shoes and Inserts (Current as of Publication Date)

Web site: http://www.medicare.gov/coverage/therapeutic-shoes-or-inserts.html

If you have Medicare Part B and you meet certain criteria, you can get the following items each year:

◆ One pair of depth-inlay shoes and 3 pairs of inserts

   OR

◆ One pair of custom-molded shoes (including inserts) if you can't wear depth-inlay shoes because of a foot deformity, and 2 additional pairs of inserts

Note: In certain cases, Medicare may also cover shoe modifications instead of inserts.

All of the following eligibility criteria must be met:

◆ You have diabetes.
◆ You have at least 1 of the following conditions in 1 foot or both feet:
—Partial or complete foot amputation
—Past foot ulcers
—Nerve damage due to diabetes with signs of problems with calluses
—Poor circulation
—Calluses that could lead to ulcers
—Deformed foot
◆ You are being treated under a comprehensive diabetes care plan and need therapeutic shoes and/or inserts because of your diabetes.

Other requirements:

◆ Therapeutic shoes and/or inserts must be prescribed by a podiatrist or other qualified doctor.
   AND
◆ The shoes and/or inserts must be fitted and provided by a doctor or other qualified individual (eg, pedorthist, orthotist, prosthetist).

American Association of Diabetes Educators©

Berlin Questionnaire

1. Complete the following:

Height _____ Age _____

Weight _____ Male/female _____

Has your weight changed? _____

2. Do you snore?

- ☐ Yes
- ☐ No
- ☐ Don't know

If you snore:

3. Your snoring is . . .

- ☐ Slightly louder than breathing
- ☐ As loud as talking
- ☐ Louder than talking
- ☐ Very loud

4. How often do you snore?

- ☐ Almost every day
- ☐ 3 or 4 times a week
- ☐ 1 or 2 times a week
- ☐ Never or almost never

5. Does your snoring bother other people?

- ☐ Yes
- ☐ No

6. Has anyone noticed that you quit breathing during your sleep?

- ☐ Almost every day
- ☐ 3 or 4 times a week
- ☐ 1 or 2 times a month
- ☐ Never or almost never

7. Are you tired after sleeping?

- ☐ Almost every day
- ☐ 3 or 4 times a week
- ☐ 1 or 2 times a month
- ☐ Never or almost never

8. Are you tired during wake time?

- ☐ Almost every day
- ☐ 3 or 4 times a week
- ☐ 1 or 2 times a month
- ☐ Never or almost never

9. Have you ever nodded off or fallen asleep while driving?

- ☐ Yes
- ☐ No

If yes, how often does it occur?

- ☐ Every day
- ☐ 3 or 4 times a week
- ☐ 1 or 2 times a week
- ☐ 1 or 2 times a month
- ☐ Never or almost never

10. Do you have high blood pressure?

- ☐ Yes
- ☐ No
- ☐ Do not know

Name _____

Date of birth _____

American Association of Diabetes Educators©

Category 1

1. Do you snore?
- [ ] Yes
- [ ] No
- [ ] Don't know

If you snore:

2. Your snoring is . . .
- [ ] Slightly louder than breathing
- [ ] As loud as talking
- [ ] **Louder than talking**
- [ ] **Very loud**

3. How often do you snore?
- [ ] **Almost every day**
- [ ] **3 or 4 times a week**
- [ ] 1 or 2 times a week
- [ ] Never or almost never

5. Does your snoring bother other people?
- [ ] **Yes**
- [ ] No

6. Has anyone noticed that you quit breathing during your sleep?
- [ ] **Almost every day**
- [ ] **3 or 4 times a week**
- [ ] 1 or 2 times a month
- [ ] Never or almost never

- [ ] **Are 2 or more above responses in bold? If so, Category 1 is positive.**

Category 2

7. Are you tired after sleeping?
- [ ] **Almost every day**
- [ ] **3 or 4 times a week**
- [ ] 1 or 2 times a month
- [ ] Never or almost never

8. Are you tired during wake time?
- [ ] **Almost every day**
- [ ] **3 or 4 times a week**
- [ ] 1 or 2 times a month
- [ ] Never or almost never

9. Have you ever nodded off or fallen asleep while driving?
- [ ] **Yes**
- [ ] No

If yes, how often does it occur?
- [ ] **Every day**
- [ ] **3 or 4 times a week**
- [ ] 1 or 2 times a week
- [ ] 1 or 2 times a month
- [ ] Never or almost never

- [ ] **Are 2 or more above responses in bold? If so, Category 2 is positive.**

Category 3

Do you have high blood pressure? [ ] **Yes**

BMI >30? [ ] **Yes**

- [ ] **Is either of the above responses in bold? If so, Category 3 is positive.**

Scoring

Number of positive categories _____

If **two or more categories are positive,** there is a high likelihood of sleep apnea.

Name _____

Date of birth _____

American Association of Diabetes Educators©

Tests to Monitor Your Baby

◆ **Amniocentesis**—A small amount of fluid is drawn from the sac that surrounds the baby using a thin needle inserted into the uterus. The fluid is analyzed to help determine if your baby has health problems. Amniocentesis can also check to see if your baby's lungs have finished developing.

◆ **Biophysical profile**—Using ultrasound, your baby's muscle tone, breathing, and movement are checked. This test also measures the amount of amniotic fluid surrounding your baby.

◆ **Chorionic villus sampling (CVS)**—Cells are removed from the placenta using a thin needle inserted either through the vagina and cervix or through the abdomen and uterus. The cells are analyzed to look for health problems.

◆ **Contraction stress test**—Also called stress test. A fetal monitor measures the baby's heart rate during contractions. This test can help the doctor decide if your baby needs to be delivered early.

◆ **Fetal echocardiogram**—The fetal echocardiogram uses ultrasound to check for problems in the baby's heart.

◆ **Maternal blood screening test**—A blood test that can tell you whether your baby is at risk for spinal cord and brain problems, Down syndrome, and other birth defects. Other names for this test are multiple marker screen test, triple screen, or quad screen.

◆ **Nonstress test**—A fetal monitor assesses the baby's heart rate when the baby is active.

◆ **Ultrasound**—Pictures of the baby inside your womb are made using sound waves. The picture is called a sonogram. Ultrasound can show the baby's size and position, body structures, and sex. It helps the doctor estimate the baby's age, monitor its growth, and look for birth defects.

Tips for Managing Diabetes While Traveling

Traveling might be on your agenda for work or for pleasure. Here are some tips that can help you manage the 7 diabetes self-care behaviors while away from home.

Healthy Eating

◆ Always keep some extra food with you in case of delays. Crackers and cheese, peanut butter, hard candy, and glucose tablets will get you through until a meal is possible.

◆ In foreign countries, avoid tap water. Drink bottled water or bottled drinks instead. Remember to ask for drinks without ice cubes. Use bottled water for brushing your teeth.

◆ Avoid food from street vendors.

Being Active

◆ On long trips, make it a point to move your legs every 1 to 2 hours. This can help lower your risk for blood clots, which can form after prolonged inactivity.

◆ When traveling for business use the hotel fitness center. If no fitness center is available, check the hotel television station for exercise programming. Take short walks during lunch or breaks in meetings.

Monitoring

◆ Check your glucose level frequently during long travel and as soon as you arrive at your destination.

◆ Take extra care to keep your meter and monitoring supplies safe from harm. The cargo compartments of buses, airplanes, and trains, as well as the trunk of a car, may be too hot or too cold for your meter and

American Association of Diabetes Educators©

358   Diabetes Education Curriculum

supplies. Carry your meter and all monitoring supplies on board with you when traveling by these modes of transportation. Bring resealable plastic bags to protect your medications and devices.

◆ Be aware of the current Transportation Safety Administration (TSA) regulations that apply to most modes of public transportation. Notify the TSA officer that you have diabetes and are carrying monitoring supplies with you. Blood glucose meters, test strips, lancets, alcohol swabs, and control solutions are allowed past the security checkpoint after screening. Sharps disposal containers or similar hard disposal containers for storing used lancets and test strips are also allowed. TSA Web site: http://www.tsa.gov. The TSA Blog includes TSA Travel Tips: Travelers with Diabetes or other Medical Conditions: http://blog.tsa.gov/2014/04/tsa-travel-tips-travelers-with-diabetes.html.

Taking Medication

◆ Before you travel to a foreign country, get a letter from your doctor that describes your diabetes management, including the need for monitoring and medications. List any allergies (medication, food, substances) that you may have. Carry signed prescriptions for all your medications in case you run out or your supplies are lost during your travel.

◆ Pack twice as much medication as you think you will need on your trip. If you take insulin, be sure to pack twice the number of syringes or pen needles you think you'll need.

◆ While traveling, keep your medication in your carry-on baggage. Don't risk losing your medication by packing it in checked luggage. The cargo compartments of buses, airplanes, and trains, as well as the trunk of a car, may be too hot or too cold for insulin.

◆ Insulin does not need to be refrigerated, but if you are planning extended time outdoors in very warm or cold weather, insulated travel packs, mini coolers, and refrigerated gel packs are good options for storing insulin.

◆ If you take insulin, be aware that it may be available in U-40 or U-80 strength in countries outside the United States. U-40 or U-80 means that there are 40 or 80 units of insulin in each milliliter of liquid (as opposed to the vials in the United States, which contain 100 units of insulin per milliliter of liquid). U-40 and U-80 insulin require a special syringe. If you take your usual number of units using U-40 or U-80 insulin, you will get a less concentrated dose.

◆ When drawing up insulin on board an airplane, remember that the cabin is pressurized. This eliminates the need to inject air into the vial prior to drawing up your dose.

◆ Always discuss international travel with your provider so that you can safely plan for your insulin needs. Many insulin users find that a daily injection of long-acting insulin plus premeal rapid-acting insulin injections provides flexibility during international travel. If you travel east, your day is shortened, so you may need less insulin than usual. If you travel west, your day is lengthened, and you may need more insulin than usual.

Reducing Risks

◆ Always carry or wear medical identification.

◆ If traveling to a foreign country, be able to ask for assistance in that language. Write these phrases on a card that you can pull out when needed. Better yet, learn how to say "I have diabetes," "I need a doctor," and "I need orange juice."

◆ For a list of doctors in other countries who speak English, you can call the International Association for Medical Assistance to Travelers at 1-716-754-4883 or http://www.iamat.org. If you don't have this list but have a medical emergency in a foreign country, contact the American Consulate, American Express, or local medical schools to get a list of doctors.

American Association of Diabetes Educators©

Module 8   *Reducing Risks*   359

- Travel time is not a good time to break in a new pair of shoes. Do not wear flip-flops! When traveling, carry an alternate pair of good-fitting shoes, especially if you will be doing lots of walking. Carry antibacterial ointment and some bandages in case you develop a blister on your feet. If you plan to swim in lakes, rivers, or the ocean, wear water shoes to protect your feet from injury.

- In case of diarrhea or upset stomach during travel, carry over-the-counter medication such as loperamide (Imodium-AD®), Pepto-Bismol®, or Kaopectate®.

- Use sunblock, SPF 30 or higher, to protect your skin if you'll be outside for an extended time. Be sure to wear sunblock on your feet, neck, and ears.

Sick-Day Management

	Type 1 Diabetes	Type 2 Diabetes
Hydration	8 ounces fluid per hour	Same
	Every third hour, consume this 8 ounces as a sodium-rich choice such as bouillon	
Self-monitoring of blood glucose	Test every 2–4 hours while blood glucose is elevated or until symptoms subside	Same
Ketones	Test every 4 hours or until negative	Determine for the individual
Medication adjustments	Continue as able	Same
	Adjust insulin doses to correct hyperglycemia, but do not stop or hold insulin if diagnosed as having type 1 diabetes melltus	
	Hold metformin during serious illness	
	Instruct patients to call their healthcare provider for specific instructions if they have not previously received them	
Food and beverage selections	Guide patients to consume 150–200 g carbohydrates daily, in divided doses	Same
	Switch to soft foods or liquids as tolerated	
	Provide patients a list of foods and beverages in portion sizes containing 15 g carbohydrate	
Contact healthcare professionals	Provide guidelines on conditions that require the patient to call:	Same
	• Vomiting more than once	
	• Diarrhea more than 5 times or for longer than 6 hours	
	• Blood glucose levels >300 mg/dL (16.65 mmol/L) on 2 consecutive measurements that are not responsive to increased insulin and fluids	
	Moderate or large urine ketones or blood ketones >10.8 mg/dL (>0.6 mmol/L)	

Immunizations

Immunization Action Coalition A nonprofit organization that works to increase immunization rates and prevent disease by creating and distributing educational materials for health professionals and the public that enhance the delivery of safe and effective immunization services. The coalition also facilitates communication about the safety, efficacy, and use of vaccines within the broad immunization community of patients, parents, healthcare organizations, and government health agencies. Services include handouts for patients and clinical staff and vaccine information statements in multiple languages. Web site: http://www.immunize.org

Vaccine Information Statements in Multiple Languages Web site: http://www.immunize.org/vis/vis_pcv.asp

American Association of Diabetes Educators©

INFORMATION SERIES FOR ADULTS

What You Need to Know About Diabetes and Adult Vaccines

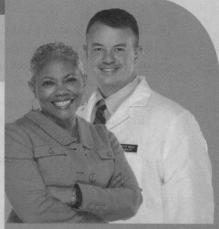

Each year thousands of adults in the United States suffer serious health problems from diseases that could be prevented by vaccines — some people are hospitalized, and some even die. People with diabetes (both type 1 and type 2) are at higher risk for serious problems from certain vaccine-preventable diseases.

Vaccines are important for you.

Diabetes, even if well managed, can make it harder for your immune system to fight infections, so you may be at risk for more serious complications from an illness compared to people without diabetes. **That's why you should talk to your healthcare professional to make sure you have all the vaccines you need.**

- Some illnesses, like influenza, can raise your blood glucose to dangerously high levels. **That's why a flu vaccine every year is important.**

- People with diabetes have higher rates of hepatitis B than the rest of the population. Outbreaks of hepatitis B associated with blood glucose monitoring procedures have occurred among people with diabetes. **That's why the hepatitis B vaccine is important for you.**

- People with diabetes are at increased risk for death from pneumonia (lung infection), bacteremia (blood infection) and meningitis (infection of the lining of the brain and spinal cord). These infections can be prevented by the pneumococcal polysaccharide vaccine. **Certain types of pneumonia can be prevented by pneumococcal vaccines.**

Vaccines are one of the safest ways to protect your health.

- **Vaccines are tested and monitored.** Vaccines are tested before being licensed by the Food and Drug Administration (FDA). The Centers for Disease Control and Prevention (CDC) and FDA continue to monitor vaccines after they are licensed.

- **Vaccine side effects are usually mild and temporary.** The most common side effects include soreness, redness, or swelling at the injection site. Severe side effects are very rare.

- **Vaccines are safe to get, even if you are taking prescription medications.** In fact, they are an important part of staying healthy especially if you have a chronic condition like diabetes.

What vaccines do you need?

Whether you have type 1 or type 2 diabetes, there are a number of vaccines that can protect your health:

- **Flu vaccine** each year to protect against seasonal flu
- **Pneumococcal vaccine** to protect against certain types of pneumococcal diseases
- **Hepatitis B vaccine** series to protect against hepatitis B

In addition all adults need:
- **Tdap vaccine** to protect against tetanus, diphtheria, and pertussis (whooping cough)
- **Zoster vaccine** to protect against shingles if you are 60 years or older

There may be other vaccines you need so be sure to talk with your healthcare professional about what's right for you.

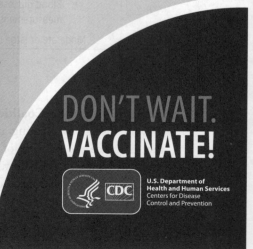

360

INFORMATION SERIES FOR ADULTS

Getting adult vaccines can be easier than you think.

You regularly see your provider for diabetes care, and that's a great place to start! He or she may carry vaccines recommended for people with diabetes.

If your provider does not offer the vaccines you need, ask for a referral so you can get the vaccines elsewhere.

Adults can get vaccines at doctors' offices, pharmacies, workplaces, community health clinics, and health departments. To find a place near you to get a vaccine, go to http://vaccine.healthmap.org.

Most health insurance plans cover recommended vaccines. Check with your insurance provider for details and for a list of vaccine providers covered by your plan. If you do not have health insurance, visit www.healthcare.gov to learn more about health insurance options.

Don't Wait. Vaccinate!

Talk with your healthcare professional to make sure you are up-to-date with the vaccines recommended for you.

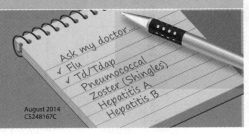

Talk with your doctor or other healthcare professional to make sure you are up-to-date with the vaccines recommended for you.

For more information on vaccines or to take an adult vaccine quiz to find out which vaccines you might need, go to www.cdc.gov/vaccines/adults.

August 2014
CS248167C

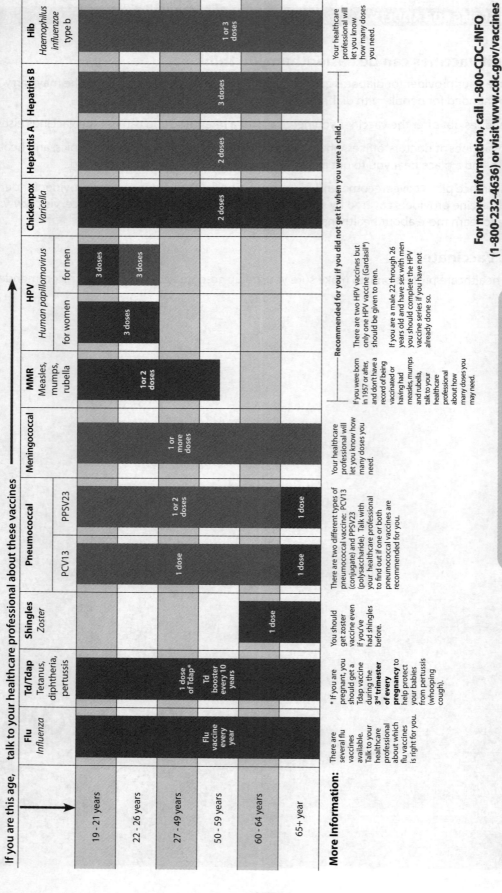

2015 Recommended Immunizations for Adults: By Health Condition

If you have this health condition, talk to your healthcare professional about these vaccines

If you have this health condition,	Flu Influenza	Td/Tdap Tetanus, diphtheria, pertussis	Shingles Zoster	Pneumococcal PCV13	Pneumococcal PPSV23	Meningococcal	MMR Measles, mumps, rubella	HPV Human papillomavirus for women	HPV for men	Chickenpox Varicella	Hepatitis A	Hepatitis B	Hib Haemophilus influenzae type b
Pregnancy		*see below	SHOULD NOT GET VACCINE				SHOULD NOT GET VACCINE			SHOULD NOT GET VACCINE			
Weakened Immune System	Flu vaccine every year	1 dose of Tdap followed by Td booster every 10 years		1 dose	1 - 2 doses	1 or more doses						3 doses	post-HSCT* recipients only
HIV: CD4 count less than 200													
HIV: CD4 count 200 or greater								3 doses through age 26 years	3 doses through age 21 years				1 or 3 doses
Kidney disease or poor kidney function													
Asplenia (if you do not have a spleen or if it does not work well)			1 dose for those 60 years or older		1 - 2 doses	1 or more doses	1 or 2 doses			2 doses		3 doses	1 or 3 doses
Heart disease Chronic lung disease Chronic alcoholism				1 dose		1 or more doses						3 doses	1 or 3 doses
Diabetes (Type 1 or Type 2)													
Chronic Liver Disease											2 doses	3 doses	

More Information:

* If you are pregnant, you should get a Tdap vaccine during the **3rd trimester of every pregnancy** to help protect your babies from pertussis (whooping cough).

There are several flu vaccines available. Talk to your healthcare professional about which flu vaccines is right for you.

You should get zoster vaccine even if you've had shingles before.

There are two different types of pneumococcal vaccine: PCV13 (conjugate) and PPSV23 (polysaccharide). Talk with your healthcare professional to find out if one or both pneumococcal vaccines are recommended for you.

Your healthcare professional will let you know how many doses you need.

If you were born in 1957 or after, and don't have a record of being vaccinated or having had measles, mumps and rubella, talk to your healthcare professional about how many doses you may need.

Recommended For You if you did not get it when you were a child.

There are two HPV vaccines but only one HPV vaccine (Gardasil®) should be given to men.

If you are a male 22 through 26 years old and have sex with men you should complete the HPV vaccine series if you have not already done so.

Your healthcare professional will let you know how many doses you need.

*Hematopoietic stem cell transplant

Recommended For You: This vaccine is recommended for you *unless* your healthcare professional tells you that you cannot safely receive it or that you do not need it.

May Be Recommended For You: This vaccine is recommended for you if you have certain other risk factors due to your age, health, job, or lifestyle that are not listed here. Talk to your healthcare professional to see if you need this vaccine.

YOU SHOULD NOT GET THIS VACCINE

If you are traveling outside the United States, you may need additional vaccines.
Ask your healthcare professional about which vaccines you may need at least 6 weeks prior to your travel.

For more information, call 1-800-CDC-INFO (1-800-232-4636) or visit www.cdc.gov/vaccines

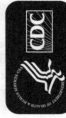

U.S. Department of Health and Human Services
Centers for Disease Control and Prevention

Treating Influenza (Flu)

Do you have Asthma, Diabetes or Chronic Heart Disease?

If so, you are at high risk of serious illness if you get the flu. In past flu seasons, as many as 80 percent of adults hospitalized from flu complications had a long-term health condition, as did about 50 percent of hospitalized children. **Asthma, diabetes and chronic heart disease were among the most common of these. Treatment with an influenza antiviral drug can mean the difference between having milder illness instead of very serious illness that could result in a hospital stay.** This fact sheet provides information about using prescription antiviral drugs to treat influenza in people at high risk for flu complications.

Why am I at greater risk of serious flu complications?

Your medical condition makes it more likely that you will get complications from the flu, like pneumonia. The flu also can make long-term health problems worse, even if they are well-managed. People with asthma or chronic congestive heart failure may experience worsening of their conditions. Diabetes (type 1 and 2) can make the immune system less able to fight the flu. Also, flu illness can raise blood sugar levels.

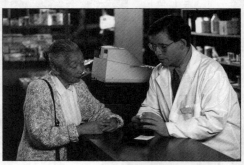

Can the flu be treated?

Yes. There are prescription medications called "antiviral drugs" that can be used to treat influenza illness. Antiviral drugs fight influenza viruses in your body. They are different from antibiotics, which fight against bacterial infections.

What should I do if I think I have the flu?

If you get the flu, antiviral drugs are a treatment option. Check with your doctor promptly if you have a high risk condition and you get flu symptoms. Symptoms can include fever, cough, sore throat, runny or stuffy nose, body aches, headache, chills and fatigue. Your doctor may prescribe antiviral drugs to treat your flu illness.

Should I still get a flu vaccine?

Yes. Antiviral drugs are not a substitute for getting a flu vaccine. While flu vaccines can vary in how they work, flu vaccination is the first and best way to **prevent** influenza. Antiviral drugs are a second line of defense to **treat** the flu if you get sick.

What are the benefits of antiviral drugs?

- When used for treatment, antiviral drugs can lessen symptoms and shorten the time you are sick by 1 or 2 days.
- **Antiviral drugs also can prevent serious flu-related complications (like pneumonia).** This is especially important for people with a high-risk health condition, like asthma, diabetes or chronic heart disease.

What are the possible side effects of antiviral drugs?

Some side effects have been associated with the use of influenza antiviral drugs, including nausea, vomiting, dizziness, runny or stuffy nose, cough, diarrhea, headache and some behavioral side effects. These are uncommon. Your doctor can give you more information about these drugs or you can check the Centers for Disease Control and Prevention (CDC) or the Food and Drug Administration (FDA) websites.

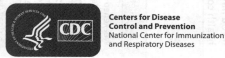

CS250831A

When should antiviral drugs be taken for treatment?

Studies show that flu antiviral drugs work best for treatment when they are started within 2 days of getting sick. However, starting them later can still be helpful, especially if the sick person has a high-risk health condition (see list below) or is very sick from the flu (for example, hospitalized patients). Follow your doctor's instructions for taking these drugs.

What antiviral drugs are recommended?

There are three antiviral drugs recommended by the CDC and approved by the FDA. These are oseltamivir (brand name Tamiflu®), zanamivir (brand name Relenza®) and peramivir (brand name Rapivab®). Tamiflu® comes as a pill or liquid, and Relenza® is an inhaled powder. (Relenza should NOT be used in anyone with breathing problems, like asthma or COPD, for example.) Rapivab® is administered intravenously by a health care provider. There are no generic flu antiviral drugs.

How long should antiviral drugs be taken?

To treat flu, Tamiflu® and Relenza® are usually taken for 5 days, although people hospitalized with the flu may need the medicine for longer than 5 days.

Can children and pregnant women take antiviral drugs?

Yes. Children and pregnant women can take antiviral drugs.

Who should take antiviral drugs?

It's very important that antiviral drugs be used early to treat the flu in:
+ People who are very sick with the flu (for example, people who are in the hospital).
+ People who are sick with the flu and have a high-risk health condition like asthma, diabetes or chronic heart disease. (See the full list of high-risk conditions).

Following is a list of all the health and age factors that are known to increase a person's risk of getting serious complications from the flu:

Asthma

Blood disorders (such as sickle cell disease)

Chronic lung disease (such as chronic obstructive pulmonary disease [COPD] and cystic fibrosis)

Endocrine disorders (such as diabetes mellitus)

Heart disease (such as congenital heart disease, congestive heart failure and coronary artery disease)

Kidney disorders

Liver disorders

Metabolic disorders (such as inherited metabolic disorders and mitochondrial disorders)

Morbid obesity

Neurological and neurodevelopmental conditions

People younger than 19 years of age on long-term aspirin therapy

People with Chronic Obstructive Pulmonary Disease (COPD)

Weakened immune system due to disease or medication (such as people with HIV or AIDS, or cancer, or those on chronic steroids)

Other people at high risk from the flu:

Adults 65 years and older

Children younger than 5 years old, but especially children younger than 2 years old d

Pregnant women and women up to 2 weeks after the end of pregnancy

American Indians and Alaska Natives

For more information visit www.cdc.gov/flu or call 800-CDC-INFO.

08/18/2014

Diabetes and Hepatitis B Vaccination

Information for Diabetes Educators

What is hepatitis B?
Hepatitis B is a contagious liver disease that results from infection with the hepatitis B virus.

When first infected, a person can develop an "acute" infection, which can range in severity from a very mild illness with few or no symptoms to a serious condition requiring hospitalization. **Acute** hepatitis B refers to the first 6 months after someone is infected with the hepatitis B virus. Some people are able to fight the virus and clear the infection. For others, the infection remains and leads to a "chronic," or lifelong, illness. **Chronic** hepatitis B refers to the illness that occurs when the hepatitis B virus remains in a person's body. Over time, the infection can cause serious damage to the liver and lead to complications such as liver failure or liver cancer.

How is hepatitis B spread?
The hepatitis B virus is usually spread when blood or other body fluids from a person infected with the hepatitis B virus enters the body of someone who is not infected. Hepatitis B can be spread through sharing needles, syringes, or other injection equipment. In addition, the hepatitis B virus can spread through sexual contact and from an infected mother to her baby during childbirth.

Why is hepatitis B relevant to people with diabetes?
Among people living with diabetes, the hepatitis B virus has been spread through contact with infectious blood. People living with diabetes are at increased risk for hepatitis B if they share blood glucose meters, fingerstick devices or other diabetes-care equipment such as syringes or insulin pens.

How infectious is the hepatitis B virus?
The hepatitis B virus is 50 – 100 times more infectious than HIV which makes it easily transmitted.

The hepatitis B virus can survive outside the body at least a week. During that time, the virus can still cause infection if it enters the body of a person who is not infected.

How has transmission occurred in healthcare facilities?
CDC has investigated numerous hepatitis B outbreaks in people with diabetes in assisted living, long-term care facilities and nursing homes. Modes of transmission are believed to have occurred from:

- Use of blood glucose meter for more than one resident without cleaning and disinfection between uses
- Failure to consistently wear gloves and perform hand hygiene between fingerstick procedures
- Use of the same fingerstick devices for more than one resident
- Cross-contamination of clean supplies with contaminated blood glucose monitoring equipment used by home health agencies
- Use of the same injection equipment such as a syringe or insulin pen for more than one person
- Failure to maintain separation of clean and contaminated podiatry equipment
- Improper sterilization of contaminated podiatry equipment
- Failure to perform environmental cleaning and disinfection between podiatry patients

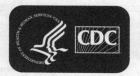

U.S. Department of Health and Human Services
Centers for Disease Control and Prevention

Continued on next page

Why should people with diabetes be vaccinated?

People living with type 1 or type 2 diabetes mellitus have higher rates of hepatitis B than the general population. Some of the cases of hepatitis B have occurred in individuals with diabetes whose equipment came in contact with infected blood, or who had contact with the virus through breaks in the skin. This has happened through improper reuse and sharing of glucose monitoring equipment or other diabetes care equipment. Transmission has occurred among people with diabetes who reside in assisted living facilities when several people received glucose monitoring in close succession.

> CDC now recommends the hepatitis B vaccine for adults with diabetes.

What is the recommendation for vaccinating adults younger than 60 years of age?

In 2011, the Centers for Disease Control and Prevention and the Advisory Committee on Immunization Practices (ACIP) released new guidelines that recommend hepatitis B vaccination for all unvaccinated adults with diabetes who are younger than 60 years of age. Vaccination should occur as soon as possible after diagnosis of diabetes; vaccination should also be given to adults diagnosed with diabetes in the past.

What is the recommendation for vaccinating adults 60 years and older?

For unvaccinated adults with diabetes who are 60 years and older, the ACIP recommends hepatitis B vaccination at the discretion of their health care provider. As with other vaccines, the effectiveness of the hepatitis B vaccine decreases with age. Decisions to vaccinate should include the patient's likelihood of acquiring hepatitis B, including the need for assisted blood-glucose monitoring, and overall health status. Hepatitis B vaccination may provide partial, if not full protection for many older adults with diabetes.

What is the recommendation for vaccinating children living with diabetes?

In the United States, the hepatitis B vaccine is now part of the routine childhood vaccination schedule. In 1991, CDC and the ACIP recommended that all children and adolescents be vaccinated for hepatitis B. Estimates of vaccine coverage among infants and children are now over 90%.

What should diabetes educators tell their patients about hepatitis B?

Diabetes educators should provide their clients or patients with the following information on how to protect themselves from getting the hepatitis B virus:

- Prevent exposure to hepatitis B and other blood borne pathogens by not sharing equipment such as blood glucose monitors or other diabetes care equipment.
- The best way to prevent hepatitis B is by getting vaccinated. CDC recommends hepatitis B vaccination for all unvaccinated adults with diabetes younger than 60 years of age.
- If you think you have already been vaccinated, confirm with your doctor.
- The hepatitis B vaccine is given as a series of 3 shots over a period of 6 months (0, 1, 6 month schedule). The entire series is needed for long-term protection.
- If you have not received the hepatitis B vaccine series talk to your doctor about getting vaccinated.

For more information visit:

- **Diabetes:** http://www.cdc.gov/diabetes/
- **Viral Hepatitis:** http://www.cdc.gov/hepatitis/
- **CDC's hepatitis B vaccination recommendation for adults with diabetes mellitus is available at** http://www.cdc.gov/mmwr/preview/mmwrhtml/mm6050a4.htm

Publication No. 220421
October 2012

www.cdc.gov/hepatitis

Diabetes And Pneumonia:
Get the Facts

Did you know that a pneumococcal (new-mo-Koc-kal) shot (or pneumonia shot) can be a lifesaver if you have diabetes? People with diabetes are about 3 times more likely to die with flu and pneumonia. Yet, only one third of them ever get a simple, safe pneumonia shot.

Pneumonia is a serious illness for anyone, but if you have diabetes, you are more likely to be sicker longer, go to the hospital, or even die. One pneumonia shot can help protect you against getting sick.

Who Should Get The Pneumonia Shot?

A pneumonia shot is recommended for anyone aged 2 or older who, because of chronic health problems (such as diabetes) or age, has a greater chance of getting and dying with pneumonia.

Extra Protection

A pneumonia shot can also protect you against other infections caused by the same bacteria. Consider the risks everyone faces:

- 1 out of 20 adults who get pneumonia (a lung infection) dies

- 2 out of 10 adults who get infection of the blood (bacteremia) die

- 3 out of 10 adults who get infection of the covering of the brain (meningitis) die

About 10,000 people die each year because of these bacterial infections. A pneumonia shot, however, can help protect you against getting these illnesses. In fact, it is about 60% effective in preventing the most serious pneumonias, meningitis, bacteremia, and death.

Is The Shot Safe?

The pneumonia shot is very safe. It does not contain any live bacteria, which means there is no way to get pneumonia from the shot.

People may have mild redness or swelling in the arm where the shot was given. This goes away in a day or two.

Where And When To Get A Shot

A pneumonia shot is available through your doctor's office, your community health clinic, hospitals, and some worksite programs. You can get it anytime during the year. For most people, one shot is enough protection for a lifetime. People under 65 who have a chronic illness or a weakened immune system should ask their doctor about getting another shot 5—10 years after their first one.

Will Insurance Cover The Shot?

The pneumonia shot is covered by Medicare Part B and by some other health insurance plans.

Remember...

You may already be planning to get a flu shot this fall— another lifesaver for people with diabetes. Ask your doctor about getting a pneumonia shot at the same time.

CDC
CENTERS FOR DISEASE CONTROL AND PREVENTION

SUPPLEMENT

Sexual Dysfunction

Table of Contents

BACKGROUND INFORMATION AND INSTRUCTIONS FOR THE EDUCATOR 371

SEXUAL DYSFUNCTION: INSTRUCTIONAL PLAN 373

    Diabetes and Sexual Concerns 373

    Male Sexual Dysfunction 373

        Causes of ED 373

        Anatomy of an Erection 373

        If There Are Problems With the Arteries 374

        If There Are Problems With the Nerves 374

        If There Are Problems With Testosterone 374

        Treatment of ED 375

    Female Sexual Dysfunction 380

        The Anatomy of Sexual Response in Women 380

        If There Are Problems With the Arteries 380

        If There Are Problems With the Nerves 380

        Treatment of Female Sexual Dysfunction 381

REFERENCES 382

SEXUAL DYSFUNCTION: RESOURCES 384

BACKGROUND INFORMATION AND INSTRUCTIONS FOR THE EDUCATOR

Sexual dysfunction is a common problem among those with diabetes. Up to 75% of men and 35% of women with diabetes experience sexual problems related to diabetic neuropathy.[1] The contributing causes of sexual dysfunction, however, go beyond neuropathy. Possible causes for sexual dysfunction are multifactorial and may involve the vascular system, glycemic control, nutrition, sex hormones, psychological factors, and medication use.

372   Diabetes Education Curriculum

Since the advent of drug therapy (eg, Viagra®) for erectile function, there is more of an openness to discuss sexuality today. Nevertheless, sexuality remains a sensitive subject. Sexual dysfunction is the most neglected complication of diabetes.[2] Many patients suffer in silence rather than discuss their experiences with sexual dysfunction with their provider. Some patients may assume that sexual dysfunction is an expected, automatic outcome of diabetes, and therefore fail to report it. Despite the fact that nearly all erectile dysfunction is organic in origin,[3] many patients are hesitant to speak up for fear their provider will suggest in so many words that "it's all in your head."[4(p2173)] Many healthcare providers, because of their own discomfort, fail to proactively discuss sexual health concerns, which is a disservice to our patients.[5]

When educating men with diabetes, it is important to explore how diabetes and its comorbidities affect their sexual health as well as their self-perceptions.[6] Communication with men about sexual dysfunction should be affirming, nonjudgmental, nonconfrontational, and confidential. Understanding the male perceptions of *control* and *masculinity* is of great significance to the diabetes educator. Valued qualities among men are independence, control, and self-reliance. The opposites of these qualities are dependence, lack of control, and relying on others. In the face of illness, there is a need to give up control, to be dependent on others for information, and to ask for help. This need, though rational, is at odds with the common perception of what it means to be a man.[7,8] For the man experiencing sexual dysfunction, the inability to perform sexually to his satisfaction is interpreted as personal failure.[6]

The diabetes educator can help normalize the situation by creating an awareness that sexual dysfunction is common. The realization that he is "not the only one" promotes help-seeking behaviors among men.[6] The physical limitations that occur in sexual dysfunction generate negative psychologic outcomes such as chronic stress, anxiety, low self-worth, depression, and difficulties with interpersonal relationships.[9]

Since less media attention has been paid to female sexual dysfunction, many women with diabetes may be unaware that diabetes can affect their sexual health. Women with diabetes are, in fact, at double the risk of their nondiabetic counterparts for having sexual problems.[10] The knowledge that they have diabetes affects sexual expression and self-esteem in many women. The common labeling of type 2 diabetes as a "lifestyle" disease and the accompanying overweight status can translate to feelings of shame and lower desirability in women.[11,12] Asking women with diabetes about any sexual problems gives them a chance to discuss their concerns, which they may have perceived as being "invisible" to the healthcare team.[13]

In the clinic setting, the sexual concerns of women with diabetes often go unaddressed, despite the high incidence of the problem. Physicians tend to ask men questions about sexual problems more often than they do women.[14] Studies find that many male physicians feel uncomfortable asking female patients questions about their sex life, considering it to be intrusive.[15,16] Other studies, however, show that most women welcome questions about sexual health from their physicians. Including questions about sexual function in routine medical assessment yields more diagnoses of sexual dysfunction and subsequent treatment.[17-19]

The diabetes educator may be the first provider to broach the subject of sexual health with patients. As such, the educator has an important opportunity to intervene in a way that leads to a significant improvement in patients' quality of life.[7,9,20]

The educator's role includes:

⧫ **Assessing patients' concerns about sexual function.** One-on-one questioning can help determine a patient's concerns. An example of a query that can normalize their concerns is *"Most men with diabetes worry that their illness will damage their sexual function. Have you had a concern?"* For the elderly patient, the educator might say, *"Many men your age start to experience sexual difficulties. If you have any concerns, I would be happy to discuss it further."* For women, the educator might say, *"Many women have found that their sexual responsiveness changed after they got diabetes. Has that been your experience?"*

⧫ **Identifying patients at risk for sexual dysfunction.** Standardized tools are available to assess for sexual dysfunction.[21,22(p822)] Such tools can be integrated into the diabetes assessment tools distributed to patients during the initial intake. (See "Sexual Health Inventory for Men" in the "Resources" section.)

American Association of Diabetes Educators©

Supplement *Sexual Dysfunction* 373

◆ **Providing education about sexual dysfunction**, correcting misconceptions, and discussing relevant treatment options for sexual dysfunction. Addressing sexuality and diabetes as a *routine topic* within the diabetes education curriculum ensures that this important aspect of life is not overlooked. The topic can be legitimized by telling patients, *"Sexuality is one important element of your quality of life."*

◆ **Serving as a bridge to needed resources** such as further medical evaluation and treatment. Completed assessment tools should be forwarded to the referring physician to ensure continuity of care. Some patients may find benefit from counseling provided by a mental health professional trained in sex therapy/counseling. For interested patients, this is a referral you can suggest to the provider. Including the patient's sex partner is essential in any further treatment and/or counseling. To avoid an awkward situation, however, do not assume that the patient's spouse is the sex partner, as this is not always the case. In one-on-one conversations, it is better to use terms such as *sex partner* rather than *wife* or *husband*.

The following is an instructional plan for including sexual dysfunction within a patient's diabetes self-management education curriculum.

SEXUAL DYSFUNCTION: INSTRUCTIONAL PLAN

Diabetes and Sexual Concerns

Diabetes is a common cause of sexual problems for both men and women. Sexual response depends on the normal release of hormones, adequate blood flow, and proper nerve function. When any of these functions is impaired, your sexual response can be affected. And when your sexual response isn't what you want it to be, your relationships and quality of life can suffer.

Being unable to enjoy sex the way you feel you should also affects how you feel about yourself. It can cause frustration and anxiety and even trigger depression in some people.[23] That's why it's important to explore any concerns you have about sexual health with your healthcare team. Treatments are available. And there are a number of actions you can take to improve or even prevent the situation.

Male Sexual Dysfunction

The most common form of sexual dysfunction in men is erectile dysfunction, or ED. The majority of men with diabetes are affected by ED at some time or other. In ED, there is a problem getting or keeping an erection that is firm enough for satisfactory intercourse.

Causes of ED

Erectile dysfunction can be caused by a number of things, including fatigue, stress, depression, medication, and pelvic trauma (see Table S.1, Medications That May Cause Sexual Dysfunction). When ED is attributed to diabetes, the main problems usually involve circulation and nerve function. High blood glucose can make circulation and nerve damage worse. That is why ED is more common in men with diabetes than in the general population. Another condition that can cause ED is low levels of the male sex hormone testosterone.

Anatomy of an Erection

It helps to have a basic understanding of what is happening to produce a normal erection. The first organ to become involved is the brain. When a man becomes sexually stimulated, the brain sends signals to other parts of the body to respond. The nerves are signaled to allow for increased blood flow into the penis, by way of the arteries. Arteries bring blood into the penis; veins let blood out of the penis. When the penis is full of arterial blood, however, it presses the penis veins shut, trapping the blood inside the penis, and it becomes firm.

American Association of Diabetes Educators©

374 Diabetes Education Curriculum

TABLE S.1 Medications That May Cause Sexual Dysfunction

Generic Name	Trade Name	Generic Name	Trade Name
Selective serotonin reuptake inhibitors (SSRIs)		*Angiotensin-converting enzyme (ACE) inhibitors*	
Sertraline	Zoloft®	Lisinopril	Prinivil®, Zestril®
Fluoxetine	Prozac®	Enalapril	Vasotec®
Paroxetine	Paxil®		
MAO inhibitors		*Beta blockers*	
Phenelzine	Nardil®	Atenolol	Tenormin®
Isocarboxazid	Marplan®	Propranolol	Inderal®
Tranylcypramine	Parnate®	Metoprolol	Lopressor®, Toprol XL®
Tricyclic antidepressants		*Calcium channel blockers*	
Amytriptyline	Elavil	Diltiazem	Cardizem®
Nortriptyline	Pamelor®, Aventyl®	Verapamil	Covera HS®, Isoptin®, Calan®, Verelan®
Benzodiazepines		Amlodipine	Norvasc®
Alprazolam	Xanax®	*Miscellaneous heart and blood pressure medications*	
Lorazepam	Ativan®	Digoxin	Lanoxin
Oxazepam	Serax®	Spironolactone	Aldactone®
Chlorazepate dipotassium	Tranxene®	Hydrochlorthiazide (HCTZ)	Esidrix®, HydroDIURIL
Diazepam	Valium®	HCTZ/triamterene	Maxzide®, Dyazide®
Clonazepam	Klonipin®	Clonidine	Catapres®
Anticonvulsants/antiepileptics		Methyldopa	Aldomet®
Phenytoin	Dilantin®	*H₂ receptor antagonist*	
Phenobarbital	———	Cimetidine	Tagamet®
Also alcohol, narcotics, and illicit drugs		*Antifungal*	
		Ketoconazole	Nizoral®

Sources: GB Brock, TF Lue, "Drug-induced male sexual dysfunction: an update," *Drug Saf* 8 (1993): 414-26; WW Finger, M Lund, MA Slagle, "Medications that may contribute to sexual disorders: a guide to assessment and treatment in family practice," *J Fam Pract* 44, no. 1 (1997): 33-43.

If There Are Problems With the Arteries . . .

When plaque builds up in the arteries, the vessels become narrower, so less blood flows through to the penis. The arteries are stiffer and are less able to expand to hold the extra blood that is needed for a full erection. Less blood in the penis means that the veins aren't pressed shut. As a result, blood flows out of the penis instead of staying trapped inside. Recent research shows that ED is a good predictor of silent heart disease.[24] For this reason, if you have ED and are unaware of problems with heart disease, ask your doctor to check on your heart health.

If There Are Problems With the Nerves . . .

The nerves that trigger increased blood flow to the penis can be damaged by long-term high blood glucose (hyperglycemia).

If There Are Problems With Testosterone . . .[25]

For reasons not fully understood, **men with diabetes are *more than twice as likely*** as other men to have low **testosterone levels.** Testosterone is the most abundant sex hormone in men. Testosterone is responsible for the

American Association of Diabetes Educators©

growth of facial hair, a deep voice, muscle mass, sex drive, sperm production, and the health of muscle and bone tissue. If a man has low testosterone levels, he may experience these symptoms:

- Low energy level/fatigue
- Loss of strength/loss of lean muscle mass
- Increased body fat
- Low sex drive
- Depressed mood
- Decreased sense of well-being
- Osteoporosis

Treatment of ED

There are lots of things you can do to lower your risk for ED, to lessen some of the problems, and to treat the symptoms. Your plan of care may differ from that of other men; treatment should be customized to each person and should focus on what is causing the problem.

Healthy Eating

- If you are overweight or obese, lose weight. Work with a dietitian to adjust your meal plan. Obese men with prediabetes or type 2 diabetes are more prone to low testosterone levels. This is because fat itself produces the hormones estrone and estradiol, which promote female sex characteristics.[26] Weight loss will help you produce a more normal amount of these hormones. In one study, weight loss among obese men was associated with improved sexual function.[27]
- Limit alcohol. Drinking more than 2 alcoholic drinks per day can damage the blood vessels, making ED worse.[23]

Being Active

Being more physically active may help reduce the risk of ED, especially if regular activity started early in life rather than later.[27,28]

Monitoring

Managing your diabetes to get the A1C to target can lower your risk for ED.[29] If you take pills for ED treatment, they will be less effective the higher your A1C goes.[30] High blood glucose over the long term damages the blood vessels as well as the nerves responsible for sexual function. Remember, an A1C below 7% also reduces the risk for many other types of complications.

Reducing Risks

- If you smoke, stop. Smoking damages the blood vessels[31] that are involved in a healthy erection.
- Get enough rest. Fatigue can cause problems with sexual response.

Healthy Coping

- The stresses of life can sometimes find their way into the bedroom. Finding healthy ways of lowering your stress can help.
- If you think you may have anxiety or depression, ask your doctor to evaluate you. Depression and anxiety can affect sexuality. And sexual problems can make depression and anxiety worse. When depression or anxiety and/or sexual problems are present, your quality of life can suffer. So it's important to address both concerns and pursue whatever treatments are right for you.
- Counseling with a healthcare professional trained in sex therapy/counseling may be helpful for any communication concerns with your partner that may be related to sexual problems.

American Association of Diabetes Educators©

Taking Medication

The following is a *detailed list of available ED medication* and treatments. For patients already taking medication to treat ED, share only the information that is relevant to them to facilitate safe and effective medication-taking behavior. Alternatively, consider providing an *overview* of the options in a more general sense for patients seeking general information about ED treatment options.

There are a variety of medications available to treat ED, such as pills, injections, and pellets that are inserted into the urethra. There are also devices that can help with getting an erection. Surgery is even an option for some men.

Oral Medication for ED

- **PDE-5 Inhibitors (phosphodiesterase-5 inhibitors).** Pills like Viagra® (sildenafil), Cialis® (tadalafil), and Levitra® (vardenafil) work by allowing more blood to flow into the penis to produce a firmer erection. If a man has a low testosterone level, however, these medications will not work.[30] Once testosterone replacement has corrected the low testosterone level, then oral medications for ED can be taken (see Table S.2, PDE-5 Inhibitors, for specific information). Most men with diabetes tend to respond to these ED medications to some extent, but they don't respond as well as those without diabetes.[32,33]

I heard that Viagra® can cause blindness. Is that true?

Temporary blindness is a *very* rare occurrence in which there is blocked blood flow to the optic nerve. It has happened in only a few cases after the use of a PDE-5 inhibitor. Although there was no evidence that it was caused by the drug itself or that it was due to some other medical problem, the US Food and Drug Administration (FDA) approved updated labeling on sildenafil (Viagra®), tadalafil (Cialis®), and vardenafil (Levitra®).[34]

Anyone who has vision problems after taking a PDE-5 inhibitor should stop taking the drug and notify his provider right away.[34] Temporary loss of hearing has also occurred after the use of PDE-5 inhibitors. FDA-approved warnings are included on the labeling of sildenafil (Viagra®), tadalafil (Cialis®), and vardenafil (Levitra®).[35] See Table S.2 for more detailed information on PDE-5 inhibitors.

- **Yohimbine.**[36] Yohimbine is a medication that comes from the bark of an evergreen plant. This pill is thought to work by increasing blood flow into the penis and preventing the blood from flowing out, producing an erection. Yohimbine is considered to be only mildly effective for ED.

  Its use is controversial among medical professionals because it has not been researched sufficiently.[37] Side effects can include dangerous fluctuations in blood pressure and heart rate, upset stomach, anxiety, flushing, and blurred vision.[38] Men with kidney disease or who take medication for depression should not take yohimbine. Brand names for ED products containing yohimbine include Actibine®, Aphrodyne®, Baron-X®, Dayto-Himbin®, Erex®, Mederek®, ProHim®, Testomar®, Yocon®, Yohimar®, Yohimbe®, Yohimex®, Yoman®, Yovital®, and Thybine®.

What about over-the-counter pills that are supposed to help with erection?

Are "male enhancement" pills available over the Internet or by mail order safe to use?

Supplement *Sexual Dysfunction* 377

TABLE S.2 PDE-5 Inhibitors: Viagra®, Cialis®, and Levitra®

	Sildenafil (Viagra®)[†]	Tadalafil (Cialis®)[‡]	Vardenafil (Levitra®)[§]
When to take	• Take about 30 minutes to 1 hour before sex	• Cialis® for Daily Use—take it the same time every day • 36-Hour Cialis®—take 30 minutes to 36 hours before sex	• Take about 1 hour before sex
How to take	• Works with or without food or alcohol • Maximum dose = 1 per day • Fastest results if taken on an empty stomach	• Works with or without food; avoid excess alcohol to prevent dizziness or low blood pressure • Cialis® for Daily Use—maximum dose = 1 per day; take same time every day • 36-Hour Cialis®—maximum dose = 1 per day	• Works with or without food • Maximum dose = 1 per day
What to expect	Should cause an erection. Will not work if you are not sexually aroused. Erection should go away after sex.		
		• Cialis® for Daily Use—May take up to 5 days before it is effective	
Side effects	• Common: headaches, facial flushing, and upset stomach • Less common: blurred vision, temporary bluish vision, and sensitivity to light	• Common: headaches, indigestion, flushing, arm and leg pain, back pain, muscle aches, and stuffy nose	• Common: headaches, indigestion, flu-like symptoms, flushing, runny nose, sinus inflammation • Less common: temporary bluish vision or trouble telling blue from green colors
Reasons NOT to take	Don't take if you are taking any medication containing nitrates, because the combination can cause a dangerous drop in blood pressure. Nitrate medications include nitroglycerin patches (Nitro-Dur®, Transderm-Nitro®), nitroglycerin ointment (Nitro-Bid®, Nitrol®), nitroglycerin pills (Nitro-Bid®, Nitrostat®), and isosorbide (Dilatrate-SR®, Isordil®, Sorbitrate®). Street drugs known as "poppers" contain nitrates (amyl nitrate or buytl nitrate) and use of PDE-5 inhibitors should be avoided.		
Other precautions	Do not take if you have heart disease so severe that sexual activity is unsafe.		
	If you take an alpha blocker medication* for high blood pressure or prostate problems, your doctor may start you on a lower dose of Viagra®.	Let your doctor know if you take an alpha blocker medication* for high blood pressure or prostate problems.	If you take an alpha blocker medication* for high blood pressure or prostate problems, your doctor may start you on a lower dose of Levitra®.
	If you develop an erection lasting more than 4 hours, get medical attention right away to avoid permanent penile damage.		

*Alpha blocker medications include alfuzosin (Uroxatral®), doxazosin mesylate (Cardura®), prazosin (Minipress®), tamsulosin (Flomax®), and terazosin (Hytrin®).

[†]http://livertox.nih.gov/Sildenafil.htm; http://www.emedexpert.com/classes/sexual.shtml.

[‡]http://livertox.nih.gov/Tadalafil.htm; http://www.emedexpert.com/classes/sexual.shtml.

[§]http://livertox.nih.gov/Vardenafil.htm; http://www.emedexpert.com/classes/sexual.shtml.

American Association of Diabetes Educators©

378   Diabetes Education Curriculum

◆ **Over-the-counter herbal supplements for ED.** There are a variety of ED products available without a prescription that can be obtained from pharmacies, mail order, and Internet companies. Many of these ED products claim to be safe and all natural. Be aware that just because an ingredient is natural does not necessarily mean it is safe for all people.

Some ED products that are available through the Internet or by mail order come from other countries and are not approved by the FDA. **ALWAYS consult your provider regarding any over-the-counter herbal supplements before taking them. Find out if the active ingredient is safe for your situation— your other medical conditions and the medications you already take.** See Table S.3, Brand Names of Male Enhancement Supplements, and Table S.4, Active Ingredients Commonly Found in Male Enhancement Supplements.

Injections for ED

Injections for ED are given directly into the base of the penis using an autoinjection pen device. The most common medication used in these injections is alprostadil (the synthetic version of prostaglandin E_1). Brand names are Caverject® and Edex®.

Injected alprostadil works by allowing more blood to flow into the penis. An erection occurs within a few minutes of injection, whether or not there is any sexual stimulation. The erection typically remains for 30 to

---

TABLE S.3   Brand Names of Male Enhancement Supplements

Be aware of the following "male enhancement" supplements, which may contain any number of herbs that claim to increase the male sexual performance. Most of the research on the efficacy of these herbs has been done in animal studies. Much of the belief in these herbs has been passed down over centuries of use as an aphrodisiac. Some of the herbs, although natural, can have unwanted side effects.

Brand Names

Avela®	MagnaRX®	ProVigro®	VigRX®
Enzyte®	ProSolution®	SizePro®	ZeneRX®
Extagen®			

TABLE S.4   Active Ingredients Commonly Found in Male Enhancement Supplements

L-arginine*—An amino acid thought to be involved in the synthesis of nitric oxide, which increases blood flow into, and prevents blood flow out of, the penis during erection. Men with genital herpes should not take supplements with L-arginine, as it will aggravate their condition.

Tongkat ali*—From the root of the *Eurycoma longifolia* tree, native to Malaysia. Known as "Asian Viagra." Supposedly increases testosterone levels. Not to be used by men with diabetes, as it can alter blood glucose levels, possibly inducing hypoglycemia. Not for use by men with heart disease, kidney disease, liver disease, sleep apnea, male breast cancer, or prostate cancer.

Horny goat weed*—An herb of the *Epimedium* family. Chinese name for herb is *yin yang huo*. Epimedium contains the flavonoid *icariin*, which is thought to increase nitric oxide levels, thus producing an erection.

Tribulus terrestris extract*—An herb with the active ingredient *protodioscin*, which is said to act as a precursor in the synthesis of sex hormones.

Cnidium monnier†—A flowering herb, *Cnidium monnier*, is purported to increase the release of nitric oxide to help produce an erection.

*WebMD, "Vitamins and supplements lifestyle guide," on the Internet at: http://www.webmd.com/vitamins-and-supplements/lifestyle-guide-11/supplement-faq.
†WebMD, "Find a vitamin or supplement: cnidium," on the Internet at: http://www.webmd.com/vitamins-supplements/ingredientmono-1098-CNIDIUM.aspx?activeIngredientId=1098&activeIngredientName=CNIDIUM.

American Association of Diabetes Educators©

60 minutes, whether or not ejaculation has taken place. Pain and bruising at the injection site are possible, as is the development of scar tissue. Priapism, a condition where the erection remains for 4 or more hours, can occur.

A small test injection should be tried in the provider's office to learn how the patient will respond to the medication.[39] Close follow-up to figure out the correct dose for each patient's needs is essential to help avoid priapism. Injections cannot be used by men taking blood thinners.

Intraurethral Suppositories for ED

Intraurethral suppositories are tiny pellets of a medication called alprostadil (the synthetic version of prostaglandin E_1). The brand name is Muse®. The pellet is inserted into the urethra (the opening in the tip of the penis) using a special applicator. It is best to insert it just after urination to provide lubrication. Commercial lubricant should not be used, as this will affect the absorption of the medication.

The pellet melts with body heat (melts at 87°F), and the medication absorbs into the tissues of the penis.[40] It is important to walk or stand upright for the next 10 minutes; lying down right away may cause dizziness. The medication dilates the arteries, allowing more blood to flow into the penis and creating an erection in about 10 minutes.

The most common side effect is discomfort and irritation from insertion. Package instructions for tips on proper insertion of the pellet should be closely followed. Research shows that intraurethral alprostadil for ED is not as effective as the injected form.[41] Intraurethral suppositories may be used twice a day.[42]

Vacuum Suction Devices (VSDs)

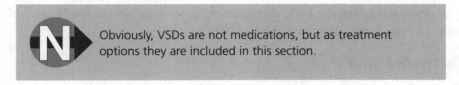

Obviously, VSDs are not medications, but as treatment options they are included in this section.

Vacuum suction devices create a vacuum to pull blood into the penis. First, the cylinder device is placed over the penis while the patient is standing or sitting. Negative pressure (suction) starts to build when the device is activated. Some devices have a lever that is pumped by hand; others are battery operated.

Once an erection is achieved, a silicone rubber ring is rolled over the device and onto the base of the penis. The ring is intended to help trap blood in the penis. Couples who have successfully used VSDs incorporate the pumping into their foreplay. The constriction ring should remain on for *no more than 30 minutes*, as it can cause skin irritation.[42]

A disadvantage of using a VSD is that the penis may feel numb and will be cold to the touch. Bruising of the penis can occur. Ejaculation may be difficult due to the constriction ring.[39] Vacuum suction devices can be used along with other forms of ED therapy, such as injections. If a man has severe circulation problems and cannot walk stairs, the VSD may not be effective.

Testosterone Replacement[25,43]

Being overweight or obese is often linked to ED. The studies that have looked at testosterone replacement are mixed. If you are not showing signs of low testosterone, there is no reason to check your testosterone level or use testosterone replacement. If ED is caused by low testosterone, then part of the treatment may be to replace the missing hormone, thus reducing symptoms. Testosterone replacement can be given in 5 ways:

1. injection
2. topical gel
3. pellets implanted under the skin
4. a buccal tablet that dissolves on the gums
5. skin patch

380   Diabetes Education Curriculum

Injections of testosterone are given in the doctor's office every 10 to 21 days. The buccal tablet is kept in place on the upper gums and replaced every 12 hours with a new one. Topical gels are rubbed onto the skin of the abdomen, upper arm, or shoulder every day. A new daily skin patch is placed on the upper arm, thigh, back, or abdomen. Care must be taken not to place a dose in the same area for longer than 1 week at a time.

Penile Prosthesis Surgery

Prosthesis surgery for ED is usually considered a last resort, if all other options have failed. A penile prosthesis consists of 3 parts:

1. 2 inflatable tubes that are implanted in the penis
2. a pump that is placed in the scrotum
3. a reservoir for fluid that is put into the abdomen

When the pump is activated, fluid goes into the tubes, creating an erection. A valve on the pump is pressed to deactivate the system, allowing the erection to subside.

Prosthesis surgery requires 2 to 4 hours on the operating table. It is an expensive surgery (at least $20,000), and recovery takes 4 to 8 weeks. Prosthetic surgery has a very high rate of success. Over 90% of erections are suitable for sexual intercourse.[44]

For men with diabetes, a penile prosthesis can be risky because of the risk of infection. To lower the risk for infection, the blood glucose level should be well controlled (A1C below 7%). There are other possible outcomes to consider. As with an organ transplant, the body may reject the prosthesis. Mechanical failure is also possible. Most prostheses last about 15 years before they need to be replaced.

Female Sexual Dysfunction

Sexual function in women can be influenced by a number of things, including fatigue, stress, depression, or medication. Diabetes is associated with sexual dysfunction in women.[10] When problems are attributed to diabetes, the main problems usually involve circulation and nerve function.

The Anatomy of Sexual Response in Women

It helps to have a basic understanding of what is happening in the body during a normal sexual response. The first organ to become involved is the brain. When a woman becomes sexually stimulated, the brain sends signals to other parts of the body to respond. The nerves are signaled to allow for increased blood flow into the pelvis and vagina by way of the arteries, producing vaginal lubrication.

If There Are Problems With the Arteries . . .

When plaque builds up in the arteries, the vessels become narrower, so less blood flows through to these areas.

If There Are Problems With the Nerves . . .

The nerves that trigger increased blood flow into the pelvis and vagina can be damaged by long-term high blood glucose (hyperglycemia). This affects arousal. Damage to sensory nerves (neuropathy) can cause decreased sensation. Symptoms of sexual dysfunction in women include[45]:

- ◆ Vaginal dryness, which can cause pain with intercourse
- ◆ Diminished vaginal/clitoral sensation
- ◆ Difficulty becoming aroused
- ◆ Difficulty achieving an orgasm

American Association of Diabetes Educators©

Treatment of Female Sexual Dysfunction
Healthy Coping

- The stresses of life can sometimes find their way into the bedroom. Finding healthy ways of lowering your stress can help.
- If you think you may have anxiety or depression, ask your doctor to evaluate you. Depression and anxiety can affect sexuality, and sexual problems can make depression and anxiety worse. When depression or anxiety and/or sexual problems are present, your quality of life can suffer. So it's important to address both concerns and pursue whatever treatments are right for you.
- Counseling with a healthcare professional trained in sex therapy/counseling may be helpful for any communication concerns with your partner that may be related to sexual problems.

Monitoring

Managing your diabetes to get the A1C to target can lower your risk for nerve damage and circulation problems. High blood glucose over the long term damages the blood vessels as well as the nerves responsible for sexual function. Remember, an A1C below 7% also reduces the risk for many other types of complications.

Taking Medication

- *Review your medication.* It's important to review all your medications, because many can cause sexual side effects. These include some medications used to treat high blood pressure, depression, heart problems, and other conditions.[46] Certain medications are also known to cause vaginal dryness. See Table S.1, Medications That May Cause Sexual Dysfunction, and Table S.5, Medications That May Cause Vaginal Dryness.

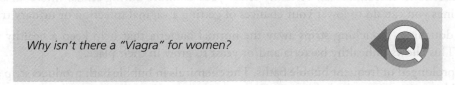

Why isn't there a "Viagra" for women?

Currently there are no approved pills to help women with sexual dysfunction. Research has been done to learn the benefit of sildenafil, the active ingredient in Viagra®, on female sexual dysfunction. Studies so far show that sildenafil shows little or no benefit to women with sexual dysfunction.[47] Research is ongoing for other ways of treating sexual dysfunction.[48,49]

- *Use a lubricant for vaginal dryness.* During and after menopause, vaginal dryness may be an ongoing problem for many women. It can cause itching and discomfort. If you have these symptoms, check with your provider first to see if you have an infection that needs treatment. To combat chronic vaginal dryness, consider a water-based lubricant that provides moisture for up to 3 days, such as Replens®. This product is as effective as a vaginal estrogen cream for women past menopause.[50] If you are past menopause, ask your provider if an estrogen vaginal cream would help.

Safe lubricants for vaginal dryness include those that are water-based or silicone-based. Lubricants can help with ongoing dryness and can help make intercourse more comfortable. These lubricants are available over the counter. Examples are:

Water-Based Vaginal Lubricants		Silicone-Based Vaginal Lubricants	
K-Y® Sensual Silk®	Maximus®—glycerin-free	Eros®	ID Millennium®
Astroglide®	Liquid Silk®—glycerin-free	Wet Platinum®	
Lubrin®	Slippery Stuff®—glycerin-free		

382 Diabetes Education Curriculum

TABLE S.5 Medications That May Cause Vaginal Dryness		
Beta-blockers*	Ortho-Cyclen	Lo/Ovral
Ativan	Calcium channel blockers*	OTC and prescription cold and allergy medications
Depo Provera	Xanax	

*See Table S.1, Medications That May Cause Sexual Dysfunction, for specific names of beta-blockers and calcium channel blockers.

Some vaginal lubricants contain *glycerin*, which breaks down to glucose. Although there are no studies to prove it, it may be wise to avoid lubricants with glycerin if you are prone to getting vaginal yeast infections.

Lubricants to Avoid

Kitchen oils and baby oil should not be used as vaginal lubricants for 2 reasons. First, these oils stay in the tissues and can harbor bacteria in the vagina. Second, they also cause damage to condoms, which puts a woman at risk for sexually transmitted diseases and/or pregnancy.

Reducing Risks

- If you smoke, stop. Smoking damages the blood vessels,[31] even those that are involved in a healthy sexual response.
- Get enough rest. Fatigue can cause problems with sexual response.
- Prevent infections. Infections can certainly affect your comfort during sexual intercourse. Here are a few simple things you can do to lower your chances of getting a vaginal infection or urinary tract infection[51]:
  —Avoid douching. Douching strips away the normal bacteria that help keep a healthy vaginal environment. This allows unhealthy bacteria and/or yeast to grow in their place.
  —Avoid prolonged or frequent bubble baths. The chemicals in bubble bath products strip away the normal vaginal bacteria, as described above.
  —Avoid using scented soaps or lotions in the vaginal area, for the same reasons described above.

REFERENCES

1. Vinik AI, Richardson D. Erectile dysfunction in diabetes. Diabetes Rev. 1998;6:16-33.
2. Rice D. Perspectives of a diabetes educator. In: Living Well With Diabetes: Male Sexual Functioning. Continuing Education Program; August 18, 1999; Orlando, Fla.
3. Klein R, Klein BE, Lee KE, Moss SE, Cruickshanks KJ. Prevalence of self-reported erectile dysfunction in people with long-term IDDM. Diabetes Care. 1996;19:135-41.
4. Marwick C. Survey says patients expect little physician help on sex. JAMA. 1999;281:2173-4.
5. Penson DF, Wessells H. Erectile dysfunction in diabetic patients. Diabetes Spectr. 2004;17:225-30.
6. Jack L Jr. A candid conversation about men, sexual health, and diabetes. Diabetes Educ. 2005;31(6):810-7.
7. Jack L Jr. Diabetes and men's health issues. Diabetes Spectr. 2004;17:206-8.
8. Broom D, Whittaker A. Controlling diabetes, controlling diabetics: moral language in the management of diabetes type 2. Soc Sci Med. 2004;58:2371-82.
9. Rice D, Jack L Jr. Use of an assessment tool to enhance diabetes educators' ability to identify erectile dysfunction. Diabetes Educ. 2006;32(3):373-80.
10. Enzlin P, Mathieu C, Vanderschueren K, Demytterene K. Diabetes mellitus and female sexuality: a review of 25 years' research. Diabetic Med. 1998;15:809-15.

American Association of Diabetes Educators©

11. Shaefer KM. Women living in paradox: loss and discovery in chronic illness. Holistic Nurs Pract. 1995;9:63-74.

12. LeMone P. The physical effects of diabetes on sexuality in women. Diabetes Educ. 1996;22:361-6.

13. Sarkadi A, Rosenqvist U. Intimacy and women with type 2 diabetes: an exploratory study using focus group interviews. Diabetes Educ. 2003;29(4):641-52.

14. House W, Pendleton L. Sexual dysfunction in diabetes: A survey of physicians' responses to patients' problems. Postgrad Med. 1986;79:227-35.

15. Temple-Smith M, Hammond J, Pyett P, Presswell N. Barriers to sexual history taking in general practice. Aust Fam Physician. 1996;25 Suppl 2:S71-4.

16. Lurie N, Margolis K, McGovern P, Mink P. Physician self-report of comfort and skill in providing preventive care to patients of the opposite sex. Arch Fam Med. 1998;7:134-7.

17. Loehr J, Verma S, Seguin R. Issues of sexuality in older women. J Womens Health. 1997;6:451-7.

18. Metz M, Seifert M. Women's expectations of physicians in sexual health concerns. Fam Pract Res J. 1988;7:141-52.

19. Driscoll C, Garner E, House J. The effect of taking a sexual history on the notation of sexually related diagnoses. Fam Med. 1986;18:293-5.

20. Schover LR. Beginning the dialogue: discussing sexual functioning. In: Living Well With Diabetes: Male Sexual Functioning. Continuing Education Program; August 18, 1999; Orlando, Fla.

21. Rosen RC, Cappelleri JC, Smith MD, et al. Constructing and evaluating the sexual health inventory for men: IIEF-5 as a diagnostic tool for erectile dysfunction. Paper presented at: VIII World Meeting on Impotence Research; 1998; Amsterdam, the Netherlands.

22. Rosen RC, Riley A, Wagner G, et al. The International Index of Erectile Function (IIEF): a multidimensional scale for assessment of erectile dysfunction. Urology. 1997;49:822-30.

23. Mayo Clinic. Erectile dysfunction: take control today (cited 2015 Jul 9). On the Internet at: http://www.mayoclinic.org/diseases-conditions/erectile-dysfunction/in-depth/erectile-dysfunction/ART-20043927.

24. Gazzaruso C, Giordanetti S, De Amici E, et al. Relationship between erectile dysfunction and silent myocardial infarction in apparently uncomplicated type 2 diabetic patients. Circulation. 2004;110:22-6.

25. American Association of Diabetes Educators. Men's Health, Low Testosterone and Diabetes: Individualized Treatment and a Multidisciplinary Approach [white paper]. Chicago: American Association of Diabetes Educators; 2008.

26. Tan RS, Pu SJ. Impact of obesity on hypogonadism in the andropause. Int J Androl. 2002;25:195-201.

27. Esposito K, Giugliano F, Di Palo C, et al. Effect of lifestyle changes on erectile dysfunction in obese men: a randomized controlled trial. JAMA. 2004;291:2978-84.

28. Derby CA, Mohr BA, Goldstein I, et al. Modifiable risk factors and erectile dysfunction: can lifestyle changes modify risk? Urology. 2000;56:302-6.

29. Romeo JH, Seftel AD, Madhun ZT, Aroon DC. Sexual function in men with type 2 diabetes associated with glycemic control. J Urol. 2000;163:788-91.

30. Thethi TK, Asafu-Adjaye NO, Fonseca VA. Erectile dysfunction. Clin Diabetes. 2005;23(3):105-13.

31. Centers for Disease Control and Prevention. Morbidity and Mortality Weekly Report. The Surgeon General's 1990 report on the health benefits of smoking cessation. Executive summary (cited 2015 Jul 9). 1990 Oct 5;39 (RR-12):viii-xv. On the Internet at: http://www.cdc.gov/mmwr/preview/mmwrhtml/00001800.htm.

32. Richardson D, Vinik A. Etiology and treatment of erectile failure in diabetes mellitus. Curr Diab Rep. 2002;2:501-9.

33. Fink HA, Mac DR, Rutks IR, et al. Sildenafil for male erectile dysfunction: a systematic review and meta-analysis. Arch Intern Med. 2002;162:1349-60.

34. US Food and Drug Administration. FDA Statement. FDA updates labeling for Viagra, Cialis, and Levitra for rare post-marketing reports of eye problems. Last updated 2005 Jul 8 (cited 2015 Jul 9). On the Internet at: http://www.fda.gov/NewsEvents/Newsroom/PressAnnouncements/2005/ucm108458.htm.

35. US Food and Drug Administration. Center for Drug Evaluation and Research. Drug safety (cited 2015 Jul 9). On the Internet at: http://www.fda.gov/NewsEvents/Newsroom/PressAnnouncements/2007/ucm109012.htm.

American Association of Diabetes Educators©

384   Diabetes Education Curriculum

36. Drugs.com. Yohimbine (cited 2015 Jul 9). On the Internet at: http://www.drugs.com/cons/yohimbine.html.

37. Morales A. Yohimbine in erectile dysfunction: the facts. Int J Impot Res. 2000;12 Suppl 1:S70-4.

38. Ruck B, Shih RD, Marcus SM. Hypertensive crisis from herbal treatment of impotence. Am J Emerg Med. 1999; 17:317-8.

39. Cohan P, Korenman SG. Erectile dysfunction. J Clin Endocrinol Metab. 2001;86(6):2391-4.

40. Padma-Nathan H, Hellstrom WJ, Kaiser FE, Lebasky RF. Treatment of men with erectile dysfunction with transurethral alprostadil. N Engl J Med. 1997;336:1-7.

41. Shabsigh R, Padma-Nathan H, Gittleman M, McMurray J, Kaufman J, Goldstein I. Intracavernous alprostadil alfadex is more efficacious, better tolerated, and preferred over intraurethral alprostadil plus optional actis: a comparative, randomized, crossover, multicenter study. Urology. 2000;55:109-13.

42. Vinik A, Richardson D. Erectile dysfunction in diabetes: pills for penile failure. Clin Diabetes. 1998;16(3):108-19.

43. Dhindsa S, Miller MG, McWhirter CL, et al. Testosterone concentrations in diabetic and nondiabetic obese men. Diabetes Care. 2010;33:1186-92.

44. Carson CC, Mulcahy JJ, Govier FE. Efficacy, safety, and patient satisfaction outcomes of the AMS 700CX inflatable penile prosthesis: results of a long-term multi-center study. J Urol. 2000;164:376-80.

45. Goldstein I, Berman J. Vasculogenic female sexual dysfunction: vaginal engorgement and clitoral erectile insufficiency syndrome. Int J Impotence Res. 1998;10 Suppl 2:S84-90.

46. Miočić J, Car N, Metelko Ž. Sexual dysfunction in women with diabetes mellitus. Diabetologia Croatica. 2008; 37(2):35-42.

47. Shields KM, Hrometz SL. Use of sildenafil for female sexual dysfunction. Ann Pharmacother. 2006;40(5):931-4.

48. Uckert S, Mayer ME, Jonas U, Stief CG. Potential future options in the pharmacotherapy of female sexual dysfunction. World J Urol. 2006;24(6):630-8.

49. Mayer ME, Bauer RM, Schorsch I, et al. Female sexual dysfunction: what's new? Curr Opin Obstet Gynecol. 2007; 19(6):536-40.

50. Grady D. Management of menopausal symptoms. N Engl J Med. 2006;355(22):2338-47.

51. WebMD. Women's health. Vaginal dryness: causes and moisturizing treatments (cited 2015 Jul 9). On the Internet at: http://organizedwisdom.com/helpbar/index.html?return=http://organizedwisdom.com/Vaginal_Dryness&url= women.webmd.com/vaginal-drynesssymptoms_signs_index.

SEXUAL DYSFUNCTION: RESOURCES

Sexuality and Diabetes.. 385

Sexual Health Inventory for Men (SHIM)... 391

Brief Sexual Symptom Checklist: Women's Version...................................... 392

American Association of Diabetes Educators©

SEXUALITY AND DIABETES

Sexuality is one of the greatest gifts we have as humans. When it works it can be wonderful and when it doesn't work it can be confusing and tremendously frustrating.

As sexual beings we are energetic and excited to test out the possibilities. If we are healthy, sex is exciting and fun and barring any anxieties, things work out and we continue to enjoy playing. Unfortunately we don't stay young forever and life may begin to take a toll with stress, aging, illness, relationship difficulties, anxiety and depression. Particularly when we throw the long term effects of diabetes in the mix, sex can become quite complicated.

WHAT DOES DIABETES AFFECT?

There are two answers to this question.

Not much if it is well controlled.

Everything if it is not well controlled.

WHAT'S NEEDED FOR GOOD SEX?

Good sex requires the right circumstances so those participating can be both excited and feel safe. We need "arousal" which requires good nerve conduction, blood flow, and the right balance of hormones. We also need our preferred stimulation which requires touch of various types. And we need the capability to respond, which again, requires all of the above. It seems simple, but we are not simple and sex is also not so simple. The most difficult aspect of this cycle is how diabetes can affect it and unfortunately it can affect all aspects of sexual pleasure.

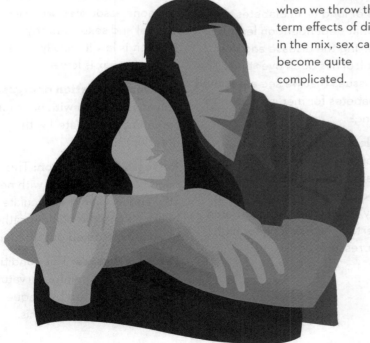

  American Association of Diabetes Educators

Developed with support from Pfizer, Inc.

sexuality and diabetes

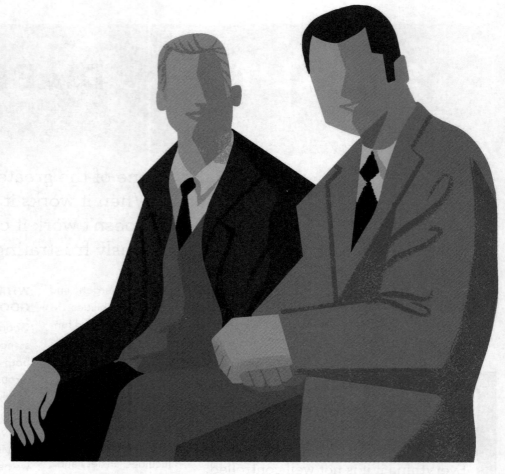

ISSUES AFFECTING MEN

Effects of long term diabetes are somewhat dependent on length of time having the disease and how the control has been over time. The sexual issues that we see associated with diabetes for men are the following:

Erectile dysfunction: This is associated with complications associated with reduced blood flow and poor nerve conduction (neuropathy). It may also be associated with certain medications for high blood pressure.

Low testosterone: This is the hormone associated with sexual arousal and sexual energy (Libido). When it is low it usually means interest in sex is lower.

Delayed ejaculation or orgasm: This is associated with neuropathy sometimes associated with anti-depressants.

Retrograde ejaculation: This condition is associated with neuropathy and is when the ejaculate backs up into the bladder rather than being ejected out the penis.

Peronies disease: This condition which causes a painful curvature of the penis is caused by plaque build up in an artery of the penis.

  American Association of Diabetes Educators

Developed with support from Pfizer, Inc.

sexuality and diabetes

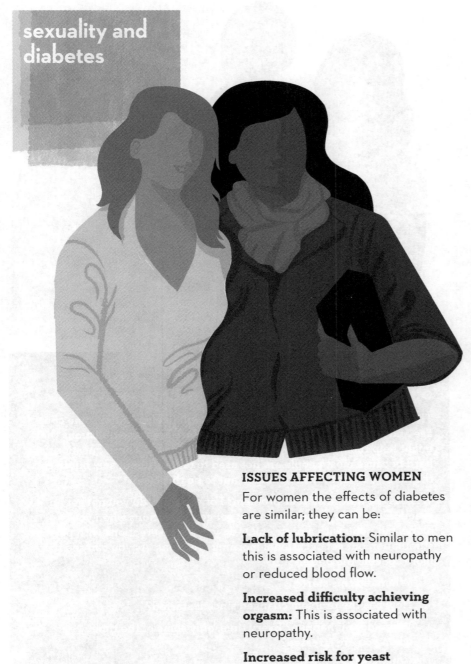

ISSUES AFFECTING WOMEN

For women the effects of diabetes are similar; they can be:

Lack of lubrication: Similar to men this is associated with neuropathy or reduced blood flow.

Increased difficulty achieving orgasm: This is associated with neuropathy.

Increased risk for yeast infections: This is due to elevated glucose levels.

For both men and women there are other factors that can have an effect on sexuality that are associated with having diabetes. Those who have diabetes run an increased risk for developing problems with depression and anxiety. These two conditions affect interest and performance with sex.

WHAT ELSE AFFECTS SEX?

Diabetes is not the only issue that affects your ability to have sex. Here is a brief list to check before you assume the cause is not if related to your diabetes.

Your relationship: Do you talk, touch, play, laugh and feel safe?

Your aging process: Are you healthy, happy with your body, how's your weight?

Health care in general: Do you smoke, drink, exercise, eat well, sleep well and manage stress?

Sex education: Do you know enough?

Medications: What do you take and can they have an effect?

If you run through this list and feel reasonably good about what you are doing to take care of yourself and you are still having any of the symptoms listed above then it may be time to see the doctor or your diabetes educator.

American Association of Diabetes Educators

Developed with support from Pfizer, Inc.

sexuality and diabetes

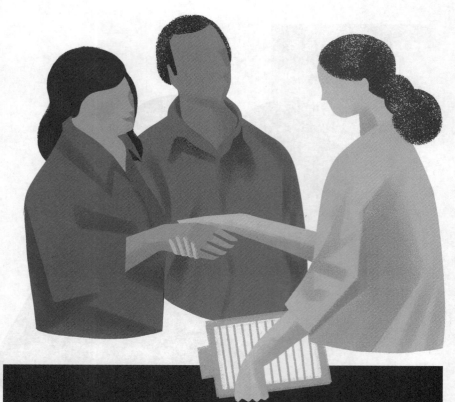

NEXT STEPS

There are different specialists who may treat sexual issues; the list below gives examples of some of those professionals you might see.

Diabetes educator

Primary Care Provider

Urologist

Obstetrician/Gynecologist

Sex therapist

Relationship therapist

As you can tell each of these will have a different set of ideas of how to go about the treatment process, so you may want to start with your diabetes educator or primary care provider to get the direction for whom to see next or what kind of treatment they might recommend.

Be assured there are treatments that can be helpful. Some will help restore functioning and some may simply help you identify a different way to play in this adult playground. Sexuality is such a special way to play, don't simply give up without knowing what might be useful and giving it a try.

QUESTIONS TO ASK YOUR HEALTHCARE PROVIDER

The visit to your healthcare professional will likely require some courage and a little reflection before you go. Here are some questions that might help them identify what is happening to you. These questions are hard because most people are not used to talking about sex, but to get the help you want it will be important to be this clear.

What is the nature of your problem? For example, do you not get an erection any time, ever? Or do you get good erections when you're alone, but none with a partner. Or do you get no erections with partner stimulation but get occasional morning erections. As you can see the more specific the better.

* When did this start?
* How has the problem changed since it started?
* When does it happen? Every time, only some of the time, when you are stressed?
* What makes a difference? More stimulation, different stimulation, more time in foreplay?
* Do you have enough foreplay?
* Does it matter how well your diabetes is controlled?
* How is your interest in sex? Has this changed?
* Do you receive the stimulation you would like? Does this make a difference?

  American Association of Diabetes Educators

Developed with support from Pfizer, Inc.

sexuality and diabetes

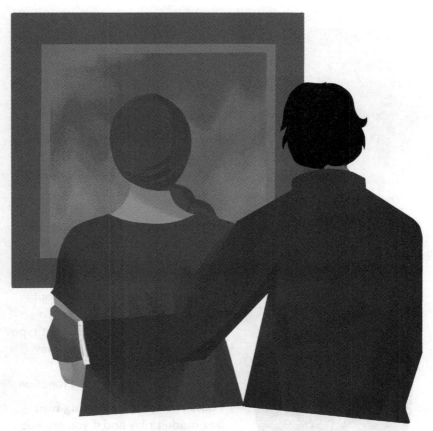

ENJOYING A HEALTHY SEX LIFE: TIPS FOR PEOPLE WITH DIABETES

Take care of your diabetes. There is evidence to suggest that sexual problems for both men and women with diabetes are similar to other complications caused by prolonged, elevated blood sugar levels. So be mindful of what you eat and drink, test regularly, and take your medications as prescribed. This will assure you are doing your part to protect this aspect of your health. In the short term make sure your blood sugar is in your target range before you start sexual play. Nothing is worse than having low blood sugar during sex, or having it be so high that it interferes with your current arousal.

Stay fit with regular exercise. Having an interest in sex and being able to engage in such a strenuous activity requires you and your heart to be in good shape. So in addition to being sexual, get some other physical activity during your week. Spend some time working your core muscles too. These muscles are very important in enhancing your sexual experience.

Use it or lose it. One of the most effective ways to maintain an interest in sex is to have sex. This old adage holds true because when we have sex certain hormones are produced that make us feel good at the time and also increase our desire to engage again sooner. If we stop having sexual play we begin to lose interest and interest may fade from both our mental and physical memory.

  American Association of Diabetes Educators

Developed with support from Pfizer, Inc.

sexuality and diabetes

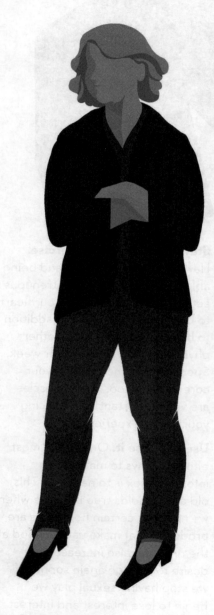

Keep your sexual play interesting. For most couples they learn what works to meet their sexual needs and then they use this activity forever. This becomes so familiar it can lead to boredom. Couples may benefit from a discussion that explores new interests or activities. This doesn't mean you get kinky, although that is a possibility, but does mean you discuss trying a different position or a different type of foreplay. Something new may restore some freshness and improve both interest and function.

Make sure you are having fun. Sex is adult play and if you are not having fun perhaps you need something to change. If sex creates anxiety, or functionally you are having a hard time getting things to work, it might be time to talk with your diabetes educator, doctor or a sex therapist. If you have enjoyed sex **don't give up hope,** go see someone who might help.

Take time to connect with your partner. Have a date night, have exercise time together, turn off the TV sit with each other and talk and touch. Too often our lives become too busy and we're always doing something. We forget that connection requires intention and attention. Have a relationship with each other on purpose. Plan it and do it because it is good for the relationship and ultimately it will be good for your sex life too.

Redefine sex, have a lot of foreplay, take your time. Because the sexual difficulties with diabetes may be primarily associated with arousal, foreplay activity may be helpful for lubrication and for erections. It can also be very pleasurable. Do not just jump into intercourse, unless you are in agreement and things work for you this way. Take time for play time, outer-course, before intercourse.

If you are having difficulty with any aspect of your sex life, see a professional to get some direction of how you might be helped. There are many treatments that can be helpful, but having someone to talk with about your concerns may be all you need. If you require more at least you have started the process. Even if you decide to not use the treatments, at least you will have the information and understand your choices.

Written by Joseph Nelson, MA, LP, CST

 American Association of Diabetes Educators

Developed with support from Pfizer, Inc.

Sexual Health Inventory for Men (SHIM)

Patient name: _____   Today's date: _____

Sexual health is an important part of an individual's overall physical and emotional well-being. Erectile dysfunction, also known as impotence, is a very common medical condition affecting sexual health. Fortunately, there are many different treatment options for erectile dysfunction. This questionnaire is designed to help you and your doctor identify whether you may be experiencing erectile dysfunction. If you are, you may choose to discuss treatment options with your doctor. Each question has several possible responses. Circle the number of the response that **best describes** your own situation. Please be sure that you select one and only one response for **each question**.

Over the past 6 months:

How do you rate your confidence that you could get and keep an erection?

Very low	Low	Moderate	High	Very high
1	2	3	4	5

When you had erections with sexual stimulation, how often were your erections hard enough for penetration (entering your partner)?

No sexual activity	Almost never or never	A few times (much less than half the time)	Sometimes (about half the time)	Most times (much more than half the time)	Almost always or always
0	1	2	3	4	5

During sexual intercourse, how often were you able to maintain your erection after you had penetrated (entered) your partner?

Did not attempt intercourse	Almost never or never	A few times (much less than half the time)	Sometimes (about half the time)	Most times (much more than half the time)	Almost always or always
0	1	2	3	4	5

During sexual intercourse, how difficult was it to maintain your erection to completion of intercourse?

Did not attempt intercourse	Extremely difficult	Very difficult	Difficult	Slightly difficult	Not difficult
0	1	2	3	4	5

When you attempted sexual intercourse, how often was it satisfactory for you?

Did not attempt intercourse	Almost never or never	A few times (much less than half the time)	Sometimes (about half the time)	Most times (much more than half the time)	Almost always or always
0	1	2	3	4	5

Score: Add the numbers corresponding to questions 1–5. If your score is 21 or less, you may be showing signs of erectile dysfunction and may want to speak with your doctor.

Sources: RC Rosen, JC Cappelleri, MD Smith, et al, "Constructing and evaluating the sexual health inventory for men: IIEF-5 as a diagnostic tool for erectile dysfunction," paper presented at the VIII World Meeting on Impotence Research (Amsterdam, 1998); RC Rosen, A Riley, F Wagner, et al, "The International Index of Erectile Function (IIEF): a multidimensional scale for assessment of erectile dysfunction," *Urology* 49 (1997): 822.

Brief Sexual Symptom Checklist: Women's Version

Patient name: _____   **Today's date:** _____

Please answer the following questions about your overall sexual function in the past **3 months** or more.

1. Are you satisfied with your sexual function?   ☐ Yes   ☐ No   If no, please continue.

2. How long have you been dissatisfied with your sexual function? _____

3a. The problem(s) with your sexual function is: (mark one or more)

  ☐ 1 Problems with little or no interest in sex
  ☐ 2 Problems with decreased genital sensation (feeling)
  ☐ 3 Problems with decreased vaginal lubrication (dryness)
  ☐ 4 Problems reaching orgasm
  ☐ 5 Problems with pain during sex
  ☐ 6 Other: _____

3b. Which problem is most bothersome? (circle one) 1 2 3 4 5 6

4. Would you like to talk about it with your doctor?   ☐ Yes   ☐ No

---

Source: D Hatzichristou, RC Rosen, G Broderick, et al, "Clinical evaluation and management strategy for sexual dysfunction in men and women," *J Sex Med* 1, no.1 (2004): 57.

APPENDIX

Diabetes Resources

Magazines—print and online

Diabetes Forecast	Published by the American Diabetes Association. Along with membership, you get 12 issues of the magazine per year. Call 1-800-DIABETES. Online version of magazine: http://www.diabetes.org/diabetes-forecast.jsp.
Diabetes Health	Call 1-800-488-8468. Online version of magazine: http://www.diabeteshealth.com.
Diabetes Wellness News	Call 1-866-293-3155. Online version of newsletter: http://www.diabeteswellness.net.
Better Homes and Gardens Diabetic Living	Available at retail centers such as grocery store checkouts, bookstores, etc.

Nonprofit associations

American Association of Diabetes Educators	http://www.diabeteseducator.org
American Diabetes Association	http://www.diabetes.org
Juvenile Diabetes and Research Foundation	http://www.jdrf.org
Academy of Nutrition and Dietetics	http://www.eatright.org
American College of Obstetricians and Gynecologists	http://www.acog.org

Government Web sites—health information for the public

Centers for Disease Control and Prevention	http://www.cdc.gov/diabetes/
National Diabetes Information Clearinghouse	http://diabetes.niddk.nih.gov
WIN—Weight-Control Information Network	http://www.win.niddk.nih.gov/index.htm
HealthFinder.gov	http://www.healthfinder.gov
National Diabetes Education Program	http://ndep.nih.gov
National Council on Aging	http://www.benefitscheckup.org/moreprograms.cfm?partner_id=0
The Special Supplemental Nutrition Program for Women, Infants, and Children (WIC)	http://www.fns.usda.gov/wic/women-infants-and-children-wic/

393

Nutrition support groups

Weight Watchers	http://www.weightwatchers.com
TOPS—Take Off Pounds Sensibly	http://www.tops.org
Overeaters Anonymous	http://www.oa.org

Patient assistance programs

RxAssist	A directory of all patient assistance programs in the United States. Search for specific medications by typing in the name of the drug or drug company. Call 401-729-3284; http://www.rxassist.org.
Community health centers	Federally funded centers that provide care to people with no insurance. To locate a community health center, call 1-888-ASK-HRSA (275-4772); http://findahealthcenter.hrsa.gov.
Free clinics	To locate a free clinic, listed by state. http://www.rxassist.org/patients/res-free-clinics.cfm.
Social service agencies	United Way referral service. http://www.211.org.
	Directory of public and private community resources and services. http://www.safetynetcenter.org.

Dental assistance programs

State dental assistance programs	http://www.dentalguideusa.org/state_dental_assistance.htm
National Donated Dental Services Program	http://dentallifeline.org

Medical assistance while traveling

International Association for Medical Assistance to Travelers	For a list of doctors in other countries who speak English: 1623 Military Rd., #279 Niagara Falls, NY 14303 Tel: 716-754-4883 http://www.iamat.org

Cultural education resources for patient education

Diabetes health information in Spanish	http://www.cdc.gov/spanish/enfermedades/diabetes.html
Diabetes—multiple languages	Includes links on diabetes education based on various languages. http://www.nlm.nih.gov/medlineplus/languages/diabetes.html.
Health Translations	A collection of handouts available in a variety of languages, including Arabic, Bosnian, Chinese, Russian, Spanish, and Vietnamese. Most are branded with logos from the following organizations: American Diabetes Association, American College of Cardiology, and the Preventive Cardiology Nurses Association. https://healthinfotranslations.org.
Healthy Roads Media	Offers a variety of resources on various health topics, including diabetes, in 11 languages. Resources available in different formats (written, audio, web-video). http://www.healthyroadsmedia.org.
National Diabetes Education Program	Contains diabetes education materials based on various languages. http://ndep.nih.gov/resources/index.aspx.
Cultural and ethnic food and nutrition education materials	Contains a list of cultural and ethnic food and nutrition education materials (books, pamphlets, and audiovisuals). http://www.nal.usda.gov/fnic/pubs/ethnic.pdf.

Recommended reading for diabetes educators on culture, language and health literacy

| Health Resources and Service Administration (HRSA): Cultural competence resources | http://www.hrsa.gov/culturalcompetence/ |

Emergency and disaster preparedness

| Centers for Disease Control and Prevention (CDC): Diabetes Care During Natural Disasters, Emergencies, and Hazards | Includes a number of resources on the following topics:
• Emergency preparedness
• Insulin, drug, and requirement advice
• Winter weather and extreme heat
• Health advice
• General hurricane recovery information
http://www.cdc.gov/diabetes/living/preparedness.html |

School personnel

| Diabetes Medical Management Plan (DMMP) | http://ndep.nih.gov/media/sample-diabetes-medical-management-plan-508.pdf
This plan should be completed by the student's personal diabetes healthcare team, including the parents/guardian. It should be reviewed with relevant school staff, and copies should be kept in a place that can be accessed easily by the school nurse, trained diabetes personnel, and other authorized personnel. |
| Hypoglycemic & Hyperglycemia Emergency Care Plans | http://ndep.nih.gov/media/sample-emergency-care-plans-for-hypoglycemia-and-hyperglycemia-508.pdf |

Index

Note: Tables, figures, and exhibits are italicized in the index.

A

A1C
 bile acid sequestrants and, 113
 cardiovascular health and, 294
 diagnostic levels of, 21
 erectile dysfunction and, 375
 female sexual dysfunction and, 381
 home monitoring results and, 195
 medication taking and, 102
 monitoring of, 172–174, 194–195, 293–294, 333, 375
 as outcome measure, 3
 pregnancy and, 327, 333
 stress management and, 252
 target levels of, 22, 102, 195, *195*, 294
AADE curriculum. *See* Diabetes education curriculum
Academy of Nutrition and Dietetics, 35, 66. *See also* Nutrition practice guidelines
Acarbose, 111–112
 contraindications to, 112
 dosage and administration of, 111
 effects on monitoring, *189*
 mechanism of action, 111
 side effects of, 112
Acceptable daily intake (ADI), of sweeteners, 46
ACE inhibitors, 300, 310
 contraindicated in pregnancy, 301, 302, 328, *328*
 recognizing (names of), *300*
Acesulfame potassium, 47, *48*, 332
Activity. *See* Physical activity
Activity scripts
 on goal setting, 245
 on problem solving, 216, 244–245

Actos. *See* Pioglitazone
Adherence. *See* Medication taking (adherence)
Adult learning, principles of, 4, 7, *8*
Advantame, *48*, 332
Advicor. *See* Lovastatin plus niacin
Aerobic activity, 78–82
 frequency and duration of, 80–81
 intensity of, 81–82
 preparing for, 80
 progressive, 81
Affirmations, 270–271, 285
Afrezza. *See* Inhaled insulin
1,5-AG (1,5-anhydroglucitriol), 174, 196
Agave nectar, 47
Aging, physical activity and, 78, 80
Air shot, 130, 162
Albiglutide, 123–125
 contraindications to, 125
 dosage and administration of, 124–125
 injection sites for, 127–128
 mechanism of action, 124
 precautions with, 125
 side effects of, 125
 storage of, 125
Albumin, urine, 309–310
Alcohol consumption, 53–55
 and blood pressure, 299
 and erectile dysfunction, 375
 and neuropathy, 315
 and nocturnal hypoglycemia, 223
 and pregnancy, 332
Alcoholism, vaccines for patients with, 363
Allergies
 to food, 57
 to tattoo ink, 322
Aloe gel, *134*

397

398 Diabetes Education Curriculum

Alogliptin, 108–110
  contraindications to, 109
  dosage and administration of, 109
  effects on monitoring, *189*
  mechanism of action, 108–109
  side effects of, 110
Alpha-glucosidase inhibitors, 111–112, *189*
Alpha lipoic acid (ALA), 132
Alprostadil, 378–379
Alternate site testing, 182–183
Alternative therapies. *See also* Complementary and
      alternative medicine
  definition of, 133
Amaryl. *See* Glimepiride
Ambivalence, in problem solving, 220–221
American Association of Clinical Endocrinologists
      (AACE)
  on self-monitoring of blood glucose, 185
  on target A1C levels, 294
  on target glucose levels, 177
American Association of Diabetes Educators (AADE),
      268, 393. *See also specific topics*
American College of Obstetricians and Gynecologists
      (ACOG)
  on hypertension, 295–296
  online resource of, 268, 393
  on target glucose levels, 177, *178*, 330, *330*
American Council of the Blind (ACB), 353
American Diabetes Association (ADA)
  on estimated average glucose, *196*
  online resource of, 268, 393
  on self-monitoring of blood glucose, 185
  on target A1C levels, 294
  on target glucose levels, 177, *178*
  on workplace rights and accommodations, 228
American Dietetic Association, 393
American Foundation for the Blind (AFB), 353
American Lung Association, 353
Americans with Disabilities Act, 228
Amitriptyline, 315
Amniocentesis, 357
Amputation, foot, 314
Amylin analogs, 126–127, *189*
Analogies, for learning, 19, 175
Anger/resentment, 255–256
Angiotensin-converting enzyme (ACE) inhibitors, 300,
      310
  contraindicated in pregnancy, 301, 302, 328, *328*
  recognizing (names of), *300*

Angiotensin receptor blockers (ARBs), 300, 310
  contraindicated in pregnancy, 301, 302, 328, *328*
  recognizing (names of), *300*
1,5-Anhydroglucitriol (1,5-AG), 174, 196
Ankle/brachial index (ABI), 296–297
Anticonvulsants, and erectile dysfunction, *374*
Antidepressants, and erectile dysfunction, *374*
Antiepileptics, and erectile dysfunction, *374*
Antihypertensive drugs, 299–303
  in pregnancy, 113, 300, 302, 328, *328*
  race/ethnicity and, 299–300, 303
  renal effects of, 300, 302, 310
Antiplatelet agents, 308–309
Antiviral drugs, for influenza, 364–365
Anxiety, 256–257
Apnea. *See* Sleep apnea
Appraisal of Diabetes (ADS), 288
ARBs (angiotensin receptor blockers), 300, 310
  contraindicated in pregnancy, 301, 302, 328, *328*
  recognizing (names of), *300*
*The Art and Science of Diabetes Self-Management
      Education Desk Reference*, 133
"Asian Viagra," *378*
Aspartame, 47–48, *48*, 332
Aspirin therapy, 308–309
Asplenia, vaccines for patients with, 363
Asthma, influenza in patients with, 364–365
Autonomic neuropathy, 316–317
  cardiovascular, 316
  physical activity and, 90
Avandia. *See* Rosiglitazone
Aventyl. *See* Nortriptyline

B

Balance training, 78, 80
Banaba, *134*
Barrier(s), 12–13
  to coping, 253
  to healthy eating, 26, 59–60
  to hyperglycemia management, 230–232
  to hypoglycemia management, 227
  to medication taking, 102, 103, 104, 136–139
  to monitoring, 174, 190–193, 206
  to physical activity, 76, 90–91
  to problem solving, 213, 215
  to risk reduction, 291, 340–341
Barrier contraceptives, *326*
Basal insulin, 114, 122
Beans, as fiber source, 50, *50*

Beck Depression Inventory (BDI), 286
Behavioral objectives, 11
  for coping, 254
  for medication taking, 104
  for monitoring, 174
  for nutrition, 27
  for physical activity, 76
  for problem solving, 215
  for risk reduction, 291
Behavior chain analysis, 246–248, 257–259
Behavior chain templates, 239, 276
Behavior change
  in coping, 272–273
  developing plan for, 4–5
  documentation of, 13
  health belief model of, 9
  in medication taking, 141
  in monitoring, 198–199
  in nutrition, 62
  as outcome, 3–5, 4, 14
  patient empowerment model of, 9
  in physical activity, 93
  in problem solving, 238
  in risk reduction, 343
  social cognitive theory of, 9–10
  theories of, 9–10
Benzodiazepines, and erectile dysfunction, 374
Berlin Questionnaire, 320, 355–356
Beta-blockers, 301, 301, 382
Beta carotene, 132
Better Homes and Gardens Diabetic Living, 393
Bilberry, 134
Bile acid sequestrants, 113, 306
Biophysical profile, 357
Birth control, 325–326, 326
Birth defects, 326, 329
Birth weight, 329
Bitter melon, 135
Black box warning, on pioglitazone and rosiglitazone, 109
Bladder dysfunction, 319
Blindness, physical activity and, 89
Blood glucose, 18–19
  alcohol and, 54
  bile acid sequestrants and, 113
  carbohydrate intake and, 34, 35, 40
  complementary and alternative medicine and, 134, 134–136
  diagnostic levels of, 21–22

dietary fiber and, 50
factors affecting, 205, 207
fasting, normal range of, 18
in gestational diabetes, 21, 22, 329–330
illness (sick day) and, 233–235, 236, 359
medications controlling. See Medication, diabetes;
  Medication taking (adherence)
nerve effects of, 315, 317
obesity and, 31
OTC medications and, 235
physical activity and, 77–78, 84–88, 86, 230
in prediabetes, 20–21
pregnancy risks and, 326, 329
renal effects of, 309–310
target levels of, 22, 176–177, 178
target levels in children, 177, 178
target levels in postpartum women, 336
target levels in pregnancy, 177, 178, 330, 330
tocolytic agents and, 114
in type 1 diabetes, 19–21
in type 2 diabetes, 20–21
vision (eye) effects of, 313
Blood glucose control
  A1C levels in, 194–195, 293–294
  legacy effect of, 195
  long-term, measuring, 174, 194–197
  medication taking and, 102–103
  nerve effects of, 315, 317
  nutrition and, 28
  problem solving for, 214–215
  renal effects of, 310
  vision (eye) effects of, 313
Blood glucose meters, 179–185
  blood sample for, 179, 181–184, 207
  control testing of, 180
  costs and insurance for, 179, 188
  memory function of, 179, 184
  recording and sharing results, 183–185
  selection of, 179
  traveling with, 181, 338, 357–358
Blood glucose monitoring, 173–194
  alternate site testing in, 182–183
  assessment tool for diabetes educator, 209
  barriers to, 174, 190–193, 206
  blood sample for, 179, 181–184, 207
  checklists for, 205
  for children, 177, 178
  continuous system for, 180
  control testing for, 180

American Association of Diabetes Educators©

400   **Diabetes Education Curriculum**

costs and insurance for supplies, 179, 188
diabetes medications and, 188, *189*
facilitators for, 174, 193–194
factors affecting, 205, 207
general guidelines for, 180–185
handouts on, 201–204
hand-washing for, 181
interpreting and responding to results of, 189–190
literature review on, 172
long-term, 174, 194–197
meals and, *187,* 188
during physical activity, 84
positive questioning about, 207
postpartum, 336
for pregnant women, 173, 177, *178,* 182, 188, 333
problem solving on, 190–193, 208
reality scenarios on, 190–193
reasons for, 176
recording and sharing results of, 183–185
resources on, 200–209
selecting meter for, 179
self-monitoring. *See* Self-monitoring of blood glucose
sexual health and, 375
storage of supplies for, 181
timing and frequency of, 185–192
traveling and, 181, 338, 357–358
Blood ketone monitoring, 235
Blood pressure, 294–303
controlling, 298–303
in diabetic children, 296
diastolic, 295
dietary approaches to, 33, 52, 299
medications for regulating, 113, 299–303
monitoring of, 196
normal, 295
obesity and, 31
physical activity and, 77, 89, 299
in pregnant diabetic women, 295–296, 328, 336
race/ethnicity and treatment of, 299–300, 303
renal effects of, 309
self-monitoring of, 297–298
sodium intake and, 28, 52–53
systolic, 295
target levels of, 295–296, 298
vision (eye) effects of, 313
weight loss and, 28
Blood pressure monitors, 297–298
Blood sample, for glucose meter, 179, 181–184, 207
BMI. *See* Body mass index

Body art, 322–323
Body mass index (BMI), 29–30
categories of, 29, *29*
for children, 29
limitations of measure, 29
online resource on, 29
in pregnancy, *29,* 29–30
Bolus insulin, 114, 122
Breakfast
carbohydrate intake in, 35
metabolic effects of, 28
Breastfeeding, care during, 336–337
Brief Medication Questionnaire, 103
Brief Sexual Symptom Checklist, for women, 392
Bydureon. *See* Exenatide, extended-release
Byetta. *See* Exenatide

C

Caffeine, 233, 299
Caiapo, *135*
Calcium channel blockers, 302, *302*
Calendar, for physical activity, 100
Calories, 33
daily needs for, 31–32, *32*
meal plan for, 32–33
per serving, 55
CAM. *See* Complementary and alternative medicine
Canaglifozin, 112–113
contraindications to, 112
dosage and administration of, 112
effects on monitoring, *189*
mechanism of action, 112
precautions with, 112
side effects of, 112
Cancer, physical activity and, 78
Candida, 321
Capsaicin cream, 315
Carbamazepine, 315
Carb counting, 34, 123
Carbohydrates, 33, 35–41. *See also specific sources*
breakfast intake of, 35
calories per gram, 33
choices of, 35, *35*
content in alcohol, 53
food label information on, 56–57
glycemic index/load of, 40
for hypoglycemia management, 223–225, 335
net, 57
pre-activity, 86–88, *87*
pregnancy and, 35

American Association of Diabetes Educators©

for pregnant women, 335
recommended intake of, 34
serving sizes of, *35*
for sick-day management, 233–234, 359
total, 56
whole-grain, *35,* 50
Cardiac denervation syndrome, *317*
Cardiac rehabilitation, 89
Cardiovascular autonomic neuropathy (CAN), 316
Cardiovascular health. *See also* Blood pressure; Heart
    disease
    aspirin therapy for, 308–309
    blood pressure and, 294–303
    lipids and, 303–307
    monitoring of, 174, 196–197, 294
    pregnancy and, 328
    risk reduction in, 294–309
    smoking cessation and, 299, 307, *308*
Cataracts, 311
Caverject (alprostadil), 378–379
Center for Epidemiological Studies Depression (CES-
    D), 287
Centers for Disease Control and Prevention (CDC),
    393
    on emergency preparedness, 395
    on immunization, 362–367
    on influenza, 364–365
    on preconception care, 325
Cervical cap, *326*
CGMS. *See* Continuous glucose monitoring system
Chickenpox vaccine, 362–363
Children
    blood pressure and diabetes in, 296
    BMI measures for, 29
    calorie needs of, 31–32, *32*
    eye health in, 312
    fish intake and mercury in, 44
    lipid levels in, 304
    meal plan for, 33
    target glucose levels for, 177, *178*
Chocolate, 225
Cholesterol, 28, 303–307
    bile acid sequestrants and, 113, 306
    in children, 304
    food label information on, 43, *46,* 55
    good *versus* bad, 43, 77, 303
    medications for lowering, 304–307, *305, 306*
    monitoring levels of, 197, 294
    nutrition and, 43–45, 305
    obesity and, 31

physical activity and, 77, 305
physiological function of, 303
pregnancy and, 328
per serving, 55
sodium per, 55
target levels of, 197, 304–305
tips for cutting, 45
Cholestyramine, 306
Chorionic villus sampling (CVS), 357
Chromium, 132
Cialis (tadalafil), 376, *377*
Cinnamon, *135*
Clinical improvement, as post-intermediate outcome,
    4, *4*
Clonidine, for pregnant patients, 302
Cnidium monnier, 378
Cognitive abilities, of patient, 214
Cold medications, 235
Colesevelam, 113, 306
Colestid. *See* Colestipol
Colestipol, 306
Color-coding, 105
Combination diabetes medications, 103, 113
Combination lipid medications, 307
Communication skills, 253
Community health centers, 268, 394
Community resources, support from, 266–267
Complementary and alternative medicine (CAM),
    133–136
    common products in, 133
    definition of, 133
    safety of, 133
    side effects and drug interactions of, 133
    used to lower blood glucose, 134, *134–136*
    users of, 133
Complementary therapies, definition of, 133
Complications. *See also specific complications*
    glycemic control and, 102–103
    long-term monitoring to prevent, 174, 194–197
    nutrition and prevention of, 27–28
    renal, 309–311
    risk reduction to prevent. *See* Risk reduction
    thoughts and feelings about, identifying, 291–292
Computer download feature, of glucose meter, 179, 184
Condoms, *326*
Confidence
    and coping, 253
    and problem solving, 220–222
Contact lenses, 312
Continuous glucose monitoring system (CGMS), 180

American Association of Diabetes Educators©

402 Diabetes Education Curriculum

Continuous positive airway pressure (CPAP), 321

Continuous quality improvement (CQI), 3–5

Contraception, 325–326, *326*

Contraction stress test, 357

Control testing, 180–181

Conviction, in problem solving, 220–221

Cool-down, after physical activity, 80

Coping, 15, 249–288

    anger/resentment *versus,* 255–256

    with anxiety, 256–257

    barriers to, 253

    behavioral objectives for, 254

    behavior chain analysis for, 257–259

    cost *versus* benefit analysis for, 259–260, 284

    definition of, 250

    with depression, 252–254, 256–257

    educator's overview of, 250–254

    with erectile dysfunction, 375

    facilitators for, 253

    with female sexual dysfunction, 381

    follow-up/outcomes measurement of, 271–273

    guilt/self-blame *versus,* 256

    handouts on, 277–282

    influences on, 250–251

    instructional plan for, 254–273

    learning objectives for, 253

    literature review on, 250

    with neuropathy, *317–319*

    positive affirmations for, 270–271, 285

    with postpartum concerns, 337

    with pregnancy, 252, 331

    resources on, 276–288

    sadness/worry *versus,* 256

    shock/denial *versus,* 255

    thoughts and feelings in, 254–257

Coping skills

    communication, 253

    decision-making, 259–260

    motivation, 259–260, 284

    problem-solving, 251–252, 257–259, 283

    relapse prevention, 260–261

    social support, 253, 262–268

    stress management, 252, 269–271

    training for, 251–253

Corn syrup, 47

Costs, of monitoring supplies, 179, 188

Cost *versus* benefit analysis, 259–260, 284

Cough medications, 235

CPAP (continuous positive airway pressure), 321

Creatinine ratio, 309–310

Cue-dose training, 103

Cultural resources, 394–395. *See also* Spanish, materials in

Culture. *See also* Spanish, materials in

    and coping, 250–251

    and nutrition, 25, 36–37, *37, 41,* 60

    and problem solving, 214

Curriculum. *See* Diabetes education curriculum

Cymbalta. *See* Duloxetine

D

Dapagliflozin, 112–113

    contraindications to, 112

    dosage and administration of, 112

    effects on monitoring, *189*

    mechanism of action, 112

    precautions with, 112

    side effects of, 112

DAWN (Diabetes Attitudes, Wishes, and Needs) study, 250, 325

Decision-making skill, 259–260

Deep breathing, 271

Dehydration, 51, 84, 233

Denial/shock, 255

Dental assistance programs, 394

Dental health, 321–322

Dentures, care of, 322

Depression

    assessment for, 252, 286–287

    clinical, 256

    coping with, 252–254, 256–257

    geriatric, 287

    and medication adherence, 103

    medication for, and erectile dysfunction, *374*

    postpartum, 287

    screening for, 252, 325

    warning signs of, 256

Dextrose, 47

Diabetes. *See* Diabetes mellitus

Diabetes 39 (assessment tool), 288

Diabetes Control and Complications Trial (DCCT), 223

Diabetes Distress Scale (DDS), 288

Diabetes education

    algorithm for, 5, *6*

    national standards for, 3, 5–6

Diabetes education curriculum. *See also specific topics and modules*

    aim of, 2

    behavioral objectives in, 11

    description of modules in, 14–15

    educator's overview of, 10–11

American Association of Diabetes Educators©

foundation of, 3–7
identifying barriers/reality scenarios in, 12–13
identifying facilitators in, 13
instructional plans in, 11–12
intended audience of, 2
learning objectives in, 11
literature review on, 10–11
methodology of, 7–10
national standard for, 5
organization of modules in, 10–14
rationale for, 2
readability of, 10
relationship to other standards, 5–7
SMART goals in, 4, 13
survival skills, 12
Diabetes educators. *See also* Diabetes education;
 Diabetes education curriculum
standards of practice for, 6–7
Diabetes Forecast, 393
Diabetes goal tracker mobile app, 352
Diabetes Health, 393
Diabetes Medical Management Plan (DMMP), 395
Diabetes mellitus, 19–22
diagnosis of, 21–22
living with, 22. *See also* Coping
pathophysiology of, understanding, 18–19
resources on, 393–395
thoughts and feelings about, 254–257
types of, 19
vaccines for patients with, 363
Diabetes mellitus, type 1, 19–20
diagnosis of, 21
insulin therapy for, 114
monitoring in, 173
necessity of medication for, 105
nutrition and, 27–28
pregnancy and, 329
Diabetes mellitus, type 2, 20
diagnosis of, 21
gestational diabetes and risk of, 337
insulin resistance in, 20
medication at onset of, 102–103
necessity of medication for, 105
obesity and, 20
physical activity for, 77–78, 78–80
prediabetes and, 20–21
pregnancy and, 329
progressive nature of, 20, 22, 105
risk factors for, 20
short-term insulin therapy for, 115

symptoms of, 20
weight loss for, 28
Diabetes Online Community (DOC), 281–282
Diabetes self-management education (DSME), *3,* 3–5, *4*
Diabetes self-management education and support
 (DSME/S)
patient-centered approach to, 5
position statement of, 5
Diabetes self-management support (DSMS), definition
 of, 5
Diabetes Wellness News, 393
Diabetic ketoacidosis (DKA), 19
blood monitoring for, 235
illnesses and risk of, 234–235
signs and symptoms of, 234
urine monitoring for, 234
Diabetic nephropathy, 309–311
monitoring for, 309–310
reducing risk of, 310–311
Diabetic neuropathy, 314–319
alpha lipoic acid for, 132
autonomic, 90, 316–317
peripheral, 89, 132, 315
physical activity and, 89
reducing risk of, 314–316
sexual dysfunction in, *318–319,* 371. *See also* Sexual
 dysfunction
Diabetic retinopathy, 311–314
pregnancy and, 312, 328
reducing risk of, 313–314
treatment of, 313
Diagnosis, 21–22
coping with. *See* Coping
prediabetes, 21
thoughts and feelings about, 254–257
Diaphragm (contraception), *326*
Diarrhea, 233–235, *236. See also* Sick-day
 management
Diastolic pressure, 295
Diet, avoidance of term, 25, 27
Dietary Approaches to Stop Hypertension (DASH), 33,
 52, 299
Dietary supplements, 133–136
used to lower blood glucose, 134, *134–136*
vitamin and minerals, 51–52, 132
Diltiazem, for pregnant patients, 302
Dinner, carbohydrate intake in, 35
Direct instruction, *versus* facilitating problem solving,
 213
Disaster conditions, risk reduction during, 339–340, 395

American Association of Diabetes Educators©

Disposable insulin delivery systems, 122
Disposal
    of lancets, 183
    of needles, 131, 169–170
Diuretics, 300–302, *301*, 310
DKA. *See* Diabetic ketoacidosis
Doctor–patient relationship, 265–266
Documentation
    of behavior change, 13
    as educator standard, 7
Donebedian, Avedis, 3
DPP-IV inhibitors, 108–110, *189*
Dry mouth, chronic, 321
DSME. *See* Diabetes self-management education
Dulaglutide, 123–125
    contraindications to, 125
    dosage and administration of, 124–125
    injection sites for, 127–128
    mechanism of action, 124
    precautions with, 125
    side effects of, 125
    storage of, 125
Duloxetine, 315
Duration of action (insulin), 116–117

E

eAG (estimated average glucose), 174, 195, *196*
Eating. *See also* Nutrition
    identifying thoughts and feelings about, 27
    insulin therapy and, 118–120
    SMART goals for, 61
Eating out, 58, *58*
Eating patterns, 33
Echocardiogram, fetal, 357
Eclampsia, 295–296
Edex (alprostadil), 378–379
Edinburgh Postnatal Depression Scale (EPDS), 287
eGFR (estimated glomerular filtration rate), 310
Elavil. *See* Amitriptyline
Emergency kit, 339–340, 395
Emotional health, assessment of, 286
Emotional state
    diabetes diagnosis and, 254–257. *See also* Coping
    exploration activity on, 257
    monitoring terminology and, 172–173
    physical activity and, 78
    stress and, 269
Empagliflozin, 112
    contraindications to, 112
    dosage and administration of, 112

    mechanism of action, 112
    precautions with, 112
    side effects of, 112
Endep. *See* Amitriptyline
End-stage renal disease, physical activity and, 90
EPAP (expiratory positive airway pressure), 321
Epimedium, 378
Erectile dysfunction (ED), *318*, 373–380
    causes of, 373
    injections of alprostadil for, 378–379
    intraurethral suppositories for, 379
    male perceptions of, 373
    medications causing, *374*
    openness about, 373
    oral medications for, 376–378, *377*
    PDE-5 inhibitors for, 376, *377*
    penile prosthesis surgery for, 380
    physical activity and, 375
    testosterone replacement for, 379–380
    treatment of, 375–380
Erection, anatomy of, 373–374
Estimated average glucose (eAG), 174, 195, *196*
Estimated glomerular filtration rate
    (eGFR), 310
Eurycoma longifolia, 378
Evaluation, as educator standard, 7
Exenatide, 123–125
    contraindications to, 125
    dosage and administration of, 124–125
    effects on monitoring, *189*
    extended-release, 123–125
    injection sites for, 127–128
    mechanism of action, 124
    precautions with, 125
    side effects of, 125
    storage of, 125
Exercise physiologist (EP), 75
Exercise prescription, 75
Expiratory positive airway pressure (EPAP), 321
Exubera, withdrawal from market, 115
Eye examinations, 311–313
    for children, 312
    general *versus* diabetic, 312–313
    for pregnant diabetic patients, 312
Eye health, 311–314
    in children, 312
    monitoring of, 174, 197, 311–313
    pregnancy and, 312, 328
Ezetimibe, 306
Ezetimibe plus simvastatin, 307

F

Facilitators, 13
    for coping, 253
    for hyperglycemia management, 232
    for hypoglycemia management, 228
    for medication taking, 104, 140
    for monitoring, 174, 193–194
    for nutrition, 26, 60–61
    for physical activity, 76, 91–92
    for problem solving, 215
    for risk reduction, 291, 341
Family feelings, identifying, 262–263
Family support, 262–265
    asking for, 263–264
    for coping, 250–251, 262–265
    for nutrition, 25
    for physical activity, 76
Farxiga. *See* Dapagliflozin
Fasting hyperglycemia profile, *187*
Fasting plasma glucose test, 21
Fat(s), 33, 43–45, 305
    calories per gram, 33
    food label information on, 43, *46, 55*
    saturated, 43, *44,* 305
    per serving, 55
    serving sizes of, *44*
    tips for cutting, 45
    trans, 43, 305
    unsaturated, 43, *44*
Female sexual dysfunction, *319,* 380–382
    assessment for, 392
    awareness of, 372
    coping with, 381
    medications causing, 381, *382*
    patient information on, 385–390
    symptoms of, 380
    unaddressed, 372
    vaginal lubricants for, *381,* 381–382
Fenofibrate, 307
Fenugreek, *135*
Fetal echocardiogram, 357
Fetal monitoring, 333–334, 335, 357
Fever, 233–235, *236. See also* Sick-day management
Fiber, dietary, 50–51, 305
    food label information on, 51, *51, 56*
    sources of, 50, *50*
Fibric acid, 304–305, 307
Financial issues/assistance, 147, 179, 188, 268, 341, 354, 394
Finger-stick monitoring, 181–182, 207

Finger tourniquet, rubber band, 182, *182*
Fish intake, 43–44, 305, 332
Fish oil, 304, 307
FITT activity plan, 75
    for aerobic activity, 80–81
    for resistance (strength) training, 82–83
5-point monitoring profile, *186*
Flavonoids, 54
Flesch–Kincaid readability statistics, 10
Flexibility training, 78, 80
Follow-up/outcomes measurement, 4–5, 13–14
    of coping, 271–273
    of medication taking, 140–142
    of monitoring, 197–199
    of nutrition, 61–62
    of physical activity, 92–93
    on problem solving, 236–238
    of risk reduction, 342–343
Food allergies, 57
Food and Drug Administration (FDA)
    on blood pressure monitors, 298
    on fiber labeling, 51, *51*
    on fish intake, 44
    on food labels, 54
    on glucose meters, 179
    on online resources, 268
    on PDE-5 inhibitors, 376
    on pioglitazone and rosiglitazone safety, 109
    on sodium labeling, 53
    on sweeteners, 46, 47
    on sweeteners in pregnancy, 331–332
Food groups, 34–54. *See also specific foods and nutrients*
Food labels, 54–57
    fat and cholesterol information on, 43, *46, 55*
    fiber information on, 50–51, *51,* 56
    sodium information on, 53, *53,* 55
Foot
    amputation of, 314
    care of, 315–316, 317
    nerve damage in, 89, 314–319
    reducing risk of problems with, 314–316
Foot health, 314–319
    alcohol consumption and, 315
    monitoring of, 174, 197, 314–315
    smoking cessation and, 315
Foot ulcers, physical activity and, 89
Footwear
    for physical activity, 84
    therapeutic, cost and coverage for, 341, 354
Fortamet. *See* Metformin

American Association of Diabetes Educators©

Frames of Mind: The Theory of Multiple Intelligences (Gardner), 7–8
Free clinics, 268, 394
Freedom from Smoking Online, 353
Free foods, 48, *49*
Frequency, of monitoring, 185–192
Frequency, of physical activity, 75
    aerobic, 80–81
    resistance (strength), 82
Friends, support from, 262
Fructosamine, 174, 196
Fructose, 47
Fruits, 36–37, *37*

G

Gabapentin, 315
Gardner, Howard, 7–8
Gastroparesis, *318*
Gauge
    of lancet, 182
    of needle, 128, 159
Gemfibrozil, 307
Geriatric Depression Scale (GDS), 287
Gestational diabetes (GDM), 21, 329–336
    blood glucose goals in, 330, *330*
    coping with, 331
    diagnosis of, 22
    insulin therapy for, 115
    management of, 330–335
    medication taking in, 334
    monitoring in, 173, 333–334
    nutrition in, 331–332
    physical activity in, 332–333
    postpartum care in, 336–337
    and risk of type 2 diabetes, 337
    risk reduction in, 335–336
Gestational hypertension, 296
Gingivitis, 321–322
Ginseng, *135*
Glasses, for vision correction, 312
Glaucoma, 311
Glimepiride, 110
    contraindications to, 110
    dosage and administration of, 110
    effects on monitoring, *189*
    mechanism of action, 110
    precautions with, 110
    side effects of, 110
Glipizide, 110
    brand names for, 110

contraindications to, 110
dosage and administration of, 110
effects on monitoring, *189*
mechanism of action, 110
precautions with, 110
side effects of, 110
Glomerular filtration rate (GFR), 310
GLP-1. *See* Glucagon-like peptide-1
Glucagon injection, 226
Glucagon-like peptide-1 (GLP-1), 108, 124
Glucagon-like peptide-1 (GLP-1) agonists, 123–125, *189*
    contraindications to, 125
    dosage and administration of, 124–125
    injection sites for, 127–128
    mechanism of action, 124
    precautions with, 125
    side effects of, 125
    storage of, 125
Glucophage. *See* Metformin
Glucophage XR. *See* Metformin
Glucose
    blood levels of. *See* Blood glucose
    definition of, 35
    metabolism of, 18–19, 114
    monitoring of. *See* Blood glucose monitoring
Glucose meters. *See* Blood glucose meters
Glucose tablets, 224, 233, 335
Glucotrol. *See* Glipizide
Glucotrol XL. *See* Glipizide
Glumetza. *See* Metformin
Glyburide, 110
    brand names for, 110
    contraindications to, 110
    dosage and administration of, 110
    effects on monitoring, *189*
    mechanism of action, 110
    precautions with, 110
    side effects of, 110
Glycemic control, medication taking and, 102–103
Glycemic index (GI), 40
Glycemic load (GL), 40
Glycomark test, 196
Glynase. *See* Glyburide
Glyset. *See* Miglitol
Goal(s)
    as educator standard, 6
    mobile app for tracking, 352
    realistic *versus* relevant, 13
    SMART, 4, 13

Index 407

Goal setting, 13
  activity script on, 245
  for healthy eating, 61
  for medication taking, 140
  for monitoring, 197
  for physical activity, 75, 92
  for problem solving, 214, 216, 218–220, 235–236
  for risk reduction, 342
  SMART, 4, 13
Government Web sites, 393
Greek yogurt, 38, *38*
Guide Dog Foundation for the Blind, Inc., 353
Guilt/self-blame, 256
Gymnema, 135

H

Haemophilus influenzae type b (Hib) vaccine, 362–363
Handouts
  on coping, 277–282
  on immunization, 360–369
  on influenza, 364–365
  on medication taking, 148–170
  on monitoring, 201–204
  on nutrition, 67–72
  on physical activity, 96–99
  on problem solving, 240–243
  on sexual health, 385–390
Hand-washing, for monitoring, 181
HDL. *See* High-density lipoprotein
Health belief model, 9
Healthcare providers, support from, 264–265
Healthcare team, *213,* 266
Healthfinder.gov, 393
Health literacy, 10, 103, 214
Health outcomes
  definition of, 3
  measurement of, 3–5, *4*
Health Resources and Service Administration (HRSA), 395
Health Translations, 394
Healthy eating. *See* Nutrition
Healthy Roads Media, 394
Hearing impairments
  erectile dysfunction drugs and, 376
  resources for people with, 354
Heart attacks
  risk factors for, 294
  rosiglitazone and, 109
Heart disease
  diabetes link to, 294

erectile dysfunction in, 374
influenza in patients with, 364–365
monitoring for, 174, 196–197, 294
physical activity and, 77, 89
reducing risk of, 294–309
vaccines for patients with, 363
Heart rate, in aerobic activity, 81–82
Henna tattoos, 322
Hepatitis A vaccine, 362–363
Hepatitis B vaccine, 323–324, 362–363, 366–367
Herbal supplements, 134
  for erectile dysfunction, 376–378
Hib vaccine, 362–363
High-density lipoprotein (HDL), 43, 77, 197, 303–307
High fructose corn syrup, 47
HIV, vaccines for patients with, 363
Honey, 46–47
Hormonal contraceptives, *326*
Horny goat weed, *378*
Hospitalization, short-term insulin therapy during, 115
HPV vaccine, 362–363
Humalog Mix 50/50 (premixed insulin), *120*
Human papillomavirus (HPV) vaccine, 362–363
Humulin 50/50 (premixed insulin), *120*
Humulin N (intermediate-acting insulin), 119–120
Humulin R (regular insulin), 118–119
Hydration, 51, 84, 233, *236,* 359
Hydrogenation, 43
Hyperemesis gravidarum, 335
Hyperglycemia. *See also* Blood glucose
  barriers to managing, 230–232
  causes of, 229
  definition of, 229
  emergency plans for, 395
  erectile dysfunction in, 374
  extreme, short-term insulin therapy for, 115
  facilitators for managing, 232
  fasting, monitoring profile of, *187*
  female sexual dysfunction in, 380
  management of, 228–232
  physical activity and, 84, 230
  in pregnancy, 335
  prevention of, 230
  problem solving for, 214–215, 228–232, 235–236
  reality scenarios on, 230–232
  signs and symptoms of, 229
  SMART goals for, 235–236
  thoughts and feelings about, identifying, 228
  treatment of, 230

American Association of Diabetes Educators©

408   Diabetes Education Curriculum

Hypertension
   classification of, 295
   controlling, 298–303
   dietary approaches to, 33, 52, 299
   medications for, 113, 299–303
   physical activity and, 89
   in pregnancy, 113, 295–296
Hypoglycemia. *See also* Blood glucose
   anxiety *versus,* 257
   backup or assistance for, 225
   barriers to managing, 227
   common causes of, *226*
   definition of, 222
   emergency plans for, 395
   facilitators for managing, 228
   glucagon injection for, 226
   guidelines for treating, *225*
   insulin therapy and, 117
   management of, 222–228
   morning sickness and, 331
   nocturnal, 223
   overtreatment of, 224
   physical activity and, 84–88
   in pregnancy, 335
   preparation for, 224
   prevention of, 225, *226*
   problem solving for, 214–215, 222–228, 235–236,
      335
   reality scenarios on, 227
   rule of 15 for, 223–225
   self-treatment of, 223–225
   signs and symptoms of, 222–223
   SMART goals for, 235–236
   thoughts and feelings about, identifying, 222
   workplace accommodations for, 228
Hypoglycemia unawareness, 183, 226
Hypotension, postural, *318*

I

Identification, medical, 84, 225
Illness
   severe, short-term insulin therapy during, 115
   sick-day management in, 214–215, 233–236,
      236, 359
Imagery, 271
Imipramine, 315
Immunization, 323–324, 359–369
   recommended for adults by age, 362
   recommended for adults by health condition,
      363

Immunization Action Coalition, 359
Implementation, as educator standard, 7
Improved health status, as long-term outcome, 4, *4*
Incontinence, *319*
Incretin mimetics, 108–110, 123–127, *189*
Indian Health Services, 267
Individualization, 5
Infections, skin, 322–323
Influenza
   treatment of, 364–365
   vaccine against, 323–324, 362–363, 364
Ingredient list, on food label, 57
Inhaled insulin, 115, 121–122
   contraindications to, 122
   dosage and dose conversion for, 121, *121*
   precautions with, 122
   rapid action of, 121
   side effects of, 122
   storage and inhaler care of, 121–122
Injected diabetes medications, 114–132. *See also specific*
      medications
   amylin analogs, 126–127
   assessment checklist for, 152–153
   glucagon, 226
   injection know-how for, 152–170
   injection materials and methods for, 128–131
   injection sites for, 127–128, 164–166
   injection technique for, 159–162
   know-how for, 152–170
   leakage of, 169
   minimizing pain/discomfort from, 168–169
   needles for, 128, 159, 169–170
   pen device for, 130, 157–158, 162
   in pregnancy, 334
   preparation using syringe and vial, 128
   pump for, 115, 122–123, 131, 157
   remembering to administer, 167
   syringes for, 128–131, 157, 159–162
   traveling with, 131, 338, 358
Injected erectile dysfunction medications, 378–379
Injection sites, 127–128, 164–166
   intramuscular, avoidance of, 128
   rotation of, 128, 164, 166
   subcutaneous, 127–128
Instructional plans, 11–12
   for coping, 254–273
   for introduction to diabetes and prediabetes,
      18–22
   for medication taking, 104–142
   for monitoring, 174–238

American Association of Diabetes Educators©

for nutrition, 27–61
for physical activity, 77–93
for problem solving, 215–238
for risk reduction, 291–343
for sexual dysfunction, 373–382
Insulin, 114–123
action of, 18–19, *116*, 116–117
basal, 114, 122
bolus, 114, 122
clear and cloudy, mixture of, 129
concentration or units of, 116
duration of action, 116–117
effects on monitoring, *189*
in gestational diabetes, 21, 329–330
inhaled, 115, 121–122
injection sites for, 127–128
intermediate-acting, *116*, 119–120
leakage, after injection, 169
long-acting, *116*, 120
medications controlling. *See* Medication, diabetes;
    Medication taking (adherence)
mixing of, 119, 128–129, 168
onset of action, 116–117
peak of action, 84, 116–117
physical activity and, 77–78, 84–85
in prediabetes, 20–21
in pregnancy, 329
premixed, 120, *120*
rapid-acting, *116*, 118
regular, 118–119
secretion of, 18–19, 114
short-acting, *116*, 118–119
side effects of, 117
source of, 116
storage of, 117–118, 167
traveling with, 131, 338, 358
in type 1 diabetes, 19–20, 114
in type 2 diabetes, 20, 114–115
Insulin analogs, 116
Insulin aspart, 116
Insulin detemir, 116
Insulin glargine, 116, 120
Insulin glulisine, 116
Insulin isophane, 119–120
Insulin lispro, 116
Insulin pump therapy, 115, 122–123, 157
advantages of, 123
in pregnancy, 334
realities of, 123
traveling and, 131, 338

Insulin resistance, 20, 105
in gestational diabetes, 21, 329–330
necessity of medication for, 105
in prediabetes, 20
in type 2 diabetes, 20
Insulin secretagogues, 110–111, *189*
Insulin sensitizers, 106–108
Insulin therapy, 20, 114–123. *See also* Insulin
assumptions *versus* facts on, 156
carb counting and, 34
eating and, 118–120
effects on monitoring, *189*
indications for, 114–115
injection know-how for, 152–170
injection materials and methods for, 128–131
injection sites for, 127–128, 164–166
minimizing pain/discomfort from, 168–169
necessity of, 105
physical activity and, 84–85
postpartum, 336–337
prefilled syringes for, 130–131
in pregnancy, 115, 334
short-term, in diabetes type 2, 115
sick-day management and, 234, *236*, 359
Insurance company resources, 268
Insurance coverage, of monitoring supplies,
    179, 188
Intelligences, multiple, 7–8, *9*
Intensity, of physical activity, 75
aerobic, 81–82
resistance (strength), 83
Intermediate-acting insulin, *116*, 119–120
International Association for Medical Assistance to
    Travelers, 358, 394
International Diabetes Federation (IDF), on sleep
    health, 320
Internet resources, 267–268, 281–282, 393–395
Intramuscular injection, avoidance of, 128
Intraurethral suppositories, for erectile
    dysfunction, 379
Intrauterine devices (IUDs), *326*
Invokana. *See* Canaglifozin
Iron, 57
"I" statements, 263–264
IUDs (intrauterine devices), *326*

J

Januvia. *See* Sitagliptin
Jardiance. *See* Empagliflozin
Jewelry, medical ID, 84, 225

American Association of Diabetes Educators©

410   Diabetes Education Curriculum

JNC8, 303
Juvenile Diabetes and Research Foundation (JDRF), 268, 393

K

Ketoacidosis. *See* Diabetic ketoacidosis
Ketones, 20. *See also* Diabetic ketoacidosis
   blood monitoring of, 235, 333
   in pregnancy, 331, 333, 335
   sick days (illness) and, 234–235, *236*, 359
   urine monitoring of, 234
Kidney disease, 309–311
   chronic, stages of, *311*
   immunization in, 363
   physical activity and, 90
Kidney function, 309
Kidney health, 309–311
   antihypertensive drugs and, 300, 302, 310
   monitoring of, 174, 197, 309–310
Kilocalories (kcals), 33
Knowles, Malcolm, 7, 136

L

Labetalol, for pregnant patients, 302
Lactose, 38, 47
Lancets
   disposal of, 183
   traveling with, 358
   use of, 182, 207
Lantus. *See* Insulin glargine
Larger than gestational age, 329
L-arginine, *378*
LDL. *See* Low-density lipoprotein
Learning
   adult, principles of, 4, 7, *8*
   analogies for, 19
   on coping, 272
   as immediate outcome, 3–4, *4*, 13
   on medication taking, 141
   on monitoring, 197–198
   on nutrition, 61–62
   on physical activity, 92–93
   on problem solving, 237
   on risk reduction, 342–343
Learning objectives, 11
   for coping, 253
   for medication taking, 104
   for monitoring, 173–174
   for nutrition, 26–27
   for physical activity, 76

   for problem solving, 214–215
   for risk reduction, 291
Legacy effect, of glucose control, 195
Lentils, as fiber source, 50, *50*
Levemir (long-acting insulin), 120
Levitra (vardenafil), 376, *377*
Lifestyle activities, for increasing physical activity, 78
Lighthouse International, 353
Linagliptin, 108–110
   contraindications to, 109
   dosage and administration of, 109
   effects on monitoring, *189*
   mechanism of action, 108–109
   side effects of, 110
Lipid(s), 303–307
   bile acid sequestrants and, 113, 306
   in children, 304
   definition of, 28
   medications for lowering, 304–307, *305, 306*
   monitoring levels of, 197, 294
   nutrition and, 28, 43–45, 305
   obesity and, 31
   physical activity and, 77, 305
   pregnancy and, 328
   target levels of, 197, 304–305
   weight loss and, 28
Lipid profile, 294
Liraglutide, 123–125
   contraindications to, 125
   dosage and administration of, 124–125
   effects on monitoring, *189*
   injection sites for, 127–128
   mechanism of action, 124
   precautions with, 125
   side effects of, 125
   storage of, 125
Listeriosis, 332
Literacy, health, 10, 103, 214
Literature review, 10–11
   on coping, 250
   on medication taking, 102
   on monitoring, 172
   on nutrition, 25
   on physical activity, 74
   on problem solving, 212
   on risk reduction, 290
Liver disease, vaccines for patients with, 363
Liver health, monitoring of, 174
Lizards, 124
Logbook, manual/electronic, 184

American Association of Diabetes Educators©

Long-acting insulin, *116,* 120
Lopid. *See* Gemfibrozil
Lovastatin plus niacin, 307
Lovaza. *See* Omega-3 fatty acids
Low-calorie sweeteners, 46–48, *48*
Low-density lipoprotein (LDL), 43, 77, 197, 303–307
Lower intestinal tract dysfunction, *318*
Lubricants, vaginal, *381,* 381–382
Lunch, carbohydrate intake in, 35
Lung disease
    influenza in patients with, 364–365
    vaccines for patients with, 363
Lyrica. *See* Pregabalin

M

Macronutrients, 33. *See also* Carbohydrates; Fat(s);
    Protein
Macular edema, 311
Male enhancement supplements, 378, *378*
Male sexual dysfunction, *318,* 373–380
    assessment for, 391
    male perceptions of, 373
    patient information on, 385–390
Masculinity, and perception of sexual dysfunction, 373
Maslow's Hierarchy of Needs, 250
Maternal blood screening test, 357
Meal plan, 32–33
    carbohydrates in, 35
    in pregnancy, 331
    protein in, 42–43
    snacks in, 49
Meals and monitoring, *187,* 188
Measles, mumps, rubella vaccine, 362–363
Meat and meat substitutes, 42, *42*
Medical clearance, for physical activity, 84
Medical identification (ID), 84, 225, 339, 358
Medical nutrition therapy (MNT), 25–26. *See also*
Nutrition
Medical sharps
    disposal of, 131, 169–170, 183
    traveling with, 358
Medicare Part B coverage, 354
Medication, antihypertensive, 299–303
    in pregnancy, 113, 300, 302, 328, *328*
    race/ethnicity and, 299–300, 303
    renal effects of, 300, 302
Medication, antiviral, for influenza, 364–365
Medication, diabetes. *See also* Medication taking
    (adherence); *specific medications*
    assistance programs for, 147, 268

combination products, 103
complementary and alternative, 133–136, *135–136*
effects on monitoring, 188, *189*
emergency supply of, 339–340, 395
injected, 114–132, 152–170, 334
necessity of, 105
oral, 105–113, 334
physical activity and, 85
postpartum, 336–337
in pregnancy, 105, 334
progression in, 103, 105
timing of, 103
traveling with, 131, 338, 358
Medication, for erectile dysfunction, 376–379, *377*
Medication, lipid-lowering, 304–307, *305, 306*
Medication, neuropathic pain, 315
Medication, OTC, blood glucose effects of, 235
Medication taking (adherence), 15, 101–170
    barriers to, 102, 103, 104, 136–139
    complexity of regimen and, 103
    cue-dose training for, 103
    educator's overview of, 102–104
    facilitators for, 104, 140
    follow-up/outcomes measurement of, 140–142
    goal setting for, 140
    handouts on, 148–170
    identifying patients at risk for problems with, 103
    instructional plan for, 104–142
    learning objectives for, 104
    at onset of diabetes type 2, 102–103
    postpartum, 336–337
    in pregnancy, 334
    reading ability/health literacy and, 103
    resources on, 147–170
    Self-Care Behaviors for, 141–142, 148–151
    sick-day management and, 234, *236,* 359
    thoughts and feelings about, identifying, 104
Meditation, 271
Mediterranean eating style, 33
Meglitinides, 111
    effects on monitoring, *189*
    examples of, *85*
    physical activity and, 85
Memory function, of glucose meter, 179, 184
Meningococcal vaccine, 362–363
Menus, restaurant, 58, *58*
Mercury, in fish, 44, 332
Metabolism
    glucose, 18–19
    nutrition and, 28

American Association of Diabetes Educators©

412 Diabetes Education Curriculum

Metformin, 106–108
  brand names for, 106
  contraindications to, 107
  for diabetes type 2, 102–103
  dosage and administration of, 106
  effects on monitoring, *189*
  mechanism of action, 106
  precautions with, 107
  sick-day management and, 234, *236*, 359
  side effects of, 107
Methyldopa, for pregnant patients, 302
Microalbumin-to-creatinine test, 310
Micronase. *See* Glyburide
Miglitol, 111–112
  contraindications to, 112
  dosage and administration of, 111
  effects on monitoring, *189*
  mechanism of action, 111
  side effects of, 112
Milk, 38, *38*
Milk thistle, *135*
Mind–body techniques, 252, 271
Minerals
intake and requirements, 51–52, 132
  in pregnancy, 331
Miscarriage, 329
MMR vaccine, 362–363
MNT. *See* Medical nutrition therapy
Mobile interface, of glucose meter, 179, 184
Molasses, 47
Monitoring, 15, 171–209
  A1C, 173–174, 194–195, 293–294, 333, 375
  alternate site testing in, 182–183
  1,5-anhydroglucitriol (1,5-AG), 174, 196
  assessment tool for diabetes educator, 209
  barriers to, 174, 190–193, 206
  behavioral objectives for, 174
  benefits of, 175
  blood glucose, 173–196. *See also* Blood glucose
    monitoring
  blood sample for, 179, 181–184, 207
  cardiovascular health, 174, 196–197, 294
  checklist for healthcare professionals, 205
  checklist for SMBG education, 205
  for children, 177, *178*
  components of, 174–175
  control testing for, 180
  costs and insurance for supplies, 179, 188
  diabetes medications and, 188, *189*

  discussing the "numbers" in, 173
  driving analogy for, 175
  estimated average glucose (eAG), 174, 195, *196*
  eye health, 174, 197, 311–313
  facilitators for, 174, 193–194
  factors affecting, 205, 207
  follow-up/outcomes measurement of, 197–199
  foot health, 174, 197, 314–315
  fructosamine, 174, 196
  general guidelines for, 180–185
  handouts on, 201–204
  hand-washing for, 181
  instructional plan for, 174–238
  interpreting and responding to results of, 189–190
  ketone, 234–235, 333
  kidney health, 174, 197, 309–310
  learning objectives for, 173–174
  literature review on, 172
  liver health, 174
  long-term, 174, 194–197
  meals and, *187,* 188
  positive questioning about, 207
  postpartum, 336
  for pregnant women, 173, 177, *178,* 182, 188,
    333–334
  problem solving on, 190–193, 208
  reality scenarios on, 190–193
  reasons for, 176
  recording and sharing results of, 183–185
  resources on, 200–209
  sexual health and, 375, 381
  SMART goals for, 197
  storage of supplies for, 181
  successful, skill sets for, 173
  terminology in, 172–173
  thoughts and feelings about, identifying, 175
  timing and frequency of, 185–192
  traveling and, 181, 338, 357–358
  weight, 174
Monitor talk, 173
Monk fruit extract, *48*
Monoamine oxidase (MAO) inhibitors, and erectile
  dysfunction, *374*
Monounsaturated fats, 43, *44*
Morning sickness, 331
Motivation
  for coping, 259–260, 284
  for physical activity, 76
Multiple intelligences, theory of, 7–8, *9*

American Association of Diabetes Educators©

Multivitamins, 52
Muscle relaxation, progressive, 271
Muse (alprostadil pellets), 379
MyPlate, 66, 71–72

N

Nagging, 263
Nateglinide, 111
    contraindications to, 111
    dosage and administration of, 111
    effects on monitoring, *189*
    mechanism of action, 111
    precautions with, 111
    side effects of, 111
National Association of State Agencies of the Deaf and
    Hard of Hearing, 354
National Center for Complementary and Alternative
    Medicine (NCCAM), 133
National Council of State Agencies for the Blind
    (NCSAB), 353
National Council on Aging, 393
National Diabetes Education Program, 393, 394
National Diabetes Information Clearinghouse, 393
National Donated Dental Services Program, 394
National Federation of the Blind (NFB), 354
National Standards for DSME Programs, 3, 5–6
Native American talking circles, 267, *267*
NCCAM. *See* National Center for Complementary and
    Alternative Medicine
Needles, for injections, 128, 159, 169–170
    gauge of, 128, 159
    traveling with, 358
    used, disposal of, 131, 169–170
NeedyMeds, 147
Neotame, *48*, 332
Nerve health, 314–319
    alpha lipoic acid and, 132
    and feet, 174, 197, 314–315
    physical activity and, 89–90
    and sexual function, *318–319*, 371. *See also* Sexual
        dysfunction
Nesina. *See* Alogliptin
Net carbs, 57
Neurological exam, preconception, 329
Neurontin. *See* Gabapentin
Neuropathy, 314–319
    alpha lipoic acid for, 132
    foot care and, 315–316, 317
    living with, *317–319*

medications for pain in, 315
    physical activity and, 89–90
    reducing risk of, 314–316
    sexual dysfunction in, *318–319*, 371. *See also* Sexual
        dysfunction
Niacin, for lowering lipid levels, 304–305, 307
Niaspan. *See* Niacin
Nocturnal hypoglycemia, 223
Nonnutritive sweeteners, 47–48, *48*
Nonprofit associations, as resource, 393
Nonstarchy vegetables, 40–41, *41*
Nonstress test, 357
Nopal, *136*
Nortriptyline, 315
Novolin 50/50 (premixed insulin), *120*
Novolin N (intermediate-acting insulin), 119–120
Novolin R (regular insulin), 118–119
Novolog Mix 50/50 (premixed insulin), *120*
NPGs. *See* Nutrition practice guidelines
NPH insulin, 119–120
    mixing with regular insulin, 129–130
Nutrient groups, 34–54. *See also specific nutrients*
Nutrition, 14, 23–72. *See also* Medical nutrition
    therapy
    barriers to healthy eating in, 26, 59–60
    blood glucose control and, 28
    blood pressure control and, 28, 33, 52, 299
    calorie intake/needs in, 31–32, *32*
    common terms in, 32–34
    complication prevention in, 27–28
    culture and, 25, 36–37, *37, 41*, 60
    eating out and, 58, *58*
    educator's overview of, 25–27
    facilitators for healthy eating in, 26, 60–61
    facts *versus* fiction about, 27
    family involvement in, 25
    fiber in, *50*, 50–51, 305
    food and nutrient groups in, 34–54
    food labels on, 43, *46*, 50–51, *51*, 53, *53*, 54–57
    free foods in, 48, *49*
    goals for, 27–32
    handouts on, 67–72
    insulin therapy and, 118–120
    learning objectives for, 26–27
    lipid levels and, 28, 43–45, 305
    literature review on, 25
    metabolic effects of, 28
    mixing and matching in, 39–41
    MyPlate guidelines on, 66, 71–72

American Association of Diabetes Educators©

414   **Diabetes Education Curriculum**

outcomes measurement of, 61–62
portion control in, 33
postpartum, 336
in pregnancy, 28, 42, 60, 61, 331–332
resources on, 65–66
Self-Care Behaviors for, 61–62, 67–70
serving size in, 33–34
sick-day, 233–234, *236*, 359
SMART goal for, 61
snacks in, 49
stress management in, 270
thoughts and feelings about, identifying, 27
traveling and, 337, 357
weight and, 28–32
Nutrition assessment, 25–26, 61–62
Nutrition Facts label, 54–57
Nutrition practice guidelines (NPGs), 25–26, 35
Nutrition support groups, 66, 394
Nutritive sweeteners, 46–47

O

Obesity, 28–32
BMI determination of, 29, *29*
needles for injections in, 128
physical activity and, 88
risk factors for conditions linked to, 31
and type 2 diabetes mellitus, 20
Obstructive sleep apnea, 320–321
OGTT. *See* Oral glucose tolerance test
Omacor. *See* Omega-3 fatty acids
Omega-3 fatty acids, 43, 305, 307
Onglyza. *See* Saxagliptin
Ongoing support, 5
Online resources, 267–268, 281–282, 393–395
Onset of action (insulin), 116–117
Oral contraceptives, *326*
Oral diabetes medications, 105–113
alpha-glucosidase inhibitors, 111–112
combination, 113
DPP-IV inhibitors, 108–110
insulin secretagogues, 110–111
insulin sensitizers, 106–108
physical activity and, 85
in pregnancy, 334
sick-day management and, 234
sodium-glucose co-transporter 2 inhibitors, 112–113
Oral erectile dysfunction medication, 376–378
Oral glucose tolerance test (OGTT), 21–22
Oscillometric blood pressure monitors, 297

Outcomes measurement, *3,* 3–5, 13–14
aggregate population, 4
behavior change in, 3–5, *4*
clinical improvement in, 4, *4*
continuum of, 3–4, *4*
of coping, 271–273
improved health status in, 4, *4*
individual patient, 4
learning in, 3–4, *4,* 13
of medication taking, 140–142
of monitoring, 197–199
of nutrition, 61–62
of physical activity, 92–93
of problem solving, 236–238
of risk reduction, 342–343
Overeaters Anonymous, 66
Over-the-counter (OTC) medications
and blood glucose level, 235
for erectile dysfunction, 376–378
Overtreatment, of hypoglycemia, 224
Overweight, BMI determination of, 29, *29*
Oxytocin, 337

P

Pamelor. *See* Nortriptyline
Pancreas
damage or destruction in, 19
in gestational diabetes, 21
insulin release from, 18–19, 114
in prediabetes, 20–21
in type 1 diabetes, 19–20
in type 2 diabetes, 20
Partially hydrogenated vegetable oil, 43
Partnership for Prescription Assistance (PPA), 147
Patient assistance programs, 147, 268, 394
Patient-centered approach, 5
Patient empowerment model, 9
Patient Health Questionnaire (PHQ), 286
Patient information (handouts)
on coping, 277–282
on immunization, 360–369
on influenza, 364–365
on medication taking, 148–170
on monitoring, 201–204
on nutrition, 67–72
on physical activity, 96–99
on problem solving, 240–243
on sexual health, 385–390
Patient progress, 5
PDE-5 inhibitors, 376, *377*

American Association of Diabetes Educators©

Peak of action (insulin), 84, 116–117
Peas, as fiber source, 50, *50*
Pedicures, 317
Peer-to-peer support groups, 266–267
Pen device
  for injections of diabetes medications, 130, 158–159,
    162
  for injections of erectile dysfunction medications,
    378
Penile prosthesis, 380
Penis, erectile function of, 373. *See also* Erectile
  dysfunction
Perceived Stress Scale (PSS-10), 287
Percent daily value, 57
Periodontal disease, 321–322
Periodontitis, 321
Peripheral arterial disease (PAD), 296–297, 315
Peripheral neuropathy, 315
  alpha lipoic acid for, 132
  physical activity and, 89
Peripheral vascular disease, physical activity and, 89
Personal care record, 292
Phenylephrine, 235
Phenylketonuria, 48
Phosphodiesterase-5 inhibitors, 376, *377*
Physical activity, 15, 73–100
  aerobic, 78–82
  balance training in, 78, 80
  barriers to, 76, 90–91
  behavioral objectives for, 76
  benefits of, 77–78
  blood glucose levels in, 84–88, *86*, 230
  blood pressure and, 77, 89, 299
  calendar for, 100
  diabetes medication and, 85
  educator's overview of, 74–76
  facilitators for, 76, 91–92
  FITT plan for, 75, 80–83
  flexibility and stretching, 78, 80
  follow-up/outcomes measurement of, 92–93
  footwear for, 84
  handouts on, 96–99
  hydration during, 84
  instructional plan for, 77–93
  late-evening, precaution in, 87
  learning objectives for, 76
  lifestyle approach to increase, 78
  lipid levels and, 77, 305
  literature review on, 74
  medical clearance for, 84

moderate, structured approach to, 80–83
motivation for, 76
obesity/orthopedic issues in, 88
postpartum, 336
in pregnancy, 332–333
preparing for, 80
progress and stages of, *75*, 75–76
promotion of, 76
recommended, for diabetes type 2 and prediabetes,
  78–80
resistance (strength), 78–79, 82–83
resources on, 95–100
safety issues in, 84–88
Self-Care Behaviors for, 92–93, 96–99
self-efficacy and, 76
setting goals for, 75, 92
sexual function and, 375
snacking before, 86–88
special considerations in, 88–90
stress management in, 270
support for, 76
timing of, 86–88
traveling and, 338, 357
understanding of and interest in, identifying, 77
Physician–patient relationship, 265–266
Pictograms, for medications, 103
Piercings, 322–323
Pioglitazone, 107–108
  cardiac risks of, 109
  contraindications to, 108
  dose and administration of, 108
  effects on monitoring, *189*
  mechanism of action, 107–108
  precautions with, 108
  side effects of, 108
Planning, educator standard, 6–7
Plaque, 294
Platelets, preeclampsia and, 336
Pneumococcal vaccine, 324, 362–363, 368–369
Polydipsia, 19
Polyunsaturated fats, 43, *44*
Polyuria, 19
Portion, definition of, 33
Portion control, 33
Positive affirmations, 270–271, 285
Postpartum concerns, 336–337
Postpartum depression, 287
Postural hypotension, *318*
Potassium, 56
PPD (para-phenylenediamine), 322–323

American Association of Diabetes Educators©

416   Diabetes Education Curriculum

Pramlintide, 126–127
    dosage and administration of, 126, *126*
    effects on monitoring, *189*
    injection sites for, 127–128
    mechanism of action, 126
    precautions with, 126–127
    side effects of, 127
    storage of, 127
Prandin. *See* Repaglinide
Prayer, 251, 271
Prazosin, for pregnant patients, 302
Preconception care, 325, 327–329
Precose. *See* Acarbose
Prediabetes, 20–21
    diagnosis of, 21
    insulin resistance in, 20
    physical activity for, 77–78, 78–80
    preventing progression of, 21
Predictability, for stress management, 270
Preeclampsia-eclampsia, 295–296, 336
Prefilled syringes, 130–131
Pregabalin, 315
Pregnancy, 325–337
    A1C levels and, 327, 333
    antihypertensive drugs in, 113, 300, 302, 328, *328*
    blood glucose and risks in, 326, 329
    blood pressure in, 113, 295–296, 300, 328, 336
    cardiovascular health in, 328
    coping skills in, 252, 331
    diabetes care in, 329–335
    diabetes in. *See* Gestational diabetes
    diabetes medication in, 105, 334
    dietary supplements in, 52
    eye health/problems in, 312, 328
    fetal monitoring in, 333–334, 335, 357
    fish intake in, 44
    hypoglycemia in, 331, 335
    immunization in, 363
    insulin therapy during, 115
    ketone levels in, 331, 333, 335
    monitoring during, 173, 177, *178*, 182, 188, 333–334
    nutrition in, 28, 42, 44, 60, 61, 331–332
    physical activity in, 332–333
    planning, for diabetic women, 327–329
    postpartum concerns in, 336–337
    preconception care for, 325, 327–329
    problem solving in, 335
    target glucose levels in, 177, *178*, 330, *330*
    thoughts and feelings about diabetes and, 327
    unplanned or unintended, preventing, 325–326, *326*

vomiting in, 331, 335
    weight gain and BMI in, *29*, 29–30
Premixed insulin, 120, *120*
Prescription labels, and medication adherence, 103
Preterm labor, 336
Priapism, 379
Priming of pen, 130, 162
Problem Areas in Diabetes Scale (PAID), 288
Problem solving, 15, 211–248
    assessment in, 212–213
    barriers to, 213, 215
    behavioral objectives for, 215
    behavior chain analysis for, 246–248, 257–259
    behavior chain templates for, 239
    confidence in, enhancing, 220–222
    conviction in, enhancing, 220–221
    for coping, 251–252, 257–259, 283
    culture and, 214
    direct instruction *versus* facilitating, 213
    educator's overview of, 212–215
    facilitators for, 215
    factors influencing, 214
    follow-up/outcomes measurement in, 236–238
    goal setting for, 214, 216, 218–220, 235–236
    handouts on, 240–243
    healthcare team for, *213*
    health literacy and, 214
    for hyperglycemia management, 214–215, 228–232, 235–236
    for hypoglycemia management, 214–215, 222–228, 235–236, 335
    instructional plan for, 215–238
    literature review on, 212
    on monitoring, 190–193, 208
    patient needs and preferences in, 213
    plan for, 217
    in pregnancy, 335
    problem identification for, 213
    resources on, 239–248
    role-playing activity for, 216, 283
    role-playing activity on, 244–245
    for sick-day management, 214–215, 233–236
    skills for, 212, 215–222
    SMART goals for, 214, 218–220, 235–236
    sorting options in, 217
    steps in, 216–218
Progressive muscle relaxation, 271
Prostaglandin E₁, for erectile dysfunction, 378–379
Protein, dietary, 33, 42–43
    calories per gram, 33

American Association of Diabetes Educators©

food label information on, 57
meat and meat substitutes for, 42, *42*
pregnancy and, 42
restricted, in kidney disease, 311
Protein, in urine (proteinuria), 309–310, 336
Protodioscin, *378*
Pseudoephedrine, 235
Psychological assessment tools, 286–288
Psychosocial care/assessment, 272, 325
Publications, as resource, 267–268, 393
Pulse, in aerobic activity, 82
Pump. *See* Insulin pump therapy

Q

Quality improvement, 3–5
Quality of life measure, 288
Questionnaire on Stress in Patients with Diabetes (QSD-R), 288
Questran. *See* Cholestyramine

R

Race/ethnicity
and blood pressure medications, 299–300, 303
and type 2 diabetes, 20
Random blood glucose test, 21
Rapid-acting insulin, *116,* 118
Readability, of curriculum, 10
Reality scenarios, 12–13
on healthy eating, 59–60
on hyperglycemia management, 230–232
on hypoglycemia management, 227
on medication taking, 137–139
on monitoring, 190–193
on physical activity, 90–91
on risk reduction, 340–341
Red blood cells, A1C levels in, 293
Registered dietitian (RD), 26, 34
Registered dietitian nutritionist (RDN), 26, 34
Regular insulin, 118–119
mixing with NPH insulin, 129–130
Relapse, 260–261
getting over, 260–261
triggers for, 260
Relapse prevention skills, 260–261
Religion, 251, 271
Relion/Novolin N (intermediate-acting insulin), 119–120
Relion/Novolin R (regular insulin), 118–119
Repaglinide, 111
contraindications to, 111
dosage and administration of, 111

effects on monitoring, *189*
mechanism of action, 111
precautions with, 111
side effects of, 111
Repetitions, in resistance training, 83
Replens (vaginal lubricant), 381
Resentment/anger, 255–256
Resistance (strength) activity, 78–79, 82–83
frequency of, 82
intensity of, 83
Resources, 14, 393–395
on coping, 276–288
on medication taking (adherence), 147–170
on monitoring, 200–209
on nutrition, 65–66
on physical activity, 95–100
on problem solving, 239–248
on risk reduction, 352–369
on sexual dysfunction, 373, 384–392
Restaurant menus, 58, *58*
Retina, 311. *See also* Diabetic retinopathy
Retinal photography, 313
Retinopathy, physical activity and, 89
Rights, workplace, 228
Riomet. *See* Metformin
Risk reduction, 15, 289–370
A1C levels and, 293–294
aspirin therapy for, 308–309
barriers to, 291, 340–341
behavioral objectives for, 291
cardiovascular, 294–309
dental, 321–322
disaster conditions and, 339–340, 395
educator's overview of, 290–291
for erectile dysfunction, 375
facilitators for, 291, 341
follow-up/outcomes measurement of, 342–343
immunization and, 323–324, 359–363
instructional plan for, 291–343
learning objectives for, 291
literature review on, 290
nerve/foot, 314–316
postpartum, 337
in pregnancy, 335–337
reality scenarios on, 340–341
renal, 309–311
resources on, 352–369
skin, 322–323
sleep and, 320–321
SMART goals for, 342

American Association of Diabetes Educators©

418   Diabetes Education Curriculum

smoking cessation for, 299, 307, *308*, 315, 320, 321, 352–353

Standards of Medical Care in Diabetes and, 291–294

for traveling, 337–339, 358–359

vision (eye), 311–314

Robert Wood Johnson Diabetes Initiative, 267

Role-playing activity, for problem solving, 216

Rosiglitazone, 107–108

cardiac risks of, 109

contraindications to, 108

dose and administration of, 108

mechanism of action, 107–108

precautions with, 108

side effects of, 108

Rotation of injection sites, 164, 166

Rubber band finger tourniquet, 182, *182*

Rule of 15, 223–225

RxAssist, 147, 268, 394

S

Saccharin, 46, 47, *48*, 332

Sadness/worry, 256

Safety

of complementary and alternative medicine, 133

of physical activity, 84–88

of sweeteners, 46

Saliva substitutes, 321

Salt (sodium intake), 28, 52–53, 55

Salt substitutes, 53

Saturated fats, 43, *44*, 305

Saxagliptin, 108–110

contraindications to, 109

dosage and administration of, 109

effects on monitoring, *189*

mechanism of action, 108–109

side effects of, 110

Saxenda. *See* Liraglutide

Sedentary person

lifestyle approach to increasing activity of, 78

progression through physical activity, *75*, 75–76

Selective serotonin inhibitors (SSRIs), and erectile dysfunction, *374*

Self-blame/guilt, 256

Self-Care Behaviors, 4, *4*

for coping, 272–273, 277–280

evaluation of, 4

for medication taking, 141–142, 148–151

for monitoring, 197–199, 201–204

for nutrition, 61–62, 67–70

for physical activity, 92–93, 96–99

for problem solving, 237–238, 240–243

for risk reduction, 290–291, 342–343

Self-efficacy

coping and, 253

physical activity and, 76

Self-forgiveness, 261

Self-management, 22. *See also* Diabetes self-management education; Self-monitoring of blood glucose

Self-monitoring of blood glucose (SMBG)

ADA guidelines on, 185

alternate site testing for, 182–183

assessment tool for diabetes educator, 209

barriers to, 174, 190–193, 206

blood sample for, 181–184, 207

checklist for education on, 205

continuous system for, 180

control testing for, 180

costs and insurance for supplies, 179, 188

diabetes medications and, 188, *189*

examples of regimens, *186–187*

facilitators for, 174, 193–194

factors affecting, 205, 207

fasting hyperglycemia profile of, *187*

5-point profile of, *186*

general guidelines for, 180–185

handouts on, 201–204

hand-washing for, 181

interpreting and responding to results of, 189–190

literature review on, 172

meal-based profile of, *187*

meals and, *187*, 188

positive questioning about, 207

problem solving on, 190–193, 208

reality scenarios on, 190–193

recording and sharing results of, 183–185

resources on, 200–209

selecting meter for, 179

7-point profile of, *186*

staggered profile of, *187*

storage of supplies for, 181

3-point profile of, *186*

timing and frequency of, 185–192

traveling with supplies for, 181, 338, 357–358

Self-monitoring of blood pressure, 297–298

Self-talk, 261, 270, 285

Sepsis, 323

Serving(s)

calories per, 55

cholesterol per, 55

American Association of Diabetes Educators©

definition of, 33
fat per, 55
number in container, 55
Serving size, 33–34
    for alcohol, 53
    for carbohydrates, 35
    everyday items as guide to, 65
    for fish, 44
    for fruit, 36, 37
    for Greek yogurt, 38
    label information on, 55
    for milk, 38
    for sweets, 39
7-point monitoring profile, 186
Sex partner, use of term, 373
Sexual dysfunction, 371–395
    assessment for, 391–392
    educator's overview of, 371–373
    educator's role in, 372–373
    female, 319, 372, 380–382
    male, 318, 373–380
    openness and discussion about, 372
    resources on, 373, 384–392
Sexual Health Inventory for Men (SHIM), 391
Sexual response, in women, 380
SF-12, 286
SF-36, 286
Sharps
    disposal of, 131, 169–170, 183
    traveling with, 358
Shingles vaccine, 324, 362–363
Shock/denial, 255
Short-acting insulin, 116, 118–119
Sick-day management, 214–215, 233–236, 236, 359
    contacting health professionals in, 236, 359
    guidelines for, 233, 359
    ketone levels and monitoring in, 234–235, 359
    medication taking in, 234, 236, 359
    nutrition in, 233–234, 236, 359
    OTC medications and blood glucose levels in, 235
    SMART goals for, 235–236
Sick-day rules, 233
Sildenafil, 376, 377, 381
"Silent heart attack," 90
Silicone-based vaginal lubricants, 381, 381
Silybum marianum, 135
Sitagliptin, 108–110
    contraindications to, 109
    dosage and administration of, 109
    effects on monitoring, 189

mechanism of action, 108–109
    side effects of, 110
Skin health, 322–323
Skin infections, 322–323
Skin-on-skin friction, 322
Sleep, 320–321
Sleep apnea, 320–321
    assessment for, 320, 355–356
    definition of, 320
    symptoms of, 320, 320
    treatment of, 320–321
Slo-Niacin. *See* Niacin
SMART goals, 4, 13
    for healthy eating, 61
    for hyperglycemia, 235–236
    for hypoglycemia, 235–236
    for medication taking, 140
    for monitoring, 197
    for physical activity, 75, 92
    for problem solving, 214, 218–220, 235–236
    realistic *versus* relevant, 13
    for risk reduction, 342
    for sick-day management, 235–236
SMBG. *See* Self-monitoring of blood glucose
Smoking cessation, 308, 352–353
    and blood pressure, 299
    and dental health, 321
    and lipid levels, 307
    and neuropathy, 315
    and sexual health, 375, 382
    and sleep apnea, 320
Snacks, 49
    insulin therapy and, 118
    pre-activity, 86–88
Social cognitive theory, 9–10
Social service agencies, 268, 394
Social support, 253, 262–268. *See also* Family
    support
    from community resources, 266–267
    from family, 262–265. *See also* Family support
    from healthcare providers, 264–265
    online, 267–268, 281–282
    talking circle for, 267, 267
Sodium, 28, 52–53
    DASH plan to reduce intake of, 33, 52
    food label information on, 53, 53
    per serving, 55
    tips for cutting intake of, 52
Sodium-glucose co-transporter 2 inhibitors, 112–113, 189

American Association of Diabetes Educators©

420 **Diabetes Education Curriculum**

Spanish, materials in, 394–395
    on coping, 279–280
    on medication taking, 150–151
    on monitoring, 203–204
    on nutrition/healthy eating, 69–70, 72
    on physical activity, 98–99
    on problem solving, 242–243
Special Supplemental Nutrition Program for Women,
    Infants, and Children (WIC), 66, 393
Spermicides, *326*
Spirituality, 251, 271
Splenda (sucralose), 47–48, *48*
Staggered monitoring profile, *187*
Standards for Outcomes Measurement of Diabetes Self-
    Management Education, *3,* 3–5, 14
Standards of Medical Care in Diabetes, 291–292
    on A1C levels, 293–294
    on ankle/brachial index, 297
    on aspirin therapy, 308
    on birth control, 326
    on blood pressure, 295
    on cardiovascular autonomic neuropathy, 316
    on disaster preparation, 339
    on eye examinations/retinopathy, 311–312
    on immunization, 323–324
    on kidney health/disease, 310
    on lipid levels, 304
    on preconception care, 325
    on pregnancy planning for diabetic women, 327
    on psychosocial assessment and care, 325
Standards of Practice for Diabetes Educators, 6–7
Starch, 36
Starlix. *See* Nateglinide
State vocational rehabilitation agencies, 354
Statins, 304–307, *305, 306*
    in pregnancy, 328, *328*
Stevia, 48, *48*
Storage
    of GLP-1 agonists, 125
    of inhaled insulin, 121–122
    of insulin, 117–118, 167
    of monitoring supplies, 181
Strength (resistance) training, 78–79, 82–83
    frequency of, 82
    intensity of, 83
Stress
    assessment tools for, 287–288
    emotional and mental symptoms of, 269
    management of, 252, 269–271

    mind–body techniques for, 252, 271
    nutrition and, 270
    physical activity and, 270
    physical symptoms of, 269
    positive affirmations and, 270–271, 285
Stressors
    definition of, 269
    inventory of, 270
Stress response, 233, 269
Stress test, in pregnancy, 357
Stretching, 78, 80
Strips, test, 179–185. *See also* Blood glucose meters
Stroke, risk factors for, 294
Subcutaneous injection, 127–128
Sucralose, 47–48, *48,* 332
Sudomotor dysfunction, *319*
Sugar
    food label information on, 56
    as sweetener, 46–47
Sugar alcohols, 47, 56
Sugar substitutes, 47–48, *48*
Sugary foods (sweets), 38–39, *39*
Sulfonylureas, 110
    effects on monitoring, *189*
    examples of, *85*
    physical activity and, 85
Supplements, dietary, 51–52, 132, 133–136
    used to lower blood glucose, 134, *134–136*
    vitamin and minerals, 51–52, 132
Support. *See* Social support
Support groups, 66, 266–267, 394
Survival skills, 12
Sweating disturbances, *319*
Sweeteners, 46–48
    nonnutritive, low-calorie, 47–48, *48*
    nutritive, 46–47
    in pregnancy, 331–332
    safety of, 46
Sweets, 38–39, *39*
Symlin. *See* Pramlintide
Syringes, 128–131, 157, 159–162
    mixing two kinds of insulin in, 128
    prefilled, 130–131
    preparation of injection using, 128
Systematic review of literature, 10–11
    on coping, 250
    on medication taking, 102
    on monitoring, 172
    on nutrition, 25

American Association of Diabetes Educators©

on physical activity, 74
on problem solving, 212
on risk reduction, 290
Systolic pressure, 295

T

Tadalafil, 376, *377*
Tai Chi, 252, 271
Talking circle, 267, *267*
Talk–sing test, 81
Tanzeum. *See* Albiglutide
Target A1C levels, 22, 102, 195, *195*, 294
Target blood glucose levels, 22, 176–177, *178*
    for children, 177, *178*
    postpartum, 336
    for pregnant women, 177, *178*, 330, *330*
Target blood pressure levels, 295–296, 298
Target heart rate, 82
Target lipid levels, 197, 304–305
Target triglyceride levels, 304
Tattoos, 322–323
Teeth, health of, 321–322
Tegretol. *See* Carbamazepine
Telehealth services, 268
Testosterone levels, 374–375
Testosterone replacement, 379–380
Test strips, 179–185. *See also* Blood glucose meters
Tetanus vaccine, 324, 362–363
Thiazolidinediones. *See* Pioglitazone; Rosiglitazone
Thioctic acid, 132
3-point monitoring profile, *186*
Thrush, 321
Time (duration), of physical activity, 75
    aerobic, 80–81
Timing, of blood glucose monitoring, 185–192
Tocolytic agents, 114
Tofranil. *See* Imipramine
Tongkat ali, *378*
TOPS–Take Off Pounds Sensibly, 66, 394
Tradjenta. *See* Linagliptin
Trans fat, 43, 305
Translations. *See* Spanish, materials in
Transportation Safety Administration (TSA), 131, 181, 338, 358
Traveling
    medical assistance during, 358, 394
    medication taking during, 131, 338, 358
    monitoring during, 181, 338, 357–358
    nutrition during, 337, 357

    physical activity during, 338, 357
    risk reduction during, 337–339, 358–359
    tips for, 357–359
Tribulus terrestris extract, *378*
Tricor. *See* Fenofibrate
Tricycle antidepressants, and erectile dysfunction, *374*
Triglycerides, 28, 197, 303–307
    medications for lowering, 304, 307
    nutrition and, 43–45
    target levels of, 304
Trulicity. *See* Dulaglutide
Tuna, mercury in, 44, 332
Type of activity, in physical activity plan, 75

U

U-40 insulin, 116, 338, 358
U-80 insulin, 338, 358
U-100 insulin, 116
U-500 insulin, 116
Ulcers, foot, physical activity and, 89
Ultrasound, fetal, 357
Units of insulin, 116
Unsaturated fats, 43, *44*
Urinary tract infections, 382
Urine, protein in, 309–310, 336
Urine albumin to creatinine ratio (UACR), 309–310
Urine ketone monitoring, 234
US Department of Agriculture (USDA), 54

V

Vaccinations, 323–324, 359–369
    recommended for adults by age, 362
    recommended for adults by health condition, 363
Vaccine information statements, 359
Vacuum suction devices (VSDs), for erectile dysfunction, 379
Vaginal bleeding or discharge, in pregnancy, 336
Vaginal dryness, 380–382, *382*
Vaginal infections, 382
Vaginal lubricants, *381*, 381–382
Vanadium, 132
Vardenafil, 376, *377*
Varicella vaccine, 362–363
Vegetables
    nonstarchy, 40–41, *41*
    starchy, 36
Viagra, 376, *377*
Vials of injected medications, 128
Victoza. *See* Liraglutide

American Association of Diabetes Educators©

Vildagliptin, *189*
Visual acuity, 312
Visual impairments
    diabetes and, 174, 197, 311–314
    erectile dysfunction drugs and, 376
    physical activity for people with, 89
    pregnancy and, 312, 328
    resources for people with, 353–354
Vitamin A, 57
Vitamin C, 57, 132
Vitamin E, 132
Vitamin supplements, 51–52, 132
    in pregnancy, 331
Vocational rehabilitation agencies, 354
Vomiting, 233–235, *236. See also* Sick-day management
    in pregnancy, 331, 335
Vytorin. *See* Ezetimibe plus simvastatin

W

Waist circumference, 29–31, *30*
Waist-to-hip ratio, 30
Warm-up, for physical activity, 80
Water
    for hydration, 84, 233
    as nutrient, 51
Water-based vaginal lubricants, 381, *381*
Water pill (diuretics), 300–302, *301,* 310
Web sites, 268, 393–395
Weight, 28–32
    calorie intake/needs and, 31–32, *32*
    healthy, determining, 29–32
    monitoring of, 31, 174
Weight gain, in pregnancy, *29,* 29–30, 331

Weight lifting, 79, 82–83
Weight loss
    GLP-1 agonist for, 124
    health benefits of, 28
    physical activity for, 77–78, 81, 88
    quick, regaining of, 28
    as symptom in type 1 diabetes, 19
    as therapy for diabetes type 2, 28
    as therapy for erectile dysfunction, 375
    as therapy for high blood pressure, 299
    as therapy for lipid reduction, 305
    as therapy for prediabetes, 21
    as therapy for sleep apnea, 320
Weight Watchers, 66, 394
WelChol. *See* Colesevelam
Whole grains, *35, 50*
Wine, 53–54
WIN–Weight-Control Information Network, 66, 393
Workplace accommodations, 228
Worry/sadness, 256

X

Xerostomia, 321

Y

Yoga, 252, 271
Yogurt, Greek, 38, *38*
Yohimbine, 376–378

Z

Zetia. *See* Ezetimibe
Zoster (shingles) vaccine, 324, 362–363
Zung Self-Rating Depression Scale, 287